ESSENTIALS OF MECHANICAL VENTILATION

NOTICE

Medicine is an ever-changing science. As new research and clinical experience broaden our knowledge, changes in treatment and drug therapy are required. The author and the publisher of this work have checked with sources believed to be reliable in their efforts to provide information that is complete and generally in accord with the standards accepted at the time of publication. However, in view of the possibility of human error or changes in medical sciences, neither the author nor the publisher nor any other party who has been involved in the preparation or publication of this work warrants that the information contained herein is in every respect accurate or complete, and they disclaim all responsibility for any errors or omissions or for the results obtained from use of such information contained in this work. Readers are encouraged to confirm the information contained herein with other sources. For example and in particular, readers are advised to check the product information sheet included in the package of each drug they plan to administer to be certain that the information contained in this work is accurate and that changes have not been made in the recommended dose or in the contraindications for administration. This recommendation is of particular importance in connection with new or infrequently used drugs.

ESSENTIALS OF MECHANICAL VENTILATION

Second Edition

DEAN R. HESS, PhD, RRT

Assistant Professor of Anaesthesia
Harvard Medical School
Assistant Director of Respiratory Care Services
Massachusetts General Hospital
Boston, Massachusetts

ROBERT M. KACMAREK, PhD, RRT

Associate Professor of Anaesthesia
Harvard Medical School
Director of Respiratory Care Services
Massachusetts General Hospital
Boston, Massachusetts

McGraw-Hill
MEDICAL PUBLISHING DIVISION

New York   Chicago   San Francisco   Lisbon   London   Madrid
Mexico City   Milan   New Delhi   San Juan   Seoul
Singapore   Sydney   Toronto

Essentials of Mechanical Ventilation

2 3 4 5 6 7 8 9 0   DOC/DOC   0 9 8 7 6 5 4 3

ISBN 0-07-135229-5

This book was set in Times Roman by Keyword Publishing Services.
The editors were Jack Farrell, Kitty McCullough, and John M. Morriss.
Project supervision was carried out by Keyword Publishing Services.
The production supervisor was Lisa Mendez.
The cover designer was Elizabeth Pisacreta.

RR Donnelly was printer and binder.

This book is printed on acid-free paper.

Library of Congress Cataloging-in-Publication Data are on file for this title at the Library of Congress.

For Susan, Terri, and Lauren—who make every day worth living and tolerate my frequent absences while pursuing professional endeavors such as writing books.

D.R.H.

For Jan, who has tolerated my long hours for years, and to Robert, Julia, Katie, and Callie, who make it all worthwhile.

R.M.K.

CONTENTS

PREFACE

Mechanical ventilation is an integral part of the care of many critically ill patients. Increasingly, it is also provided at sites outside the ICU and outside the hospital – including extended care facilities and the home. A thorough understanding of the essentials of mechanical ventilation is requisite for respiratory therapists and critical care physicians. A general knowledge of the principles of mechanical ventilation is also required of critical care nurses and primary care physicians whose patients occasionally require ventilatory support.

Why a second edition of this book? Since the publication of the first edition of this book, important high-level evidence related to mechanical ventilation has been published. Most important has been the results of the ARDSnet trial, demonstrating for the first time that a strategy limiting tidal volume and airway pressure improves mortality. Protection of the lungs from injury is now accepted as a primary goal of mechanical ventilation, with other goals such as normalization of blood gases assuming less importance. It has also been accepted that strategies that improve survival are more important than strategies that simply improve physiology (e.g., blood gases). In fact, the primary criterion used to judge a ventilation strategy is its effect on mortality.

Equally important knowledge has been gained related to weaning from mechanical ventilation, where we have learned that the process of ventilator discontinuation can be shortened through the use of protocols stressing spontaneous breathing trials. Numerous new ventilator modes have been introduced in recent years, with little evidence to guide their use. Despite the significant advances in the evidence base for mechanical ventilation, some areas remain controversial such as recruitment maneuvers and the appropriate setting of PEEP in patients with acute lung injury.

This book is intended to be a practical guide to adult mechanical ventilation. We have written this book from our perspective of over 60 years' experience as clinicians, educators, researchers, and authors. We have made every attempt to keep the topics current and with a distinctly clinical focus. As in the first edition, we have kept the chapters short, focused, and practical. We have added learning objectives to make the book more useful for students and we have added numerous decision algorithms as a guide to the application of mechanical ventilation for a variety of clinical problems.

As with the first edition, the book is divided into four parts. Part One, *Principles of Mechanical Ventilation*, describes basic principles of mechanical ventilation and then continues with issues such as indications for mechanical ventilation, appropriate physiologic goals, and weaning from mechanical ventilation. Part Two, *Ventilator Management*, gives practical advice for ventilating patients with a variety of diseases. Part Three, *Monitoring During Mechanical Ventilation*, discusses blood gases, hemodynamics, mechanics, and waveforms.

In the final part, *Topics in Mechanical Ventilation*, we discuss issues such as airway management, positioning, sedation and paralysis, and miscellaneous ventilatory techniques.

This is a book about mechanical ventilation and not mechanical ventilators. We do not describe the operation of any specific ventilator (although we do discuss some modes specific to some ventilator types). Ventilator function is covered sufficiently in available respiratory care equipment books and in the product literature provided by manufacturers. We have tried to keep the material covered in this book generic and it is, by and large, applicable to any adult mechanical ventilator. We do not cover issues related to pediatric and neonatal mechanical ventilation. Because these topics are adequately covered in pediatric and neonatal respiratory care books, we decided to limit the focus of this book to adult mechanical ventilation. Although we provide a short bibliography at the end of each chapter, we have specifically tried to make this a practical book and not an extensive reference book.

This book is written for all clinicians caring for mechanically ventilated patients. We believe that it is unique and hope you will enjoy reading it as much as we have enjoyed writing it.

Dean R. Hess, PhD, RRT
Robert M. Kacmarek, PhD, RRT

ABBREVIATIONS

AARC	American Association for Respiratory Care
A/C	assist/control ventilation
ACCP	American College of Chest Physicians
AG	anion gap
ALI	acute lung injury
ALS	amyotrophic lateral sclerosis
AMV	assisted mechanical ventilation
APF	acute pulmonary failure
APRV	airway pressure-release ventilation
ARDS	acute respiratory distress syndrome
ASV	adaptive support ventilation
ATC	automatic tube compensation
auto-PEEP	end-expiratory alveolar pressure above set PEEP level
BE	base excess
BEE	basal energy expenditure
BIPAP	biphasic positive airway pressure
BIS	bispectral index
BSA	body surface area
BUN	blood urea nitrogen
C	compliance
Ca_{O_2}	arterial oxygen content
$C(a-\bar{v})O_2$	arterial to mixed venous oxygen content difference
Cc'_{O_2}	pulmonary end-capillary oxygen content
CDCP	Centers for Disease Control and Prevention
CI	cardiac index
C_L	lung compliance
CMV	continuous mandatory ventilation
CNS	central nervous system
COHb	carboxyhemoglobin
COPD	chronic obstructive pulmonary disease
CPAP	continuous positive airway pressure
Cpc	compliance of patient circuit
CPP	cerebral perfusion pressure
CPR	cardiopulmonary resuscitation
Crs	compliance of respiratory system
CSF	cerebrospinal fluid
CSV	continuous spontaneous ventilation
$C\bar{v}_{O_2}$	mixed venous oxygen content
CVP	central venous pressure
Cw	chest wall compliance

$\dot{D}_{O_2}$	oxygen delivery
DPG	diphosphoglycerate
ΔPaw	change in airway pressure
ΔPpl	change in pleural pressure
ECG	electrocardiogram
EPAP	expiratory positive airway pressure
f_b	respiratory frequency
$F\bar{E}_{CO_2}$	fractional mixed expired carbon dioxide
$F\bar{E}_{O_2}$	fractional mixed expired oxygen
FEV_1	forced expiratory volume in 1 s
$F_{I_{O_2}}$	fractional inspired oxygen
FRC	functional residual capacity
f/V_T	rate-tidal volume ratio; rapid shallow breathing index
Hb	hemoglobin
O_2Hb	oxyhemoglobin; hemoglobin oxygen saturation
HCO_3^-	bicarbonate
HFJV	high-frequency jet ventilation
HFO	high-frequency oscillation
HFPPV	high-frequency positive pressure ventilation
HFV	high-frequency ventilation
HIV	human immunodeficiency virus
HR	heart rate
I:E ratio	inspiratory:expiratory ratio
ICP	intracranial pressure
ICU	intensive care unit
ILV	independent lung ventilation
IMV	intermittent mandatory ventilation
IPAP	inspiratory positive airway pressure
IPPB	intermittent positive pressure breathing
ISB	isothermic saturation boundary
Kcal	kilocalories
K_E	inverse of time constant; $1/(R_E \times C)$
LPVS	lung protective ventilation strategy
LVSWI	left ventricular stroke work index
MAP	mean systemic arterial pressure
MDI	metered-dose inhaler
metHb	methemoglobin
MI	myocardial infarction
MIC	maximum insufflation capacity
MIP	maximum inspiratory pressure
MMV	mandatory minute ventilation
MODS	multiple organ dysfunction syndrome
MPAP	mean pulmonary artery pressure
NPPV	noninvasive positive pressure ventilation
NO	nitric oxide

N_2O	nitrous oxide
NPE	neurogenic pulmonary edema
OI	oxygenation index
OVP	operational verification procedure
$P_{0.1}$	airway pressure change in the first 100 ms (0.1 s) of inspiration with an occluded airway
$P(A\text{-}a)_{O_2}$	alveolar-arterial oxygen pressure difference
$P(a\text{-}et)_{CO_2}$	gradient between Pa_{CO_2} and Pet_{CO_2}
Pa_{CO_2}	partial pressure of carbon dioxide in arterial blood
PA_{CO_2}	partial pressure of carbon dioxide in lungs
PA_{O_2}	partial pressure of oxygen in lungs
Palv	alveolar pressure
Pa_{O_2}	partial pressure of oxygen in arterial blood
PAOP	pulmonary artery occlusion pressure
PAP	pulmonary artery pressure
PAV	proportional assist ventilation
$\bar{P}aw$	mean airway pressure
Pb	barometric pressure
PBW	predicted body weight
PCIRV	pressure-controlled inverse-ratio ventilation
PCV	pressure-controlled ventilation
PCV+	alternative for BIPAP on some ventilators
PCWP	pulmonary capillary wedge pressure
$P\bar{E}_{CO_2}$	partial pressure of carbon dioxide in mixed expired gas
PEEP	positive end-expiratory pressure
$PEEP_{tot}$	total PEEP
Pel	elastic pressure
Pes	esophageal pressure
Pet_{CO_2}	end-tidal P_{CO_2}
$Pexp_{CO_2}$	measured mixed expired P_{CO_2}
pHi	gastric intraluminal pH
P_{H_2O}	water vapor pressure
PI_{max}	maximum inspiratory pressure
PIP	peak inspiratory pressure
PLV	partial liquid ventilation
POC	point-of-care
P_{plat}	end-inspiratory plateau pressure
P_{O_2}	pressure of oxygen
P_R	resistive pressure
PRVC	pressure-regulated volume control
PSV	pressure-support ventilation
P_T	pressure required to deliver a volume of gas to the lungs
Ptc_{CO_2}	transcutaneous carbon dioxide pressure
Ptc_{O_2}	transcutaneous oxygen pressure
$P\bar{v}_{CO_2}$	mixed venous P_{CO_2}

$P\bar{v}_{O_2}$ mixed venous P_{O_2}
PVR   pulmonary vascular resistance
PVRI   pulmonary vascular resistance index
$\dot{Q}$ blood flow
$\dot{Q}s$ shunted blood flow
$\dot{Q}s/\dot{Q}_T$ shunt fraction
$\dot{Q}_T$ total cardiac output
R   resistance
RC   respiratory time constant
R_E expiratory airways resistance
REE   resting energy expenditure
RI   respiratory index
R_I inspiratory airways resistance
RQ   respiratory quotient
RSBI   rapid shallow breathing index
RVSWI   right ventricular stroke work index
RV   residual volume
Sa_{O_2} arterial oxygen saturation
SBT   spontaneous breathing trial
Sc'_{O_2} end-capillary oxygen saturation
SCCM   Society of Critical Care Medicine
SID   strong ion difference
SIMV   synchronized intermittent mandatory ventilation
Sjv_{O_2} jugular venous bulb oxygen saturation
S_{O_2} oxygen saturation
Sp_{O_2} oxygen saturation measured by pulse oximetry
SV   stroke volume
SVI   stroke volume index
SVN   small-volume nebulizer
$S\bar{v}_{O_2}$ mixed venous oxygen saturation
SVR   systemic vascular resistance
T_E expiratory time
TGI   tracheal gas insufflation
THAM   an intravenously administered buffer
T_I inspiratory time
T_T total cycle time
UUN   urine urea nitrogen
$\bar{v}$ mixed venous
$\dot{V}$ flow
$\dot{V}_A$ alveolar ventilation
VAP   ventilator-associated pneumonia
VAPS   volume-assured pressure-support ventilation
VC   vital capacity
$\dot{V}_{CO_2}$ carbon dioxide production
VCV   volume-controlled ventilation

$\dot{V}_D$	dead-space ventilation
$\int V dt$	volume
$\int P\dot{V}\, dt$	work-of-breathing
V_D/V_T	ratio of dead space to tidal volume
$\dot{V}_E$	expired minute ventilation
$\dot{V}_{E(peak)}$	peak expiratory flow
Vi	initial volume of the lung unit
VILI	ventilator-induced lung injury
$\dot{V}_{O_2}$	oxygen consumption
$\dot{V}_{pk.}$	peak flow
$\dot{V}/\dot{Q}$	ventilation-perfusion ratio
VS	volume support
Vt	volume of a lung unit at time t
V_T	tidal volume
V_{Texp}	tidal volume leaving expiration valve
work/L	work-of-breathing normalized to tidal volume
ZEEP	zero end-expiratory pressure

PRINCIPLES OF MECHANICAL VENTILATION

CHAPTER ONE

PHYSIOLOGIC EFFECTS OF MECHANICAL VENTILATION

INTRODUCTION

MEAN AIRWAY PRESSURE

PULMONARY EFFECTS
   Shunt
   Ventilation
   Atelectasis
   Barotrauma
   Ventilator-Induced Lung Injury
   Pneumonia
   Hyperventilation and Hypoventilation
   Oxygen Toxicity

CARDIAC EFFECTS

RENAL EFFECTS

GASTRIC EFFECTS

NUTRITIONAL EFFECTS

NEUROLOGIC EFFECTS

HEPATOSPLANCHNIC EFFECTS

AIRWAY EFFECTS

SLEEP EFFECTS

PATIENT-VENTILATOR DYS-SYNCHRONY

MECHANICAL MALFUNCTIONS

POINTS TO REMEMBER

ADDITIONAL READING

OBJECTIVES

1. List the factors affecting mean airway pressure during positive pressure ventilation.
2. Describe the effects of positive pressure ventilation on shunt and dead space.
3. Discuss the roles of alveolar over-distention and collapse on ventilator induced lung injury.
4. List factors contributing to ventilator-associated pneumonia.
5. Describe the cardiac effects of positive pressure ventilation.
6. Discuss the physiologic effects of positive pressure ventilation on the pulmonary, cardiac, renal, hepatic, gastric, and neurologic systems.
7. Describe methods that can be used to minimize the harmful effects of positive pressure ventilation.

INTRODUCTION

Mechanical ventilation is used to provide artificial support of lung function. Ventilators currently employed in adult acute care use positive pressure to inflate the lungs. The principles of mechanical ventilation are governed by the Equation of Motion, which states that the amount of pressure required to inflate the lungs depends upon resistance, compliance, tidal volume, and inspiratory flow (Figure 1-1). Although positive pressure is responsible for the beneficial effects of mechanical ventilation, it is also responsible for many deleterious side effects. Correct use of mechanical ventilation requires a thorough understanding of both its beneficial and adverse physiologic effects. Due to the homeostatic interactions between the lungs and other body systems, mechanical ventilation can affect nearly every organ system of the body. This chapter discusses the beneficial and adverse physiologic effects of mechanical ventilation.

MEAN AIRWAY PRESSURE

During normal spontaneous breathing, intrathoracic pressure is negative throughout the ventilatory cycle. Intrapleural pressure varies from about -5 cm H_2O during exhalation to -8 cm H_2O during inhalation. Alveolar pressure fluctuates from $+1$ cm H_2O during exhalation to -1 cm H_2O during inhalation. The decrease in intrapleural pressure during inhalation facilitates lung inflation and venous return. The maximal static transpulmonary pressure that can be generated during spontaneous inspiration is about 35 cm H_2O (transpulmonary pressure is the difference between intra-alveolar pressure and intrapleural pressure).

Thoracic pressure fluctuations during positive pressure ventilation are opposite to those that occur during spontaneous breathing. During positive pressure ventilation, the mean intrathoracic pressure is usually positive, particularly if

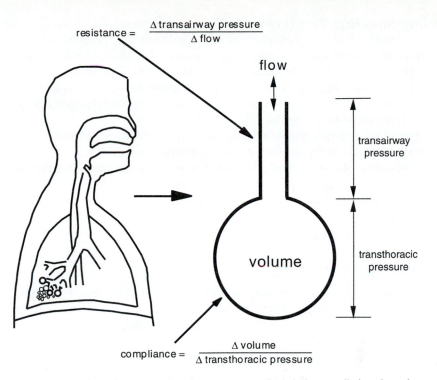

$$\text{resistance} = \frac{\Delta \text{ transairway pressure}}{\Delta \text{ flow}}$$

flow

transairway
pressure

volume

transthoracic
pressure

$$\text{compliance} = \frac{\Delta \text{ volume}}{\Delta \text{ transthoracic pressure}}$$

Figure 1-1 Equation of Motion. Note that the pressure required during ventilation depends upon resistance, compliance, inspiratory flow, and tidal volume. (From CHATBURN RL. Classification of mechanical ventilators. *Respir Care* 1992; 37:1009–1025.)

positive end-expiratory pressure (PEEP) is used. Intrathoracic pressure increases during inhalation and decreases during exhalation. Thus, venous return is greatest during exhalation and venous return may be decreased if expiratory time is too short or expiratory alveolar pressure is too high.

Many of the beneficial and adverse effects associated with mechanical ventilation are related to mean airway pressure. Mean airway pressure is the average pressure applied to the airway during the ventilatory cycle. Thus, it is related to both the amount and duration of pressure applied. A number of factors affect the magnitude of mean airway pressure.

- Inspiratory pressure level. An increase in peak inspiratory pressure increases mean airway pressure. During volume ventilation, peak inspiratory pressure is determined by the tidal volume setting, inspiratory flow setting, airway resistance, respiratory system compliance, and PEEP. During pressure ventilation, the peak inspiratory pressure is set.
- Expiratory pressure level. Airway pressure during exhalation is determined by the PEEP setting.

- Inspiratory:Expiratory (I:E) ratio. The longer the inspiratory phase relative to the expiratory phase, the higher will be the mean airway pressure. Mean airway pressure is particularly affected by an inversed I:E ratio, in which inspiratory time exceeds expiratory time. An end-inspiratory breath-hold (inspiratory hold) will prolong inspiration and increase mean airway pressure. An increase in respiratory rate will increase mean airway pressure if the inspiratory time remains constant due to the effect on I:E ratio.
- Inspiratory pressure waveform. Ventilatory techniques that produce a rectangular wave of pressure during the inspiratory phase will produce a higher mean airway pressure than those that produce an ascending ramp of pressure.

PULMONARY EFFECTS

Shunt

Shunt refers to perfusion (blood flow) without ventilation (Figure 1-2). Pulmonary shunt occurs when blood flows from the right heart to the left heart without participating in gas exchange. The result of shunt is hypoxemia. Shunt can be either capillary shunt or anatomic shunt. Capillary shunt results when blood flows past unventilated alveoli. Examples of capillary shunt are atelectasis, pneumonia, pulmonary edema, and acute respiratory distress syndrome (ARDS). Anatomic shunt occurs when blood flows from the right heart to the left heart and completely bypasses the lungs. This occurs with congenital cardiac defects. Total shunt is the sum of the capillary and anatomic shunt.

Positive pressure ventilation usually decreases shunt and improves arterial oxygenation. An inspiratory pressure that exceeds the alveolar opening pressure expands a collapsed alveolus, and an expiratory pressure greater than alveolar closing pressure prevents its collapse. By maintaining alveolar recruitment with an adequate expiratory pressure setting, arterial oxygenation is improved. However,

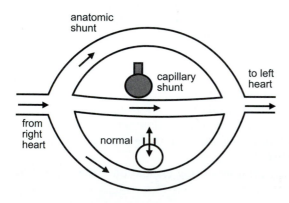

Figure 1-2 Schematic illustration of anatomic shunt and capillary shunt.

if positive pressure ventilation produces over-distention of some lung units, this may result in redistribution of pulmonary blood flow to unventilated regions (Figure 1-3). In this case, positive pressure ventilation paradoxically results in hypoxemia.

Although positive pressure ventilation may improve capillary shunt, it may worsen anatomic shunt. An increase in alveolar pressure may increase pulmonary vascular resistance, which could result in increased flow through the anatomic shunt, decreased flow through the lungs, and worsening hypoxemia. Thus, mean airway pressure should be kept as low as possible if an anatomic right-to-left shunt is present.

A relative shunt effect can occur with poor distribution of ventilation, such as might result from airway disease. With poor distribution of ventilation, some alveoli are under-ventilated relative to perfusion (shunt-like effect and low ventilation-perfusion ratio), whereas other alveoli are over-ventilated (dead space effect and high ventilation-perfusion ratio). Positive pressure ventilation may improve the distribution of ventilation, particularly by improving the ventilation of previously under-ventilated areas of the lungs.

Ventilation

Ventilation is the movement of gas in and out of the lungs. Tidal volume (V_T) is the amount of gas breathed with a single breath, and minute ventilation is the volume of gas breathed in one minute ($\dot{V}_E$). Minute ventilation is the product of tidal volume (V_T) and respiratory frequency (f_b):

$$\dot{V}_E = V_T \times f_b$$

Ventilation can be either dead space ventilation ($\dot{V}_D$) or alveolar ventilation ($\dot{V}_A$). Minute ventilation is the sum of dead space and alveolar ventilation:

$$\dot{V}_E = \dot{V}_D + \dot{V}_A$$

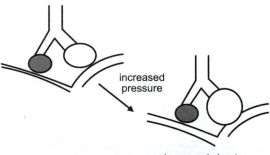

increased
pressure

increased shunt
increased dead space

Figure 1-3 Alveolar over-distention, resulting in redistribution of pulmonary blood flow to unventilated units and an increased shunt.

Alveolar ventilation participates in gas exchange (Figure 1-4), whereas dead space ventilation does not. In other words, dead space is ventilation without perfusion. Anatomic dead space is the volume of the conducting airways of the lungs, and is about 150 mL in normal adults. Alveolar dead space refers to alveoli that are ventilated but not perfused, and is increased by any condition that decreases pulmonary blood flow. Total physiologic dead space fraction (V_D/V_T) is normally about one third of the $\dot{V}_E$. Mechanical dead space refers to the rebreathed volume of the ventilator circuit, and acts as an extension of the anatomic dead space. Due to the fixed anatomic dead space, a low tidal volume increases the dead space fraction and decreases alveolar ventilation. An increased dead space fraction will require a greater minute ventilation to maintain alveolar ventilation (and Pa_{CO_2}).

Because mechanical ventilators provide a tidal volume and respiratory rate, any desired level of ventilation can be provided. The level of ventilation required depends upon the desired Pa_{CO_2}, alveolar ventilation, and tissue CO_2 production ($\dot{V}_{CO_2}$). This is illustrated by the following relationships:

$$Pa_{CO_2} \propto \dot{V}_{CO_2}/\dot{V}_A$$

and

$$Pa_{CO_2} = \left(\dot{V}_{CO_2} \times 0.863\right)/\left(\dot{V}_E \times [1 - V_D/V_T]\right).$$

A higher $\dot{V}_E$ will be required to maintain Pa_{CO_2} if $\dot{V}_{CO_2}$ is increased, such as occurs with fever and sepsis. If dead space is increased, a higher $\dot{V}_E$ is required to maintain the same level of $\dot{V}_A$ and Pa_{CO_2}. If this level of ventilation is undesirable due to its injurious effects on the lungs and hemodynamics, Pa_{CO_2} can be allowed to increase (permissive hypercapnia). Poor distribution of ventilation produces a dead space effect if some alveoli are over-ventilated relative to perfusion. Mechanical ventilation can produce over-distention of normal alveoli, resulting in alveolar dead space. Mechanical ventilation can also distend airways, increasing anatomic dead space.

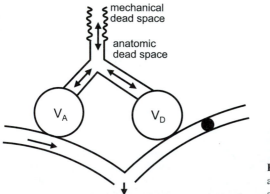

Figure 1-4 Schematic illustration of mechanical dead space, anatomic dead space, and alveolar dead space.

Atelectasis

Atelectasis is a common complication of mechanical ventilation. This can be the result of a low lung volume or airway obstruction due to mucus plugging. Use of PEEP to maintain lung volume can be effective in preventing atelectasis. Secretion clearance techniques such as suctioning and bronchoscopy may be used to prevent mucus plugging. Sigh breaths may prevent atelectasis if their magnitude, duration, and frequency are great enough. Breathing 100% oxygen can produce absorption atelectasis, and should be avoided if possible.

Barotrauma

Barotrauma is pulmonary injury resulting from alveolar over-distention. Barotrauma can lead to pulmonary interstitial emphysema, pneumomediastinum, subcutaneous emphysema, and pneumothorax (Figure 1-5). Pneumothorax is of greatest clinical concern, because it can progress rapidly to life-threatening tension pneumothorax. Pneumomediastinum and subcutaneous emphysema rarely have major clinical consequences.

Ventilator-Induced Lung Injury

Alveolar over-distention due to high peak inflation volume (volutrauma) produces acute lung injury. Alveolar over-distention is associated with high peak alveolar pressures. Because localized over-distention is not easy to monitor, it is inferred from high peak alveolar pressure. Peak alveolar pressure should be kept < 30 cm H_2O. Peak alveolar pressure during mechanical ventilation is best reflected by the end-inspiratory plateau pressure. Alveolar over-distention can be minimized by limiting the tidal volume (e.g., 6 mL/kg in patients with ARDS). Ventilator-induced lung injury can also result from alveolar collapse

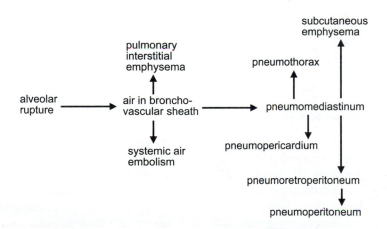

Figure 1-5 Barotrauma-related injuries that can occur as the result of alveolar rupture.

(atelectrauma). The pressure at the junction between an open and a collapsed alveolus may exceed 100 cm H_2O. Furthermore, cyclical opening of an alveolus during inhalation and closure during exhalation may be injurious to the lungs. This injury is ameliorated by optimal lung recruitment and an expiratory pressure to avoid alveolar de-recruitment. Ventilating the lungs in a manner that promotes alveolar over-distention and de-recruitment increases inflammation in the lungs (biotrauma). Inflammatory mediators (cytokines, chemokines) may translocate into the pulmonary circulation, resulting in systemic inflammation. How the lungs are ventilated may thus play a role in systemic inflammation.

Pneumonia

Nosocomial pneumonia occurs commonly in mechanically ventilated patients, and may have an incidence of 10–20 cases per 1000 ventilator days. Ventilator-associated pneumonia is often due to Gram-negative bacteria. For many years, it was believed that ventilator-associated pneumonia was acquired from contaminants delivered by the ventilator. It is now recognized that bacteria causing ventilator-associated pneumonia often originate from the oropharynx or gastrointestinal tract of the patient. The stomach and oropharynx presumably serve as a reservoir for Gram-negative bacteria that then colonize the lower respiratory tract due to aspiration around the artificial airway.

The ventilator circuit frequently contains contaminated condensate. The organisms present in this condensate almost always arise from the patient. This condensate is a potential contaminate for the clinician and should be handled as contaminated waste. Although it was once believed that frequent ventilator circuit changes were necessary to prevent ventilator-associated pneumonia, it is now recognized that the ventilator is relatively unimportant in the genesis of pneumonia.

Techniques that prevent bacterial colonization of the stomach may be useful to prevent ventilator-associated pneumonia. Stress ulcer prophylaxis that maintains gastric acidity may decrease the risk of pneumonia. Subglottic aspiration of secretions above the cuff of the endotracheal tube is useful. An adequate airway cuff pressure to minimize aspiration of secretions, yet minimize tracheal trauma, should be used (e.g., 20–25 mm Hg). If not medically contraindicated, the head of the bed of the mechanically ventilated patient should be elevated to minimize gastric reflux.

Hyperventilation and Hypoventilation

Hyperventilation lowers Pa_{CO_2} and increases arterial pH. This may be desirable when intracranial pressure is elevated, but otherwise should be avoided because of the injurious effects of over-distention. These effects include acute lung injury, barotrauma, and decreased cardiac output. Hyperventilation results in respiratory alkalosis, which can cause hypokalemia, decreased ionized calcium, and decreased oxygen release from hemoglobin (left shift of the oxyhemoglobin dissociation curve). Relative hyperventilation can occur when mechanical ventilation is provided for patients with chronic compensated respiratory acidosis. If a normal Pa_{CO_2} is established in such patients, the result is an elevated pH.

Hypoventilation raises Pa_{CO_2} and decreases pH. It has become increasingly recognized that hypercapnia during mechanical ventilation may not be harmful, and might be less injurious than the traumatic effects of high levels of ventilation to normalize the Pa_{CO_2}. A modest elevation of Pa_{CO_2} (50–70 mm Hg) is probably not by itself injurious. Respiratory acidosis may not be desirable, but pH levels as low as 7.20 are well tolerated by most patients.

Oxygen Toxicity

A high inspired oxygen concentration is considered toxic. What is less clear is the level of oxygen that is toxic. Oxygen toxicity is probably related to $F_{I_{O_2}}$ as well as the amount of time that the elevated $F_{I_{O_2}}$ is breathed. Although the clinical evidence is weak, it is commonly recommended that an $F_{I_{O_2}} > 0.6$ be avoided, particularly if breathed for a period > 48 hours. High $F_{I_{O_2}}$ levels can result in a higher than normal Pa_{O_2}. A high Pa_{O_2} may produce an elevation in Pa_{CO_2} due to the Haldane Effect (i.e., unloading CO_2 from hemoglobin), due to improving blood flow to low-ventilation lung units (i.e., relaxing hypoxic pulmonary vaso-constriction), and suppression of ventilation (less likely). However, this is usually not an issue during mechanical ventilation, because ventilation can be controlled. A high Pa_{O_2} can produce retinopathy of prematurity in neonates, but this is not known to occur in adults.

CARDIAC EFFECTS

It is well known that positive pressure ventilation may decrease cardiac output, resulting in hypotension and potential tissue hypoxia. This effect is greatest with high mean airway pressure, high lung compliance, and low circulating blood volume. Positive pressure ventilation affects cardiac performance in several ways.

- An increase in intrathoracic pressure decreases venous return and right heart filling, which may reduce cardiac output. With spontaneous breathing, venous return to the right atrium is greatest during inhalation, when the intrathoracic pressure is lowest. During positive pressure ventilation, venous return is greatest during exhalation. Thus, prolongation of inhalation relative to exhalation decreases venous return.
- Positive pressure ventilation increases pulmonary vascular resistance. The increase in alveolar pressure, particularly with PEEP, has a constricting effect on the pulmonary vasculature. The increase in pulmonary vascular resistance decreases left ventricular filling and cardiac output. Increased right ventricular afterload can result in right ventricular hypertrophy, with ventricular septal shift and compromise of left ventricular function.

- Positive pressure ventilation may decrease left ventricular afterload. This may be due to the increasing pleural pressure assisting left ventricular ejection by decreasing left ventricular transmural pressure. This effect may result in an increased cardiac output in patients with left ventricular dysfunction.

The cardiac effects of positive pressure ventilation can be ameliorated by lowering the mean airway pressure. When high mean airway pressure is necessary, circulatory volume loading and administration of vasopressors may be necessary to maintain cardiac output and arterial blood pressure.

RENAL EFFECTS

Urine output can decrease secondary to mechanical ventilation. This is partially related to decreased renal perfusion due to decreased cardiac output, and may also be related to elevations in plasma antidiuretic hormone and reductions in atrial natriuretic peptide that occur with mechanical ventilation. Fluid overload frequently occurs during mechanical ventilation. This is due to decreased urine output, excessive intravenous fluid administration, and elimination of insensible water loss from the respiratory tract due to humidification of the inspired gas.

GASTRIC EFFECTS

Patients being mechanically ventilated may develop gastric distention (meteorism). This is presumably due to gas leaking around the cuff of the artificial airway and aerophagia. Use of a gastric tube decompresses the stomach. Stress ulcer formation and gastrointestinal bleeding can also occur in mechanically ventilated patients, and stress ulcer prophylaxis should be provided. Agents that maintain gastric acidity may be useful to prevent ventilator-associated pneumonia.

NUTRITIONAL EFFECTS

Appropriate nutritional support is problematic in mechanically ventilated patients. Underfeeding can result in respiratory muscle catabolism, and increases the risk of pneumonia and pulmonary edema. Overfeeding increases metabolic rate and thus the ventilation requirement. Overfeeding with carbohydrates increases $\dot{V}_{CO_2}$, further increasing the ventilation requirement. In some mechanically ventilated patients, indirect calorimetry is useful to assess caloric requirements.

NEUROLOGIC EFFECTS

In patients with head injury, positive pressure ventilation may increase intracranial pressure. This is related to a decrease in venous return, which increases intracranial blood volume and pressure. If high mean airway pressure is used, cerebral perfusion can be severely compromised due to arterial hypotension with an associated increased intracranial pressure. In head injured patients, low mean airway pressures, and particularly low PEEP levels, should be used whenever possible. This can be difficult, however, when the treatment of a head injured patient is required in the presence of significant lung disease.

HEPATOSPLANCHNIC EFFECTS

PEEP can reduce portal blood flow. However, the clinical importance of the effects of positive pressure ventilation on hepatosplanchnic perfusion is unclear.

AIRWAY EFFECTS

Critically ill patients are usually mechanically ventilated through an endotracheal or tracheostomy tube. This puts these patients at risk for all of the complications of artificial airways such as laryngeal edema, tracheal mucosal trauma, contamination of the lower respiratory tract, sinusitis, loss of the humidifying function of the upper airway, and communication problems. Some patients are mechanically ventilated by nasal or oronasal mask. Complications of this include leaks, gastric insufflation, and skin breakdown (particularly over the bridge of the nose).

SLEEP EFFECTS

Mechanically ventilated patients do not demonstrate normal sleep patterns. The severity of sleep deprivation in these patients is of similar magnitude to that associated with excessive daytime sleepiness and cognitive impairment in ambulatory sleep deprived patients. This may produce delirium, patient-ventilator dyssynchrony, and sedation-induced ventilator dependency.

PATIENT-VENTILATOR DYS-SYNCHRONY

"Fighting the ventilator" can be due to lack of synchrony between the breathing efforts of the patient and the ventilator. This may be due to poor trigger sensitivity, incorrect inspiratory flow or time setting, inappropriate tidal volume, or inappropriate mode. Patient-ventilator dys-synchrony can also be due to auto-PEEP. If patient-ventilator dys-synchrony cannot be corrected by changing the ventilator settings, sedation and paralysis may be needed. Patient-ventilator dys-synchrony can be detected by observing the patient, or by evaluation of the ventilator waveforms. Patient-ventilator dys-synchrony can result in exhaustion. At the other extreme, excessive sedation and paralysis can result in respiratory muscle dysfunction secondary to disuse.

MECHANICAL MALFUNCTIONS

A variety of mechanical complications can occur during mechanical ventilation. These include accidental disconnection, leaks in the ventilator circuit, loss of electrical power, and loss of gas pressure. The mechanical ventilator system should be monitored frequently to prevent mechanical malfunctions.

POINTS TO REMEMBER

- Many beneficial and adverse effects of mechanical ventilation are related to mean airway pressure.
- Positive pressure ventilation usually improves arterial P_{O_2} and P_{CO_2}, but may increase shunt and deadspace under some conditions.
- Atelectasis, barotrauma, acute lung injury, pneumonia, hypoventilation or hyperventilation, and oxygen toxicity are pulmonary complications of positive pressure ventilation.
- Positive pressure ventilation can produce adverse cardiac effects, renal effects, nutritional effects, neurologic effects, hepatic effects, and airway effects.
- Patient-ventilator dys-synchrony commonly occurs, and should be corrected by use of appropriate ventilator settings or sedation.

ADDITIONAL READING

COOK D, DE JONGHE B, BROCHARD L, BRUN-BUISSON C. Influence of airway management on ventilator-associated pneumonia: evidence from randomized trials. *JAMA* 1998; 279:781–787.
COOPER AB, THORNLEY KS, YOUNG GB, ET AL. Sleep in critically ill patients requiring mechanical ventilation. *Chest* 2000; 117:809–818.
DE BACKER, D. The effects of positive end-expiratory pressure on the splanchnic circulation. *Intensive Care Med* 2000; 26:361–363.
DREYFUSS D, SAUMON G. Ventilator-induced lung injury. *Am J Respir Crit Care Med* 1998; 157:294–323.
FESSLER HE. Heart-lung interactions: applications in the critically ill. *Eur Respir J* 1997; 10:226–237.
HURFORD WE. Cardiopulmonary interactions during mechanical ventilation. *Int Anesthesiol Clin* 1999; 37:35–46.
KACMAREK RM. Ventilator-associated lung injury. *Int Anesthesiol Clin* 1999; 37:47–64.

KEITH RL, PIERSON DJ. Complications of mechanical ventilation. A bedside approach. *Clin Chest Med* 1996; 17:439–451.

KOLLEF MH. The prevention of ventilator-associated pneumonia. *N Engl J Med* 1999; 340:627–634.

MATLU GM, FACTOR P. Complications of mechanical ventilation. *Respir Care Clin N Am* 2000; 6:213–252.

SLUTSKY AS, TREMBLAY L. Multiple system organ failure: is mechanical ventilation a contributing factor? *Am J Respir Crit Care Med* 1998; 157:1721–1725.

TWO

VENTILATOR-INDUCED LUNG INJURY

INTRODUCTION

BAROTRAUMA

OXYGEN TOXICITY

VOLUTRAUMA
 Chest-Wall Compliance
 Pre-Existing Injury

ATELECTRAUMA

BIOTRAUMA

TRANSLOCATION OF CELLS

OTHER MECHANISM

VENTILATOR-INDUCED LUNG INJURY AND MULTIPLE ORGAN DYSFUNCTION
SYNDROME

POINTS TO REMEMBER

ADDITIONAL READING

OBJECTIVES

1. Discuss the primary factors that contribute to the development of ventilator-induced lung injury.
2. Describe mechanisms whereby PEEP modifies ventilator-induced lung injury.
3. Discuss the effect of an inappropriate ventilatory pattern on inflammatory mediator response and the translocation of cells and molecules.

4. Describe the proposed relationship between ventilator-induced lung injury and multiple organ dysfunction syndrome (MODS).
5. Discuss the clinical outcomes data to support the use of lung protective ventilatory strategies.

INTRODUCTION

Mechanical ventilation is life saving, it improves gas exchange, alters pulmonary mechanics and decreases the work of the cardiopulmonary system. In spite of these beneficial effects there are numerous side effects associated with mechanical ventilation:

- increased shunting and dead-space
- decreased cardiac output and renal blood flow
- increased likelihood of nosocomial pneumonia
- increased intracranial pressure.

However, the concern that has received increasing attention over the last ten years is ventilator-induced lung injury (VILI). It has become increasingly clear that the inappropriate application of mechanical ventilation can induce patient injury (Table 2-1) similar to ARDS. In addition, inappropriate application of the mechanical ventilator has been implicated in the induction or extension of multiple system organ failure.

BAROTRAUMA

Historically, the injury most associated with mechanical ventilation was barotrauma. The disruption of the alveolar capillary membrane allows air to dissect along facial planes accumulating within the pleural space or other compartments, or the development of subcutaneous emphysema (Figure 2-1). It is reasonable to assume that the higher the ventilating pressure, the greater the likelihood of barotrauma. Early reports on ARDS and asthma where unlimited peak airway pressure was applied resulted in a higher incidence of barotrauma than more recent

Table 2-1 Types of injury induced by mechanical ventilation

- Barotrauma
- Oxygen toxicity
- Volutrauma
- Atelectrauma
- Biotrauma

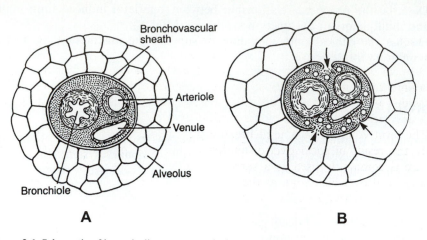

Bronchovascular
sheath

Arteriole

Venule

Alveolus

Bronchiole

A

B

Figure 2-1 Schematic of how air dissects across the lung parenchyma, resulting in barotrauma. (From MAUNDER RJ, PIERSON DJ, HUDSON LD. Subcutaneous and mediastinal emphysema: pathophysology, diagnosis, and management. *Arch Intern Med* 1984; 144:1447–1453.)

case series where high pressure and over-distention of the lungs was avoided. But no clear, specific relationship between applied pressure and barotrauma is available. Many clinicians agree that barotrauma occurs in lungs ventilated with high alveolar pressures and large tidal volumes. The specific volume and pressure required to develop barotrauma is most likely patient-specific.

OXYGEN TOXICITY

High concentrations of inhaled oxygen results in the formation of oxygen free radicals (e.g., superoxide, hydrogen peroxide, hydroxyl ion). These free radicals can cause ultra-structural changes in the lung similar to acute lung injury. In animal models, inhalation of 100% oxygen causes death within 48 to 72 hours. Human volunteers breathing 100% oxygen develop inflammatory airway changes and bronchitis within 24 hr. There is also laboratory data to suggest that exposure to bacterial endotoxin, inflammatory mediators and sub-lethal levels of oxygen ($\leq 85\%$) protect the lung from further injury when inspiring a high F_{IO_2}.

Concern for oxygen toxicity should never prevent the use of a high F_{IO_2} in a patient who is hypoxemic. An F_{IO_2} of 1.0 should be administered during suctioning, transport, periods of instability and whenever uncertain about the Pa_{O_2}. However, F_{IO_2} should be lowered to the level resulting in a Pa_{O_2} of 60 to 80 mm Hg as soon as possible. The target F_{IO_2} is ≤ 0.60. Few clinicians feel the concern of oxygen toxicity is greater than the concern of tissue hypoxia. An exception is the patient treated with bleomycin. The combination of bleomycin and oxygen results in injury to the lungs. In this setting, the lowest F_{IO_2} (≤ 0.40) should be used, tolerating a Pa_{O_2} as low as 50 mm Hg.

VOLUTRAUMA

The term volutrauma refers to lung parenchymal damage, caused by mechanical ventilation, and similar to early ARDS (Figure 2-2). Volutrauma is VILI manifested by an increase in the permeability of the alveolar capillary membrane, the development of pulmonary edema, the accumulation of neutrophils and proteins, the disruption of surfactant production, the development of hyaline membranes, and a decrease in compliance of the respiratory system (Table 2-2).

The term volutrauma is used because the induced injury appears to be primarily the result of local over-distention of the lung parenchyma. Clinically, pressure is commonly used as a surrogate for volume since it is impossible to measure local over-distention at the bedside. However, it is the over-distending volume that causes injury. The specific pressure that has been used as a surrogate for local over-distention is the peak alveolar pressure, or end-inspiratory plateau pressure. A plateau pressure > 30 cm H_2O increases the likelihood of VILI.

Chest-Wall Compliance

For an over-distending volume to be delivered to a local lung unit, a high transpulmonary pressure must be present (i.e., the difference between inside and outside the alveolus). The greater the difference between alveolar and pleural

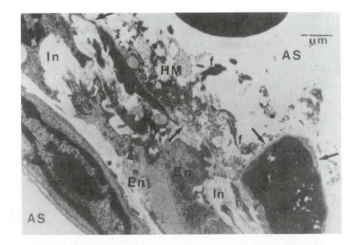

Figure 2-2 Electron microscopic view of the cross section of the alveolar-capillary complex of a rat ventilated with large volumes at a peak pressure of 45 cm H_2O with zero PEEP. Markedly altered alveolar septum with three capillaries. At the right side, the epithelial lining is destroyed, denuding the basement membrane (arrows). Hyaline membrane (HM) composed of cell debris and fibrin (f) are present. Two endothelial cells (En) of another capillary are visible inside the interstitium (In). At the lower left side, a monocyte fills the lumen of a third capillary with a normal blood-air barrier. (From DREYFUSS, ET AL. *Am Rev Respir Dis* 1985; 132:880–884.)

Table 2-2 The spectrum of lung injury induced by mechanical ventilation

Atelectasis
Alveolar hemorrhage
Alveolar neutrophil infiltration
Alveolar macrophage accumulation
Decreased compliance
Detachment of endothelial cells
Denuding of basement membranes
Emphysematous changes
Gross pulmonary edema
Hyaline membrane formation
Interstitial edema
Increased interstitial albumin levels
Interstitial lymphocyte infiltration
Intracapillary bleeding
Pneumothroax
Severe hypoxemia
Subcutaneous emphysema
Systemic gas embolism
Tension cyst formation
Type II pneumocyte proliferation

pressure, the greater the distention of the lungs. The chest-wall has a major role in determining over-distending alveolar pressures. The more compliant the chest wall, the greater the transpulmonary pressure and the greater the distention of the lung for a given alveolar pressure. When the chest wall is stiff, high alveolar pressure can be applied with less risk of over-distention because the transpulmonary pressure is lower. That is, a stiff chest wall (e.g., abdominal distention, massive fluid resuscitation, chest wall deformity, chest wall burns) protects the lung from VILI. With a stiff chest wall, end-inspiratory plateau pressures > 30 cm H_2O may be applied with less risk of lung injury.

Pre-Existing Injury

Pre-existing lung injury increases the likelihood of VILI. As a result, the use of lung protective ventilator strategies are most necessary for patients with previously injured lungs. In fact, improved survival has been reported in acute lung injury/acute respiratory distress syndrome (ALI/ARDS) patients who were ventilated with a V_T of 6 mL/kg.

ATELECTRAUMA

Another mechanism for the development of VILI is the recruitment and de-recruitment of unstable lung units (atelectrauma) during each ventilatory cycle.

The mechanism responsible for the injury associated with atelectrauma is controversial. However, many investigators believe it is a result of stress at the interface of stable and unstable lung units (Figure 2-3). It has been mathematically estimated that > 100 cm H_2O of stress is created across a collapsed lung unit when 30 cm H_2O distending pressure is applied to an adjacent distended lung unit. As illustrated in Figure 2-4, when PEEP is applied the effect of a given distending pressure is attenuated and the extent of VILI reduced. The method

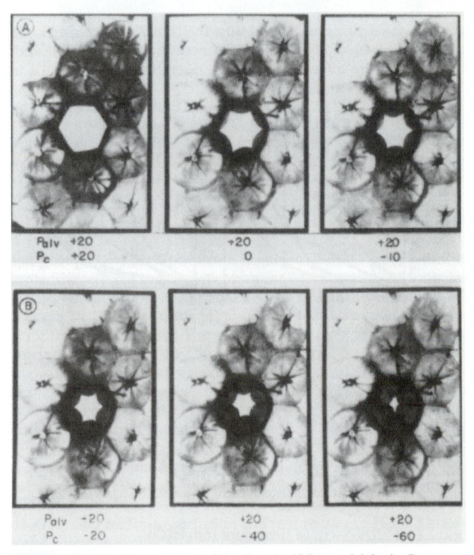

Figure 2-3 Illustration of the stress across a fully collapsed and fully expanded alveolus. P_{alv} – pressure inside surrounding alveolar units. P_c – pressure inside central alveolus. (From MEAD J, TAKISHIMA T, LEITH D. Stress distribution in lungs: a model of pulmonary elasticity. *J Appl Physiol* 1970; 28:596–608.)

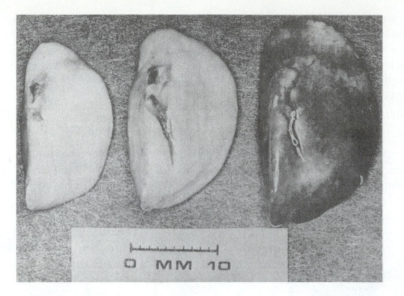

Figure 2-4 Comparison of lungs excised from rats ventilated with peak pressure of 14 cm H_2O, zero PEEP; peak pressure of 45 cm H_2O, 10 cm H_2O PEEP and peak pressure 45 cm H_2O, zero PEEP (left to right). The perivascular groove is distended with edema in the lungs from rats ventilated with peak pressures of 45 cm H_2O. The lung ventilated at 45 cm H_2O, zero PEEP is grossly hemorrhaged. (From WEBB and TIERNEY *Am Rev Respir Dis* 1974; 110:556–565.)

used to determine the amount of PEEP in ALI/ARDS that prevents de-recruitment in a given alveolar unit is controversial. However, it is becoming increasingly clear that the ideal PEEP level prevents de-recruitment at end-exhalation.

BIOTRAUMA

Another type of cellular injury, referred to as biotrauma, has been identified. Over-distending tidal volumes and repetitive opening and closing of unstable lung units result in the activation of inflammatory mediators within the lung. Numerous types of pro-inflammatory (cytokines, chemokines) and anti-inflammatory mediators are activated by injurious ventilatory patterns. These mediators increase edema formation, neutrophil migration, and relaxation of vascular smooth muscle. As with the development of volutrauma, the application of PEEP attenuates the level of inflammatory response.

TRANSLOCATION OF CELLS

Bacteria instilled into the lungs of otherwise healthy animals produces bacteremia when inappropriate ventilatory patterns are employed. If appropriate PEEP and low peak alveolar pressures are used, translocation of bacteria is minimized. The levels of systemic inflammatory mediators are also related to ventilatory pattern. Ventilatory patterns with low PEEP and high peak alveolar pressures increase systemic inflammatory mediator response compared to a lung protective ventilation strategy (LPVS).

OTHER MECHANISMS

Preliminary and controversial animal data suggests a role for vascular volume, ventilator rate and body temperature on VILI. High vascular infusion volumes, rapid respiratory rates and high body temperature appear to cause a greater injury than normal infusion volumes, normal respiratory rates, and normal body temperature. However, no patient data is currently available to support this animal data.

VILI AND MODS

It has been suggested that inappropriate ventilatory patterns (e.g., high peak alveolar pressure and low PEEP) not only cause VILI but may also cause or extend multiple organ dysfunction syndrome (MODS). If an inappropriate approach to mechanical ventilation causes lung injury, disrupts the alveolar-capillary membrane to the extent that cells move from the lung into the systemic circulation, and causes activation of pulmonary inflammatory mediators, then it is reasonable to speculate that inflammatory mediators originating from the lungs can affect other organ systems (Figure 2-5). Although speculative, based on the currently available evidence this appears a reasonable hypothesis. What is certain is that large distending tidal volumes causing high peak alveolar pressure with PEEP levels that do not prevent de-recruitment should be avoided.

POINTS TO REMEMBER

- The higher the airway pressure, the larger the tidal volume, and the more severe the disease, the greater the likelihood for barotrauma.
- Oxygen toxicity should never prevent the appropriate administration of oxygen to avoid tissue hypoxemia.
- Volutrauma is caused by large V_T, high peak alveolar pressure, and low PEEP.
- PEEP prevents derecruitment and attenuates volutrauma.
- Transpulmonary pressure determines the level of over-distention.
- Inflammatory mediators are activated by inappropriate ventilatory strategies.

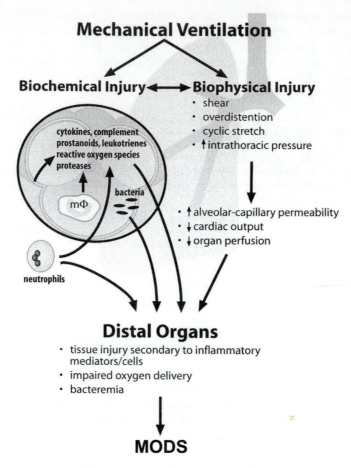

Figure 2-5 Postulated mechanism whereby mechanical ventilation may contribute to MODS. (From SLUTSKY and TREMBLAY *Am J Respir Crit Care Med* 1998; 157:1721–1725.)

- MODS may be caused or extended by inappropriate ventilatory patterns.
- VILI can be avoided by a lung protective ventilation strategy: small V_T (4 to 8 mL/kg), low peak alveolar pressure (< 30 cm H_2O) and sufficient PEEP to prevent de-recruitment (10 to 15 cm H_2O).

ADDITIONAL READING

THE ACUTE RESPIRATORY DISTRESS SYNDROME NETWORK. Ventilation with lower tidal volumes as compared with traditional tidal volumes for acute lung injury and the acute respiratory distress syndrome. *N Engl J Med* 2000; 342:1301–1308.

DREYFUS D, SAUMON G. Ventilator-induced lung injury. *Am J Respir Crit Care Med* 1998; 157:294–323.

KACMAREK RM. Ventilator associated lung injury. *Int Anesthesiol Clin* 1999; 37:47–64.

MARINI JJ, EVANS TW. Round table conference: acute lung injury. *Intensive Care Med* 1998; 24:878–883.

MEAD J, TAKISHIMA T, LEITH D. Stress distribution in lungs: a model of pulmonary elasticity. *J Appl Physiol* 1970; 28:596–608.

NAHUM A, HOYT J, SCHMITZ L, ET AL. Effects of mechanical ventilation strategy on dissemination of intratracheally instilled *Escherichia coli* in dogs. *Crit Care Med* 1997; 25:1733–1743.

RANIERI VM, SUTER PM, TORTORELLA C, ET AL. Effect of mechanical ventilation on inflammatory mediators in patients with acute respiratory distress syndrome: a randomized controlled trial. *JAMA* 1999; 282:54–61.

SLUTSKY A, TREMBLAY L. Multiple system organ failure: Is mechanical ventilation a contributing factor? *Am J Respir Crit Care Med* 1998; 157:1721–1725.

WEBB HH, TIERNEY D. Experimental pulmonary edema due to intermittent positive pressure ventilation with high inflation pressures, protection by positive end-expiratory pressure. *Am Rev Respir Dis* 1974; 110:556–565.

THREE

OVERVIEW OF THE MECHANICAL VENTILATOR SYSTEM AND CLASSIFICATION

THE VENTILATOR SYSTEM
    Pneumatic System
    Electronic System

CLASSIFICATION OF MECHANICAL VENTILATORS
    Control Variables
    Phase Variables
    Conditional Variables

BREATH TYPES DURING MECHANICAL VENTILATION

EQUATION OF MOTION AND PATIENT-VENTILATOR INTERACTION

POINTS TO REMEMBER

ADDITIONAL READING

OBJECTIVES

1. Compare the pneumatic and electronic control of the ventilator.
2. Describe the control variables, phase variables, and conditional variables used to classify ventilator function.
3. Define spontaneous and mandatory breath types.
4. Use the Equation of Motion to describe patient-ventilator interaction.

INTRODUCTION

Current generation mechanical ventilators are sophisticated life support devices. The ventilator must be reliable, flexible, and relatively easy to use by the skilled clinician. This chapter briefly describes the ventilator system, and then discusses ventilator classification, and breath types during mechanical ventilation, in more detail.

THE VENTILATOR SYSTEM

Because ventilators deliver gases to the patient, they must have a pneumatic component. First generation ventilators were typically pneumatically powered, using gas pressure to power the ventilator as well as to ventilate the patient. Current generation ventilators are electronically controlled with the aid of a microprocessor. A generic block diagram of a ventilator is shown in Figure 3-1.

Pneumatic System

The pneumatic system is responsible for delivery of a gas mixture to the patient. Room air and 100% oxygen are typically delivered to the ventilator at 50 lb/in^2. The ventilator reduces this pressure and mixes these gases to provide a prescribed $F_{I_{O_2}}$. A variety of techniques can be used to control inspiratory flow into the ventilator circuit. The ventilator circuit not only delivers gas to the patient, but also filters, warms, and humidifies the inspired gas. During exhalation, gas flows through the expiratory limb of the circuit, through a filter, through the exhalation valve, and into the atmosphere. The exhalation valve closes during inspiration to allow inflation of the lungs and is responsible for controlling PEEP. Traditionally, the exhalation valve was closed completely during the inspiratory phase. Some newer generation ventilators feature an active exhalation valve during pressure

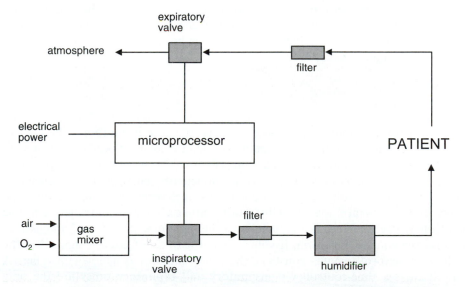

Figure 3-1 A simplified generic block diagram of the ventilator system.

control ventilation, meaning that it opens if the pressure exceeds the set pressure during the inspiratory phase.

Ventilator pneumatic systems can be either single circuit or double circuit. With single circuit ventilators, the gas that powers the pneumatic system is the same gas that is delivered to the patient. With double circuit ventilators, the gas delivered to the patient is separate from the gas that powers the pneumatics. Ventilators can be positive pressure or negative pressure generators. Positive pressure ventilators apply a positive pressure to the airway. Negative pressure ventilators apply a negative pressure to the chest wall. Critical care ventilators are typically positive pressure generators. Negative pressure ventilators are used infrequently, but may be used in some homecare applications.

Electronic System

Most current generation mechanical ventilators are microprocessor controlled. The microprocessor controls the inspiratory and expiratory valves. The microprocessor also controls information flow from the monitoring system of the ventilator (e.g., pressure, flow, volume) and the display of that information. The ventilator alarms are also controlled by the microprocessor.

CLASSIFICATION OF MECHANICAL VENTILATORS

Ventilator classification describes how the ventilator works. Classification schemes are general enough to be applied to any ventilator system. In this book, specific ventilator brands are not discussed. However, the classification scheme used here should be applicable to any commercially available ventilator. Many ventilators feature multiple modes and can be classified differently, depending upon the mode that is used.

Control Variables

The ventilator manipulates a control variable to cause inspiration. The control variable remains constant as the ventilatory load changes. Specific control variables are pressure, volume, flow, and time (Figure 3-2). A ventilator is a pressure-controller if the pressure waveform is not affected by changes in resistance and compliance. If the volume waveform remains unchanged with changes in resistance and compliance, the ventilator can be either a volume-controller or a flow controller. The ventilator is a volume controller if volume is measured and used to control the volume waveform. If volume is not used as a feedback signal, but the volume waveform remains constant, then the ventilator is a flow-controller. A ventilator is a time-controller if inspiratory and expiratory times are the only variables that are controlled.

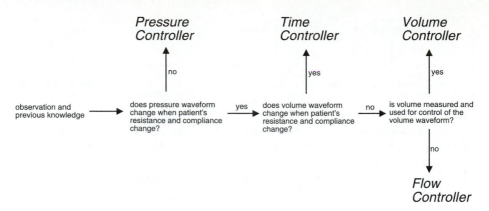

Figure 3-2 Criteria used to determine the control variable during inspiration. (From CHATBURN RL. Classification of mechanical ventilators. *Respir Care* 1992; 37:1009–1025.)

Phase Variables

Phase variables are used to initiate some phase of the ventilatory cycle. Specifically, these are the trigger, limit, and cycle (Figure 3-3). The trigger variable causes inspiration to begin. Inspiration can be time-triggered, in which the ventilator initiates inspiration at some clinician-determined interval. For example, the ventilator will initiate inspiration every three seconds if the rate is set at 20/min. Initiation of inspiration can also be triggered by the patient. Patient-triggering can be recognized by the ventilator as a pressure signal or as a flow signal (Figure 3-4). Pressure triggering occurs when patient effort causes a drop in airway pressure to a clinician preset level (sensitivity setting). Flow triggering occurs when the patient's inspiratory flow reaches a clinician preset level. The limit variable is the pressure, volume, or flow that cannot be exceeded during inspiration. Inspiration is not necessarily terminated when the limit variable is reached. The cycle variable is the pressure, volume, flow, or time that terminates inspiration. First-generation ventilators were typically pressure-cycled. With pressure support ventilation, the cycle is usually flow. With volume-controlled ventilation, the cycle is volume or time. With pressure-controlled ventilation, the ventilator is time-cycled. The baseline variable is what is controlled during the expiratory phase, and is the PEEP or continuous positive airway pressure (CPAP) setting.

Conditional Variables

Conditional variables are those that are examined by the ventilator's control logic and invoke an action if a threshold is met. Examples include the synchronization of mandatory and spontaneous breaths (synchronized intermittent mandatory ventilation) and the delivery of sigh breaths.

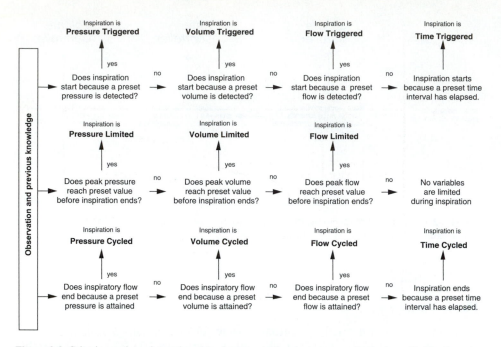

Figure 3-3 Criteria used to determine the phase variables during a mechanical ventilation breath. (From CHATBURN RL. Classification of mechanical ventilators. *Respir Care* 1992; 37:1009–1025.)

BREATH TYPES DURING MECHANICAL VENTILATION

Two clinically different breath types can be provided during mechanical ventilation: mandatory or spontaneous breaths (Figure 3-5). A spontaneous breath is both initiated and terminated by the patient. If the ventilator determines either the beginning and/or the end of the breath, the breath is mandatory.

EQUATION OF MOTION AND PATIENT-VENTILATOR INTERACTION

The interactions between ventilator and patient can be described by the Equation of Motion, which states that the pressure required to deliver a volume of gas into the lungs (P_T) is determined by the elastic (P_E) and resistive (P_R) properties of the respiratory system:

$$P_T = P_E + P_R.$$

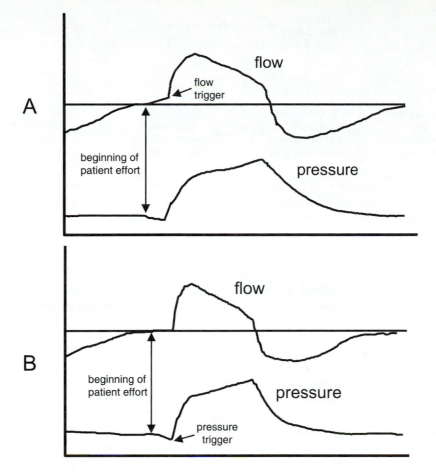

Figure 3-4 Flow (A) and pressure (B) triggering. With flow-triggering, the ventilator responds to a change in flow. With pressure-triggering, the ventilator responds to a decrease in airway pressure.

The elastic properties of the respiratory system are determined by compliance (C) and tidal volume (V_T), and the resistive properties of the lungs are determined by flow ($\dot{V}$) and airways resistance (R):

$$P_E = V_T/C \quad \text{and} \quad P_R = \dot{V} \times R.$$

Therefore

$$P_T = V_T/C + \dot{V} \times R.$$

Thus, the Equation of Motion states that the pressure required to deliver a breath is determined by tidal volume, compliance, flow, and resistance.

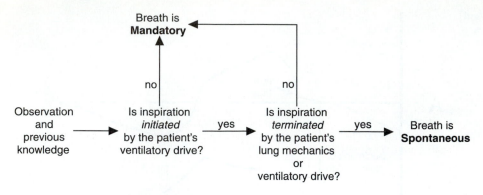

Figure 3-5 Criteria to determine breath types during mechanical ventilation. (From CHATBURN RL. Classification of mechanical ventilators. *Respir Care* 1992; 37:1009–1025.)

The pressure required to deliver the breath is determined by the pressure applied to the proximal airway (P_{airway}) and the pressure generated by the respiratory muscles (P_{muscle}):

$$P_T = P_{airway} + P_{muscle}.$$

During volume-controlled ventilation, flow and volume delivery from the ventilator are fixed. If the patient generates an inspiratory effort (P_{muscle}) during volume-controlled ventilation, the airway pressure drops – a common sign of patient-ventilator dys-synchrony. During pressure-controlled ventilation, P_{airway} is fixed. If the patient generates an inspiratory effort during pressure-controlled ventilation, flow and volume delivery increase – this should improve patient-ventilator synchrony.

POINTS TO REMEMBER

- The ventilator system consists of a pneumatic component and electronic component.
- The variable that the ventilator manipulates to cause inspiration is the control variable.
- Phase variables initiate a phase of the ventilatory cycle (inspiration or expiration).
- Two clinically different breath types that can be delivered during mechanical ventilation are mandatory breaths and spontaneous breaths.
- The Equation of Motion can be used to describe the effects of patient-ventilator interactions.

ADDITIONAL READING

AMERICAN ASSOCIATION FOR RESPIRATORY CARE. Consensus statement on the essentials of mechanical ventilators – 1992. *Respir Care* 1992; 37:1000–1025.

BRANSON RD, CHATBURN RL. Technical description and classification of modes of ventilator operation. *Respir Care* 1992; 37:1026–1044.

CHATBURN RL. Classification of mechanical ventilators. *Respir Care* 1992; 37:1009–1025.

CHATBURN RL. Classification of mechanical ventilators. In: BRANSON RD, HESS DR, CHATBURN RL. *Respiratory Care Equipment*, 2nd edition. Philadelphia, Lippincott, 1999.

CHATBURN RL, PRIMIANO FP. A new system for understanding modes of mechanical ventilation. *Respir Care* 2001; 46:604–621.

CHAPTER FOUR

TRADITIONAL MODES OF MECHANICAL VENTILATION

OBJECTIVES

1. Contrast pressure and volume controlled modes of ventilation.
2. Compare continuous mandatory ventilation, continuous spontaneous ventilation, and synchronized intermittent mandatory ventilation.
3. Compare continuous positive airway pressure and pressure support ventilation.
4. Compare full and partial ventilatory support.

INTRODUCTION

The relationship between breath types and phase variables is referred to as a mode of ventilation. During mechanical ventilation, the mode is one of the principal ventilator settings. Although many modes are available, the choice of mode is usually based on clinician preference or institutional bias. This chapter describes traditional ventilator modes (Table 4-1), which include continuous mandatory ventilation (CMV), continuous spontaneous ventilation, and synchronized intermittent mandatory ventilation (SMV).

VOLUME VERSUS PRESSURE CONTROLLED VENTILATION

The two general approaches to mechanical ventilatory support are volume control and pressure control. Although the term volume control is usually used, in reality the ventilator controls the inspiratory flow. The important variables for volume-controlled ventilation are shown in Figure 4-1. During pressure-controlled ventilation, the inspiratory flow decreases as the alveolar pressure approaches the pressure applied to the airway. The important variables affecting pressure-controlled ventilation are illustrated in Figure 4-2.

CONTINUOUS MANDATORY VENTILATION

A minimal rate is set by the clinician with this mode (Figure 4-3). The patient can trigger the ventilator at a more rapid rate, but every breath delivered is a mandatory breath type. Note that the mandatory breaths can be either volume-controlled or pressure-controlled. CMV is commonly called assist/control (A/C) ventilation – the terms CMV and A/C are used interchangeably.

Table 4-1 Ventilator modes

Mode	Mandatory breath Control variable	Spontaneous breath Control variable	Name
Continuous mandatory ventilation (CMV)	Volume	None	Volume-controlled continuous mandatory ventilation (VC CMV)
	Pressure	None	Pressure-controlled continuous mandatory ventilation (PC CMV)
Continuous spontaneous ventilation (CSV)	None	Pressure	Continuous positive airway pressure (CPAP) or pressure support ventilation (PSV)
Synchronized intermittent mandatory ventilation (SIMV)	Volume	Pressure	Volume-controlled synchronized mandatory ventilation (VC SIMV)
	Pressure	Pressure	Pressure-controlled synchronized intermittent mandatory ventilation (PC SIMV)

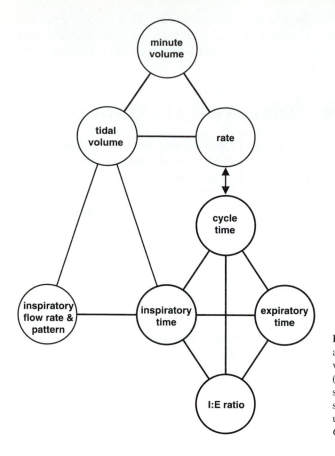

Figure 4-1 Important variables and their interaction during volume controlled ventilation. (Adapted from PERRY DG. A simplified diagram for understanding the operation of volume preset ventilators. *Respir Care* 1977; 22:42–49.)

CONTINUOUS SPONTANEOUS VENTILATION

With CSV, every breath is a spontaneous type. That is, every breath is triggered and cycled by the patient. The two most common forms of CSV are continuous positive airway pressure (CPAP) and pressure support ventilation (PSV).

Continuous Positive Airway Pressure

This is a spontaneous breathing mode – no mandatory breaths are delivered (Figure 4-4). A clinician-determined level of positive pressure is maintained throughout the ventilatory cycle. However, it is possible to set CPAP = zero, in which the pressure applied to the airway is ambient. The CPAP mode is most commonly used to evaluate extubation readiness. It is interesting to note that the performance of many current generation ventilators is such that a small level of

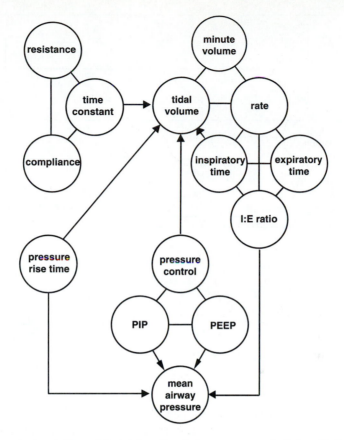

Figure 4-2 Important variables and their interaction during pressure controlled ventilation. (Adapted from CHATBURN RL, LOUGH MD. Mechanical ventilation. In: LOUGH MD, DOERSHUK CF, STERN RC, editors. *Pediatric Respiratory Therapy*. St. Louis, Mosby-Year Book, 1985.)

PSV (1–2 cm H_2O) is applied during CPAP. Ventilator performance during CPAP is better with flow-triggering than with pressure-triggering. For that reason, flow-triggering is recommended when CPAP is used.

Pressure Support Ventilation

With PSV, the patient's inspiratory effort is assisted by the ventilator at a preset level of inspiratory pressure. Inspiration is triggered and cycled by patient effort. During PSV, the patient determines the respiratory rate, inspiratory time, and tidal volume (Figure 4-5). Current generation ventilators provide backup ventilation (volume-controlled or pressure-controlled CMV) should apnea occur during PSV. PSV is normally flow cycled. Secondary cycling mechanisms with PSV are pressure and time. In other words, PSV will cycle to the expiratory phase when the

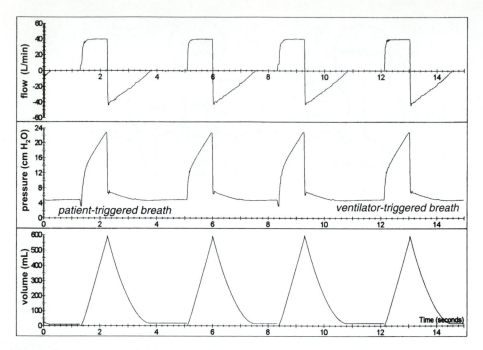

Figure 4-3 Volume-controlled continuous mandatory ventilation. Note that the breath can be triggered by the patient or the ventilator. After the breath is triggered, every breath type is mandatory.

flow decreases to a ventilator-determined level, when the pressure rises to a ventilator-determined level, or the inspiratory time reaches a ventilator-determined limit. The flow at which the ventilator cycles to the expiratory phase can be either a fixed absolute flow, a flow based on the peak inspiratory flow, or a flow based on peak inspiratory flow and elapsed inspiratory time. Newer generation ventilators allow the clinician to adjust the termination flow at which the ventilator cycles to a level appropriate for the patient. Newer generation ventilators also allow adjustment of rise time at the beginning of the pressure support breath. Rise time refers to the amount of time required to reach the pressure support level at the beginning of inspiration.

SYNCHRONIZED INTERMITTENT MANDATORY VENTILATION

SIMV is a ventilator mode in which mandatory breaths are delivered at a set rate with volume-control or pressure-control. Between the mandatory breaths, the patient is allowed to breathe spontaneously. Although older SIMV systems have been associated with a high imposed work-of-breathing, this has improved in the current generation of ventilators. The ventilator delivers the mandatory breaths in *synchrony* with the patient's inspiratory effort (Figure 4-6). If no

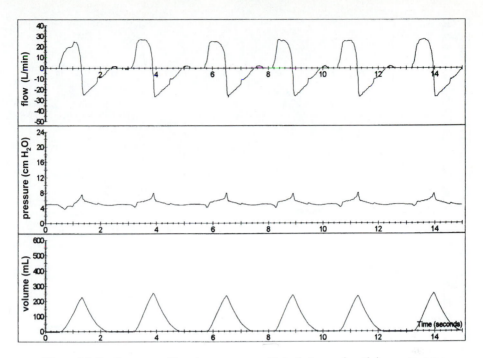

Figure 4-4 Continuous positive airway pressure. Note that every breath is spontaneous.

inspiratory effort is detected, the ventilator delivers a mandatory breath at the scheduled time. This is usually achieved by use of an assist window (Figure 4-7). This window opens at intervals determined by the set SIMV rate, and remains open for a manufacturer-specific period of time. If a patient-generated breathing effort is detected while this window is open, a mandatory breath is delivered. If no patient effort is detected in the time that the window is open, the ventilator delivers a mandatory breath. With SIMV, the spontaneous breaths can be pressure-supported (Figure 4-8).

FULL VERSUS PARTIAL VENTILATORY SUPPORT

Mechanical ventilation can be referred to as full or partial ventilatory support. With full ventilatory support, the ventilator does all of the ventilation for the patient; the patient does *not* trigger the ventilator or breathe spontaneously. This can be achieved as the result of the patient's primary disease process (e.g., quadriplegia), pharmacologic therapy (e.g., paralysis), or use of a minute ventilation high enough to suppress the patient's spontaneous breathing efforts (e.g., hyperventilation). Full ventilatory support can be achieved using CMV or SIMV. Full ventilatory support

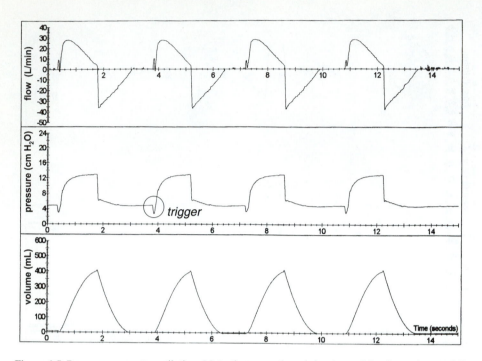

Figure 4-5 Pressure support ventilation. Note that every breath is triggered by the patient and flow cycled.

is often preferred for patients who are critically ill to decrease the oxygen cost of breathing and achieve control of the patient's ventilatory pattern.

With partial ventilator support, some of the work-of-breathing is provided by the ventilator and the remainder is provided by the patient. Partial ventilatory support is commonly used during weaning from mechanical ventilation. Partial ventilatory support is also preferred by clinicians who believe that this form of ventilation maintains respiratory muscle tone, allows the patient to maintain some control of the ventilatory pattern, and improves patient comfort. Partial ventilatory support can be achieved with CMV, SIMV, and PSV. With CMV, most of the work-of-breathing is usually provided by the ventilator. With SIMV and PSV, the balance between the work-of-breathing provided by the patient and that provided by the ventilator can be set by the clinician.

POINTS TO REMEMBER

- With CMV, all breaths are mandatory.
- All breaths are spontaneous with continuous positive airway pressure.

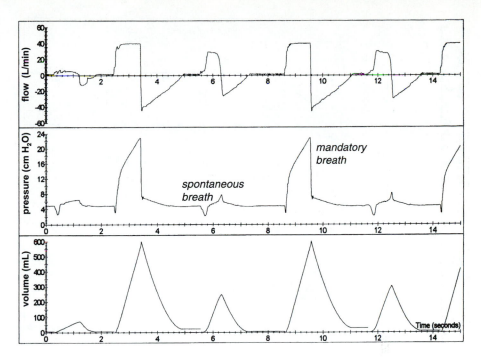

Figure 4-6 Synchronized intermittent mandatory ventilation illustrating mandatory and spontaneous breaths. The mandatory breaths are volume-controlled.

- The patient's inspiratory effort is assisted by a preset level of inspiratory pressure during pressure support ventilation.
- With synchronized intermittent mandatory ventilation, both spontaneous and mandatory breaths can be delivered and the ventilator breaths are synchronized to patient effort.
- With full ventilatory support, the ventilator does all of the breathing for the patient.

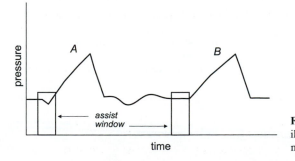

Figure 4-7 Pressure waveform for SIMV, illustrating the assist window for synchronization of mandatory breaths.

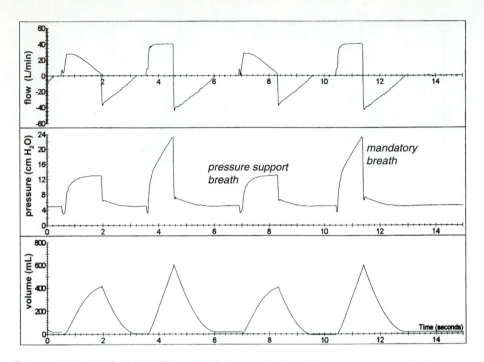

Figure 4-8 Synchronized intermittent mandatory ventilation with pressure support for the spontaneous breaths. The mandatory breaths are volume-controlled.

- With partial ventilatory support, some of the work is provided by the ventilator and the remainder is provided by the patient.

ADDITIONAL READING

AMERICAN ASSOCIATION FOR RESPIRATORY CARE. Consensus statement on the essentials of mechanical ventilators – 1992. *Respir Care* 1992; 37:1000–1008.

BRANSON RD, CHATBURN RL. Technical description and classification of modes of ventilator operation. *Respir Care* 1992; 37:1026–1044.

CAMPBELL RS, BRANSON RD. Ventilatory support for the 90s: Pressure support ventilation. *Respir Care* 1993; 38:526–537.

HESS D, BRANSON RD. New modes of ventilation. In: HILL NS, LEVY MM. *Ventilator management strategies for critical care.* New York, Marcel Dekker, 2001.

MACINTYRE NR. Clinically available new strategies for mechanical ventilatory support. *Chest* 1993; 104:560–565.

CHAPTER FIVE

NEW MODES OF MECHANICAL VENTILATION

OBJECTIVES

1. Compare approaches to dual control modes.
2. Describe Automode.
3. Describe the control of airway pressure during proportional assist ventilation.
4. Describe automatic tube compensation.
5. Compare approaches to airway pressure release ventilation.
6. Discuss the rationale for mandatory minute ventilation.

INTRODUCTION

With each generation of ventilators, new modes and variations on previous modes become available. There now exist numerous ventilator modes from a variety of manufacturers. The purpose of this chapter is to describe the technical aspects of new modes of ventilation that have recently become available. Although they have been heavily promoted by their manufacturers, the clinical role of many of these modes remains unproven. Use of these modes is often based upon their availability and clinician bias, rather than evidence that they are superior to traditional modes.

DUAL CONTROL MODES

Dual control modes allow the ventilator to control pressure or volume based on a feedback loop. However, it is important to remember that the ventilator is controlling only pressure or volume, not both at the same time. These modes are classified as dual control within a breath or dual control breath-to-breath (Table 5-1). Dual control within a breath is a mode where the ventilator switches from pressure control to volume control during the breath. Dual control breath-to-breath is simpler because the ventilator operates in either the pressure support or pressure control mode, with the pressure limit increasing or decreasing to maintain a clinician selected tidal volume.

Dual Control Within a Breath

The proposed advantage of this mode is a reduced work-of-breathing while maintaining a minimum minute volume and tidal volume. This approach operates

Table 5-1 Dual-controlled modes

Type	Manufacturer; Ventilator	Name
Dual control within a breath	VIASYS Healthcare; Bird 8400Sti and Tbird	Volume-assured pressure support
	VIASYS Healthcare; Bear 1000	Pressure augmentation
Dual control breath-to-breath: pressure-limited flow-cycled ventilation	Siemens; Servo 300	Volume support
	Cardiopulmonary Corporation; Venturi	Variable pressure support
Dual control breath-to-breath: pressure-limited time-cycled ventilation	Siemens; Servo 300	Pressure-regulated volume control
	Hamilton; Galileo	Adaptive pressure ventilation
	Drager; Evita 4	Autoflow
	Cardiopulmonary Corporation; Venturi	Variable pressure control
Dual control breath-to-breath: SIMV	Hamilton; Galileo	Adaptive support ventilation

during mandatory breaths or pressure supported breaths to combine the high initial flow of a pressure-controlled breath with the constant volume delivery of a volume-controlled breath. Common names for this approach are volume-assured pressure support and pressure augmentation. The breath is patient or ventilator triggered. The ventilator then attempts to reach the pressure support setting as quickly as possible. This portion of the breath is pressure controlled and associated with a high variable flow. As this pressure is reached, the ventilator determines the volume that has been delivered from the ventilator, compares this to the desired tidal volume, and determines if the desired tidal volume will be delivered.

If the delivered tidal volume and set tidal volume are equal, the breath is a pressure support breath (Figure 5-1). If the patient's inspiratory effort is low, the breath changes from a pressure controlled to a volume-controlled breath. Flow remains constant, increasing the inspiratory time until the tidal volume has been delivered. During this time the pressure rises above the pressure support setting. If pressure reaches the high-pressure alarm setting, the breath is pressure cycled. A similar condition can occur if there is a decrease in lung compliance or increase in airway resistance. Because this breath has the possibility of a prolonged inspiratory time, there are secondary cycle characteristics for these breaths (e.g., an inspiratory time of three seconds). Finally, the breath can allow the patient a tidal volume larger than the set volume. Because the pressure limit remains the same, this breath is also a pressure support breath (i.e., it is pressure controlled and flow cycled). If the pressure support is set too high, or if the minimum tidal volume is set too low, the volume guarantee is negated. If the peak flow setting is too high, all the breaths will be volume-controlled. If the peak flow is set too low, the switch from pressure control to volume control will occur late in the breath and inspiratory time may be prolonged.

Dual Control Breath-to-Breath: Pressure-Limited Flow-Cycled Ventilation

This mode is a closed-loop control of pressure support ventilation. Common names are volume support and variable pressure support. Tidal volume is used as feedback control to adjust the pressure support level. All breaths are patient triggered, pressure limited, and flow-cycled (Figure 5-2). A test breath with a low pressure is applied. The delivered tidal volume (exiting the ventilator) is measured and compliance is calculated. The following three breaths are delivered at 75% of the pressure support calculated to deliver the set tidal volume. The ventilator then attempts to maintain a constant delivered tidal volume. From breath-to-breath the maximum pressure change is < 3 cm H_2O and can range from 0 cm H_2O above PEEP to 5 cm H_2O below the high pressure alarm setting. Since all breaths are pressure support breaths, the breath is flow-cycled.

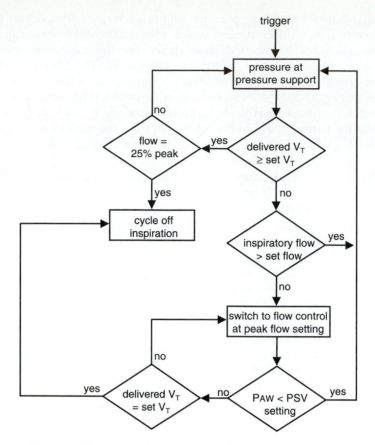

Figure 5-1 Control logic for volume-assured pressure-support mode.

There are several potential issues with this mode. Auto-PEEP may occur if the pressure level increases in an attempt to maintain tidal volume in a patient with airflow obstruction. In the patient with a high ventilatory demand, ventilator support will decrease, which could be the opposite of the desired response. If the minimum set tidal volume exceeds ventilatory demand, the patient may remain at that level of support and weaning may be delayed.

Dual Control Breath-to-Breath: Pressure-Limited Time-Cycled Ventilation

This mode is closed-loop pressure controlled ventilation. Tidal volume is a feedback control for continuously adjusting the pressure control (Figure 5-3). All breaths are patient or ventilator triggered, pressure controlled, and time cycled. The ventilator delivers a test breath and calculates total system compliance. The next three breaths are delivered at 75% of the pressure control necessary to

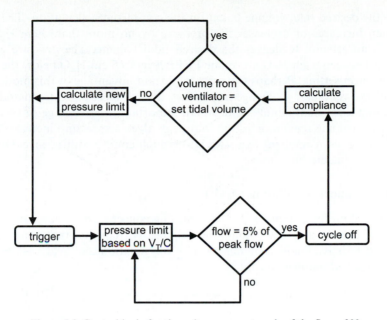

Figure 5-2 Control logic for the volume support mode of the Servo 300.

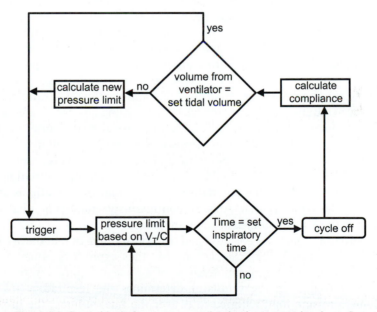

Figure 5-3 Control logic for pressure-regulated volume control and autoflow.

achieve the desired tidal volume based on the compliance calculation. The venti-lator then increases or decreases the pressure by no more than 3 cm H_2O per breath in an attempt to deliver the desired tidal volume. The pressure control fluctuates between 0 cm H_2O above the PEEP level to 5 cm H_2O below the upper pressure alarm setting. Perhaps the most important advantage of this mode is the ability of the ventilator to change inspiratory flow to meet patient demand while maintaining a constant minute volume. An important disadvantage of this mode is that tidal volume remains constant and peak alveolar pressure increases as the lungs become less compliant (e.g., ARDS), which could result in alveolar over-distention and acute lung injury.

Adaptive Support Ventilation (ASV)

ASV is based on the minimal work-of-breathing concept, which suggests that the patient will breathe at a tidal volume and respiratory frequency that minimizes the elastic and resistive loads while maintaining oxygenation and acid base balance. This is described mathematically as:

$$\text{respiratory rate} = \left(\sqrt{1 + 4\pi^2 RC \times (\dot{V}_A/\dot{V}_D)} - 1 \right)/(2\pi^2 RC)$$

where RC is the respiratory time constant, $\dot{V}_A$ is alveolar ventilation and $\dot{V}_D$ is dead space ventilation. The ASV algorithm uses this formula and patient weight to adjust a number of ventilator variables. The ventilator attempts to deliver 100 mL/min/kg of minute ventilation for an adult and 200 mL/min/kg for chil-dren. This can be adjusted by setting the % minute volume control from 20 to 200%, which allows the clinician to provide full ventilatory support or encourage spontaneous breathing and facilitate weaning.

When connected to the patient, the ventilator delivers a series of test breaths and measures system compliance, airways resistance, and auto-PEEP. The input of body weight allows the ventilator's algorithm to choose a required minute volume. The ventilator then uses the clinician input and measured respiratory mechanics to select a respiratory frequency, inspiratory time, I:E ratio, and pres-sure limit for mandatory and spontaneous breaths. Lung mechanics are measured on a breath-to-breath basis and ventilator settings are altered to meet the desired targets. If the patient breathes spontaneously, the ventilator will apply pressure support breaths and encourage spontaneous breathing. However, spontaneous and mandatory breaths can be combined to meet the minute ventilation target. The pressure limit of both the mandatory and spontaneous breaths is adjusted continuously. This means that ASV is continuously employing dual control breath-to-breath of mandatory and spontaneous breaths.

The ventilator adjusts the I:E ratio and inspiratory time of mandatory breaths to prevent auto-PEEP by calculation of the expiratory time constant (compliance × resistance) and maintenance of sufficient expiratory time. If the patient is not triggering, the ventilator determines the respiratory frequency, tidal volume, pressure limit required to deliver the tidal volume, the inspiratory time, and the I:E ratio. If the patient is triggering, the number of mandatory breaths decreases and the ventilator chooses a pressure support that maintains a tidal volume sufficient to assure alveolar ventilation based on a dead space calculation of 2.2 mL/kg. ASV can provide pressure-limited time-cycled ventilation, add dual control of those breaths on a breath-to-breath basis, allow for mandatory breaths and spontaneous breaths (dual control SIMV + PSV), and eventually switch to pressure support with dual control breath-to-breath (variable pressure with pressure supported breaths). During mandatory breath delivery, the ventilator sets inspiratory time and I:E ratio.

AUTOMODE

AutoMode allows the ventilator to switch between mandatory and spontaneous breathing modes. AutoMode combines volume support (VS) and pressure-regulated volume control (PRVC) into a single mode. If the patient is paralyzed, the ventilator will provide PRVC. All breaths are mandatory breaths that are ventilator triggered, pressure controlled, and time cycled; the pressure control increases or decreases to maintain the set tidal volume. If the patient breathes spontaneously for two consecutive breaths, the ventilator switches to VS. In this case, all breaths are patient triggered, pressure limited, and flow cycled. If the patient becomes apneic for 12 seconds in the adult setting (eight seconds in the pediatric setting or five seconds in the neonatal setting), the ventilator switches back to PRVC. The change from PRVC to VS is accomplished at equivalent peak pressures. AutoMode also switches between pressure control and pressure support or volume control to VS. In the volume control to VS switch, the VS pressure limit will be equivalent to the pause pressure during volume control. If an inspiratory pause pressure is not available, the pressure level is calculated as:

$$(PIP - PEEP) \times 50\% + PEEP.$$

PROPORTIONAL ASSIST VENTILATION

Proportional assist ventilation (PAV) was designed to increase (or decrease) airway pressure in proportion to patient effort. This is accomplished by a positive feedback control that amplifies airway pressure proportionally to instantaneous inspiratory flow and volume. Unlike other modes of ventilatory support, which deliver a preset tidal volume or inspiratory pressure at the airway, with PAV the amount of support changes with patient effort, assisting ventilation with a uniform proportionality between ventilator and patient (Figure 5-4). To the extent that inspiratory effort is a reflection of ventilatory demand, this form of support may result in a more physiologic breathing pattern. Patient effort determines the ventilating pressure.

PAV is a positive feedback controller where respiratory elastance and resistance are the feedback signal gains, defined as K_1 (cm H_2O/L) and K_2

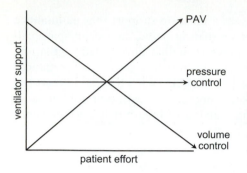

Figure 5-4 Airway pressure with increasing patient effort for PAV, pressure control, and volume control ventilation. Note that the amount of ventilator assist increases with patient effort for PAV, decreases for volume control, and remains constant for pressure control.

(cm $H_2O/L/s$), respectively. In such a system, the pressure at the airway is adjusted according to the equation:

$$P_{AW} = K_1 \times V + K_2 \times \dot{V}$$

where P_{AW} is the total pressure applied at the airway, V is inspiratory volume, and $\dot{V}$ is inspiratory flow. This equation is derived from the Equation of Motion of the respiratory system. For the airway pressure to be amplified in proportion to the pressure developed by the respiratory muscles, K_1 and K_2 must be set to < 100% of the patient's elastance and resistance. If K_1 and K_2 are ≥ 100% of elastance and resistance, runaway occurs in which the ventilator continues to add pressure to the airway after the end of the patient's inspiratory effort.

Because flow decreases and volume increases throughout inspiration, flow assist is greatest at the beginning of inspiration and volume assist is greatest at the end of inspiration. Because flow and volume vary breath-by-breath, the airway pressure during PAV varies breath-by-breath (Figure 5-5). Thus, PAV allows the respiratory rate, inspiratory time, and inspiratory pressure to vary. This is in contrast to the fixed pressure of PSV and the fixed pressure and inspiratory time of PCV.

The measurement of elastance and resistance in a spontaneously breathing patient is difficult. If impedance is overestimated, the ventilator output (pressure) will exceed the pressure required to overcome respiratory system impedance. The result is a runaway condition. The difficulty in measuring elastance and resistance is further complicated by their fluctuations in mechanically ventilated patients. The PAV algorithm also assumes that elastance and resistance characteristics are linear. For patients with respiratory failure, the non-linearity of these variables may result in inappropriate ventilation with PAV. One method for selecting the correct settings for PAV uses the runaway method. The volume assist is set at 2 cm H_2O/L (with a flow assist of 1 cm $H_2O/L/s$) and raised in 2 cm H_2O increments until runaway occurs. The patient's elastance is estimated as this level of volume assist minus 1 cm H_2O/L. The flow assist is set at 1 cm $H_2O/L/s$ (with a volume assist of 2 cm H_2O/L) and raised in 1 cm $H_2O/L/s$ increments until run-

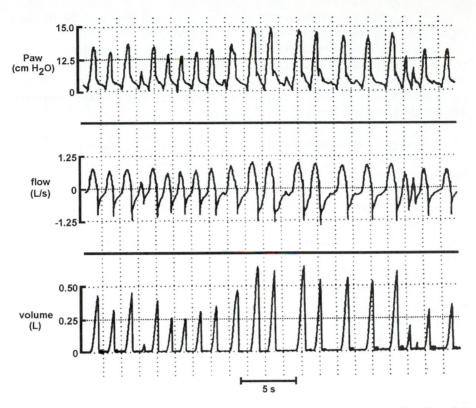

Figure 5-5 Airway pressure, flow and volume waveforms for proportional assist ventilation. Note that the airway pressure varies with the inspiratory flow and volume demands of the patient. (From MARANTZ S, ET AL. Response of ventilator-dependent patients to different levels of proportional assist. *J Appl Physiol* 1996; 80:397–403.)

away occurs. The patient's airways' resistance is estimated as the flow assist minus 1 cm $H_2O/L/s$.

AUTOMATIC TUBE COMPENSATION

Although pressure support is used to overcome endotracheal tube resistance, variable inspiratory flow and changing demands of the patient cannot be met by a single level of pressure support. The resistance of the endotracheal tube creates a condition where early in the breath when ventilator flow is high, tracheal pressure remains low and under-compensation for imposed work occurs. Late in the breath, pressure support overcompensates, prolonging inspiration which may exacerbate over-inflation. Automatic tube compensation (ATC) continuously calculates tracheal pressure in intubated mechanically ventilated patients to allow breath-by-breath compensation of endotracheal tube resistance.

ATC uses the known resistance of the endotracheal tube and the measurement of flow to calculate tracheal pressure (Figure 5-6). ATC compensates for endotracheal tube resistance via closed loop control of calculated tracheal pressure. This mode uses the known resistive coefficients of the tracheal tube (tracheostomy or endotracheal) and measurement of instantaneous flow to apply pressure proportional to resistance throughout the total respiratory cycle. The equation for calculating tracheal pressure is:

$$\text{tracheal pressure} = \text{proximal airway pressure} - (\text{tube coefficient} \times \text{flow}^2)$$

Most of the interest in ATC revolves around eliminating the imposed work-of-breathing during inspiration. However, during expiration there is also a flow dependent pressure drop across the tube. ATC compensates for this flow resistive component and may reduce expiratory resistance. ATC reduces PEEP during exhalation to facilitate compensation of expiratory resistance of the endotracheal tube.

Incomplete compensation for endotracheal tube resistance may occur because *in vivo* endotracheal tube resistance is greater than *in vitro* resistance. Additionally, kinks and accumulation of secretions in the tube change the resistive coefficient and results in incomplete compensation. Whether endotracheal tube resistance poses a clinical concern for increased work-of-breathing in adults is controversial. The imposed work-of-breathing through the endotracheal tube is modest at a usual minute ventilation for the tube sizes most commonly used for adults. Similar outcomes have been reported when spontaneous breathing trials were conducted with low-level pressure support or with a T-piece. It has also been reported that the work-of-breathing during a two-hour spontaneous breathing trial with a T-piece is similar to the work-of-breathing immediately following extubation. Although prolonged spontaneous breathing through an endotracheal tube is not desirable due to the resistance of the tube, this may

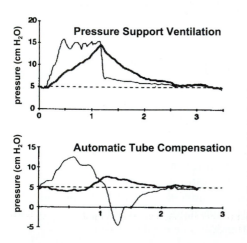

Figure 5-6 Pressure waveforms from the trachea (heavy lines) and the proximal airway (light lines) during pressure support ventilation and automatic tube compensation. Note that the tracheal pressure fluctuated very little during automatic tube compensation. (From FABRY B, ET AL. Breathing pattern and additional work-of-breathing in spontaneously breathing patients with different ventilatory demands during inspiratory pressure support and automatic tube compensation. *Intensive Care Med* 1997; 23:545–552.)

not be important for short periods of spontaneous breathing to assess extubation readiness.

AIRWAY PRESSURE-RELEASE VENTILATION

Airway pressure-release ventilation (APRV) produces alveolar ventilation as an adjunct to CPAP. Airway pressure is transiently released to a lower level, after which it is quickly restored to re-inflate the lungs (Figure 5-7). For a patient with no spontaneous breathing efforts, APRV is similar to pressure-controlled ventilation. Unlike pressure-controlled ventilation, APRV allows spontaneous breathing at any time during the respiratory cycle. This is because the exhalation valve is active during this mode. Traditionally, the exhalation valve is completely closed during the inspiratory phase of the ventilator. With newer generation ventilators, the exhalation valve opens when the set peak inspiratory pressure is exceeded during pressure controlled ventilation.

Because peak inspiratory pressure during APRV does not exceed the CPAP level, the hazards associated with high airway pressure may be minimized (e.g., alveolar over-distention, hemodynamic compromise). Because the patient is allowed to breathe spontaneously at both levels of CPAP, the need for sedation may also be decreased. The evidence to support these potential benefits is, however, presently weak. Tidal volume for the APRV breath depends on lung compliance, airways resistance, the magnitude of the pressure release, the duration of the pressure release, and the magnitude of the patient's spontaneous breathing efforts. Of concern is the potential for alveolar dere-

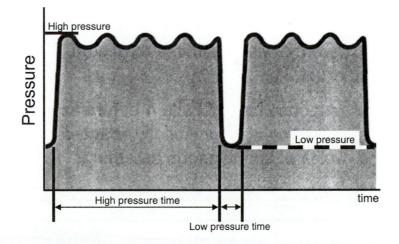

Figure 5-7 Pressure waveform for APRV. Note that the patient can breathe at both levels of pressure and that the pressure release is brief (courtesy of Dräger).

cruitment during the release of pressure with APRV. Biphasic positive airway pressure (BIPAP) is a modification of APRV. Unlike APRV, the I:E ratio used with BIPAP is not reversed. BIPAP (also called Bilevel or PCV+ on some ventilators) is also partially synchronized to the patient's inspiratory efforts. PSV can be used with Bilevel (Figure 5-8). Bilevel can be used to provide sigh breaths during PSV. For this approach, an inspiratory pressure of 20 to 30 cm H_2O is applied for 1 to 3 seconds at a rate of 2 to 4 breaths per minute.

MANDATORY MINUTE VENTILATION

Mandatory minute ventilation (MMV) is a mode intended to guarantee minute ventilation during weaning. If the patient's spontaneous ventilation does not match the target minute ventilation set by the clinician, the ventilator supplies the difference between the patient's minute ventilation and the target minute ventilation. If the patient's spontaneous minute ventilation exceeds the target, no ventilator support is provided. MMV is thus a form of closed loop ventilation in which the ventilator adjusts its output according to the patient's response. MMV is only available on a few ventilator types used in the United States and its value to facilitate weaning is unclear. MMV can be provided by altering the rate or the tidal volume delivered from the ventilator. Some ventilators increase

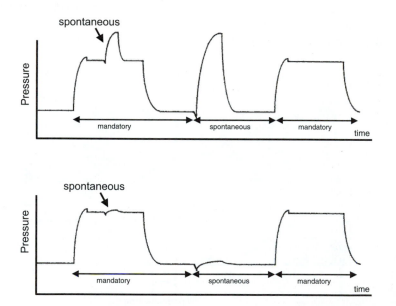

Figure 5-8 Pressure waveforms for Bilevel mode with pressure support (top) and without pressure support (bottom). (From CHATBURN RL, PRIMIANO FP. A new system for understanding modes of mechanical ventilation. *Respir Care* 2001; 46:604–621.)

the mandatory breath rate if the minute ventilation falls below the target level, whereas others increase the level of pressure support when the minute ventilation falls below the target level.

POINTS TO REMEMBER

- Dual control within a breath is a mode where the ventilator switches from pressure control to volume control during the breath.
- Dual control breath-to-breath increases or decreases the pressure limit to maintain a clinician selected tidal volume.
- Adaptive support ventilation is based on the minimal work-of-breathing concept.
- Automode allows the ventilator to switch between mandatory and spontaneous breathing modes.
- Proportional assist ventilation increases or decreases airway pressure in proportion to patient effort.
- Automatic tube compensation compensates for endotracheal tube resistance via closed loop control of calculated tracheal pressure.
- Airway pressure release ventilation produces alveolar ventilation as an adjunct to CPAP.
- Mandatory minute ventilation is a mode intended to guarantee minute ventilation during weaning.

ADDITIONAL READING

AMERICAN ASSOCIATION FOR RESPIRATORY CARE. Consensus statement on the essentials of mechanical ventilators – 1992. *Respir Care* 1992; 37:1000–1008.

BRANSON RD, CAMPBELL RS, DAVIS K. New modes of ventilatory support. *Int Anesthesiol Clin* 1999; 37:103–125.

BRANSON RD, CHATBURN RL. Technical description and classification of modes of ventilator operation. *Respir Care* 1992; 37:1026–1044.

BRANSON RD, DAVIS K. Dual control modes: combining volume and pressure breaths. *Respir Care Clin N Am* 2001; 7:397–408.

CAMPBELL RS, BRANSON RD, JOHANNIGM JA. Adaptive support ventilation. *Respir Care Clin N Am* 2001; 7:425–440.

GAY PC, HESS DR, HILL NS. Noninvasive proportional assist ventilation for acute respiratory insufficiency. Comparison with pressure support ventilation. *Am J Respir Crit Care Med* 2001; 164:1606–1611.

GRASSO S, RANIERI VM. Proportional assist ventilation. *Respir Care Clin N Am* 2001; 7:465–474.

GUTTMANN J, HABERTHUR C, MOLS G. Automatic tube compensation. *Respir Care Clin N Am* 2001; 7:475–502.

HESS D, BRANSON RD. New modes of ventilation. In: HILL NS, LEVY MM. *Ventilator management strategies for critical care.* New York, Marcel Dekker, 2001.

HESS D, BRANSON RD. Ventilators and weaning modes. *Respir Care Clin N Am* 2000; 6:407–435.

MACINTYRE NR. Clinically available new strategies for mechanical ventilatory support. *Chest* 1993; 104:560–565.

MacIntyre NR, Gropper C, Westfall T. Combining pressure-limiting and volume-cycling features in a patient-interactive mechanical breath. *Crit Care Med* 1994; 22:353–357.

Patroniti N, Foti G, Cortinovis B, et al. Sigh improves gas exchange and lung volume in patients with acute respiratory distress syndrome undergoing pressure support ventilation. *Anesthesiology* 2002; 96:788–794.

Quan SF, Parides GC, Knoper SR. Mandatory minute volume (MMV) ventilation: An overview. *Respir Care* 1990; 35:898–905.

Wrigge H, Zinserling J, Hering R, et al. Cardiorespiratory effects of automatic tube compensation during airway pressure release ventilation in patients with acute lung injury. *Anesthesiology* 2001; 95:382–389.

Younes M. Proportional assist ventilation, a new approach to ventilatory support. *Am Rev Respir Dis* 1992; 145:114–120.

CHAPTER SIX

FLOWS, WAVEFORMS, AND I:E RATIOS

OBJECTIVES

1. Apply the concept of time constant to the physiology of mechanical ventilation.
2. Compare constant-flow and decreasing flow patterns during volume controlled ventilation.
3. Describe the effect of respiratory mechanics on the airway pressure waveform during volume controlled ventilation.
4. Describe the effect of resistance and compliance on flow during pressure controlled ventilation.

5. Describe the effect of rise time adjustment during pressure controlled and pressure support ventilation.
6. Describe the effect of adjustable termination flow during pressure support ventilation.
7. Discuss the role of sigh breaths during mechanical ventilation.
8. Discuss the physiologic effects of I:E ratio manipulations.

INTRODUCTION

Present generation microprocessor-controlled ventilators allow the clinician to choose among various inspiratory flow waveforms. This chapter describes the technical and physiologic aspects of various inspiratory waveforms during mechanical ventilation.

TIME CONSTANT

An important principle for understanding pulmonary mechanics during mechanical ventilation is that of the time constant. The time constant determines the rate of change in the volume of a lung unit that is passively inflated or deflated. It is expressed by the relationship:

$$Vt = Vi \times e^{-t/\tau}$$

where Vt is the volume of a lung unit at time t, Vi is the initial volume of the lung unit, e is the base of the natural logarithm, and τ is the time constant. The relationship between Vt and τ is illustrated in Figure 6-1. Note that the volume change is nearly complete in five time constants.

For respiratory physiology, τ is the product of resistance and compliance. Lung units with a higher resistance and/or a higher compliance will have a longer time constant and require more time to fill and to empty. Conversely, lung units with a lower resistance and/or compliance will have a lower time constant and thus require less time to fill and to empty. A simple method to measure the

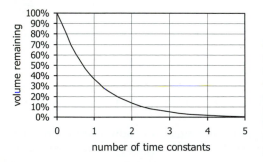

Figure 6-1 The time constant function for lung emptying. After one time constant, 37% of the volume remains in the lungs, 13% remains after two time constants, 5% remains after three time constants, 2% remains after four time constants, and < 1% remains after five time constants. The value of each time constant equals the product of resistance and compliance.

expiratory time constant is to divide the expired tidal volume by the peak expiratory flow during passive positive pressure ventilation:

$$\tau = V_T/\dot{V}_{E(peak)}$$

where V_T is the expired tidal volume and $\dot{V}_{E(peak)}$ is the peak expiratory flow. Although this is a useful index of the global expiratory time constant, it treats the lung as a single compartment model and thus does not account for time constant inhomogeneities in the lungs.

FLOW WAVEFORMS

Volume Controlled Ventilation

The flow, pressure, and volume waveforms produced with a constant flow pattern are shown in Figure 6-2. This is often called rectangular-wave ventilation due to the shape of the flow waveform. Ideally, this form of ventilation should produce a nearly constant gas flow during inspiration. However, the flow may taper during inspiration if the driving pressure from the ventilator is low and the peak airway pressure is high. With the constant flow pattern, the volume (per unit time) is delivered into the lungs equally throughout inspiration. In other words, volume delivery into the lungs at the beginning of inspiration is the same as that at the end of inspiration. Note that airway pressure increases linearly

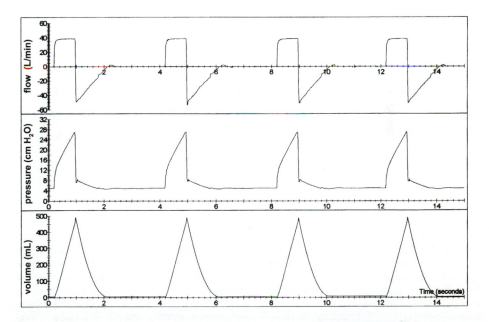

Figure 6-2 Flow, pressure, and volume waveforms with constant flow, volume controlled ventilation.

throughout inspiration, following an initial rapid pressure increase due to the resistance through the endotracheal tube. The effect of resistance and compliance on the airway pressure waveform during constant flow volume ventilation is shown in Figure 6-3.

During volume controlled ventilation, the inspiratory flow can also be set to a descending ramp. With descending ramp, flow is greatest at the beginning of inspiration and decreases to a lower flow at the end of inspiration. Typical flow, pressure, and volume waveforms with a descending ramp are shown in Figure 6-4. Due to the decrease in flow during the inspiratory phase, note that most of the tidal volume is delivered early during inspiration, and the pressure waveform approaches that of a rectangular wave. A descending ramp flow lengthens the inspiratory time, unless the peak flow is increased. The descending ramp flow can be provided in several ways (Figure 6-5). With a complete ramp, flow decreases to zero at end-inspiration. With 50% ramp, the flow at end-inspiration is half of the initial flow. Flow can also taper to a fixed, manufacturer-specific, level at the end of inspiration (e.g., 5 L/min).

Pressure Controlled Ventilation

Typical pressure, flow, and volume waveforms during pressure ventilation are shown in Figure 6-6. Note the rectangular pressure waveform and descending (exponential) flow pattern. Also note that most of the tidal volume is delivered

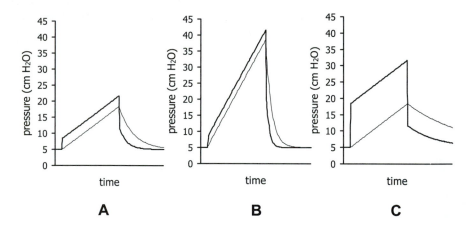

Figure 6-3 Airway pressure waveforms during constant flow volume ventilation. In each case, the tidal volume is 0.675 L, flow is 40 L/min, and PEEP is 5 cm H_2O. The heavy line represents airway pressure and the lighter line represents alveolar pressure. A. Resistance of 5 cm $H_2O/L/s$ and compliance of 50 mL/cm H_2O. B. Resistance of 5 cm $H_2O/L/s$ and compliance of 20 mL/cm H_2O. Compared to the left panel, peak inspiratory pressure increases, alveolar pressure increases, but the difference between airway pressure and alveolar pressure does not change. C. Resistance of 20 cm $H_2O/L/s$ and compliance of 50 mL/cm H_2O. Compared to the left panel, peak inspiratory pressure increases, alveolar pressure is unchanged, and the difference between airway pressure and alveolar pressure is increased.

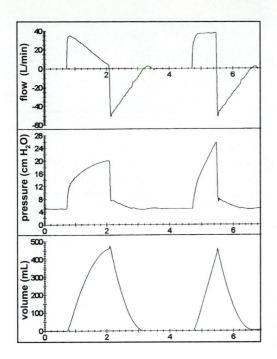

Figure 6-4 Waveforms for descending ramp and constant flows. Note the differences in the shape of the pressure waveform and peak inspiratory pressure.

early in the inspiratory phase. During pressure ventilation, flow is determined by the pressure applied to the airway (i.e., the pressure control or pressure support setting), airways resistance, and the time constant (Figure 6-7):

$$\dot{V} = (\Delta P/R) \times (e^{-t/\tau})$$

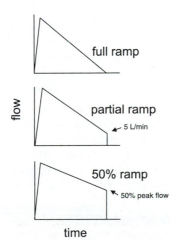

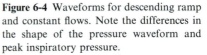

Figure 6-5 Full and partial descending ramp flow with volume controlled ventilation.

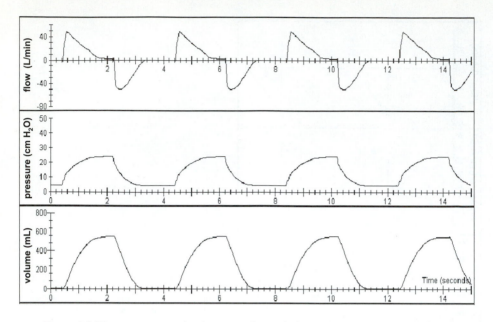

Figure 6-6 Flow, pressure, and volume waveforms during pressure controlled ventilation.

where ΔP is the pressure applied to the airway above PEEP, R is airways resistance, t is the elapsed time after initiation of the inspiratory phase, e is the base of the natural logarithm, and τ is the product of airways resistance and respiratory system compliance (the time constant of the respiratory system). The length of zero flow time at the end of inspiration is determined by the inspiratory time; a longer inspiratory time results in more zero flow time.

With newer generation ventilators, it is possible to adjust the time required for the ventilator to reach the peak inspiratory pressure (rise time). The rise time controls the flow at the beginning of the inspiratory phase (Figure 6-8). With a faster rise time, flow is greater at the beginning of inspiration, which may relieve dyspnea in patients with a high respiratory drive.

An inverse ratio can be used in conjunction with pressure-controlled ventilation. This results in pressure-controlled inverse ratio ventilation (PCIRV). In the past, this mode has been popular in some hospitals to treat patients with severe oxygenation failure. Its physiologic effect is to increase mean airway pressure and it is commonly associated with auto-PEEP. In practice, a descending ramp flow pattern with an end-inspiratory zero flow period (inspiratory pause) can be produced using either pressure-controlled or volume-controlled ventilation. Inverse ratio ventilation can also be provided using either pressure-controlled or volume-controlled strategies. The clinical results are determined by the flow pattern, rather than the use of volume-controlled or pressure-controlled ventilation strategies per se. The benefits of PCIRV on lung function are unclear and have risks such as hemodynamic compromise.

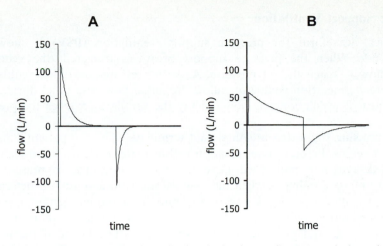

A   **B**

Figure 6-7 During pressure controlled ventilation, the inspiratory flow pattern is determined by airways resistance and respiratory system compliance. A. Airways resistance of 10 cm $H_2O/L/s$ and respiratory system compliance of 20 mL/cm H_2O. The inspiratory time is 1.5 s and the resulting tidal volume (the area under the flow curve) is 400 mL. B. Airways resistance of 20 cm $H_2O/L/s$ and respiratory system compliance of 50 mL/cm H_2O. The inspiratory time is 1.5 s and the resulting tidal volume (the area under the flow curve) is 775 mL.

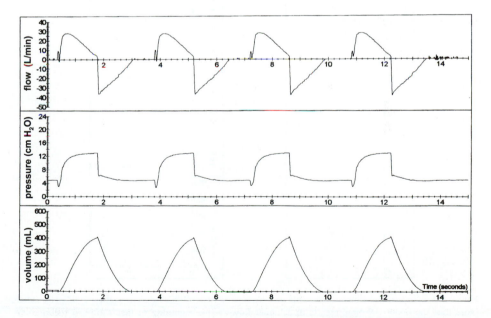

Figure 6-8 Flow, pressure, and volume waveforms for pressure support ventilation.

Pressure Support Ventilation

The typical waveform for pressure support ventilation (PSV) is shown in Figure 6-9. When the pressure support breath is triggered, the ventilator delivers flow to reach the set pressure. As with pressure-controlled ventilation, some current generation ventilators allow the initial flow (rise time) during PSV to be adjusted, which controls how quickly the ventilator reaches the pressure target.

The pressure-supported breath should terminate when the patient's inspiratory effort ceases. Premature termination will increase inspiratory muscle workload and delayed termination will increase the load on expiratory muscles. The inspiratory phase terminates when the flow decreases to a ventilator-determined level (e.g., usually 25% of peak flow or 5 L/min). To avoid unintentional prolongation of inspiration, redundant systems are used to terminate inspiration. These are typically time and pressure based. Inspiration is terminated if the time or pressure criteria are met before the termination flow criteria. These redundant features are particularly important if a leak is present in the system or if the patient's respiratory mechanics result in a long inspiratory phase (e.g., COPD). Some current generation ventilators allow adjustment of the flow at which the ventilator cycles to the expiratory phase (Figure 6-10). This may be advantageous in patients with COPD (e.g., high resistance and high compliance) or if a leak is present.

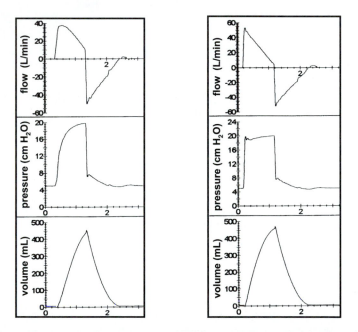

Figure 6-9 Effect of rise time adjustments of waveforms; left – 40% rise time; right – 100% rise time. Note that the faster rise time results in a higher flow at the beginning of inspiration, a rectangular pressure waveform, and a slightly higher tidal volume.

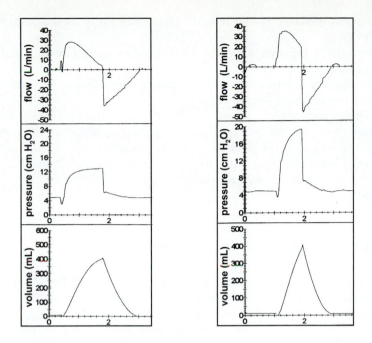

Figure 6-10 Effect of changes in flow termination criteria during pressure support ventilation. Left: Termination flow of 10%. Right: Termination flow of 40%.

EXPIRATORY FLOW

Expiratory flow is determined by alveolar driving pressure (Palv), airways resistance, the elapsed expiratory time, and the time constant of the respiratory system:

$$\dot{V} = -\,(Palv/R) \times (e^{-t/\tau}).$$

By convention, expiratory flow is negative and inspiratory flow is positive. Also note that end-expiratory flow is present if airways resistance is high and expiratory time is not sufficient (Palv is positive at end-exhalation). This indicates the presence of air-trapping (auto-PEEP).

PHYSIOLOGIC EFFECTS OF WAVEFORM MANIPULATIONS

The clinical usefulness of inspiratory waveform manipulations is controversial. The choice of waveform is usually one of clinician bias, rather than the desire to achieve a specific therapeutic goal. The following generalizations can be made regarding inspiratory waveform manipulations.

- Mean airway pressure is higher with descending ramp flow and lower with constant flow.
- Peak inspiratory pressure is lower with descending ramp flow and higher with constant flow.
- Gas distribution is improved with descending ramp flow. The result may be improved oxygenation and ventilation.
- Mean airway pressure is increased with an end-inspiratory plateau pressure. An end-inspiratory plateau pressure may improve distribution of ventilation. During the period of the plateau pressure, gas from areas of the lungs with low airway resistance (low time constants) may be redistributed to areas of the lungs with high airway resistance (high time constants); this is called pendelluft.

EFFECT OF FLOW PATTERNS ON I:E RATIO

When an inspiratory flow pattern is changed from constant flow to descending ramp flow during volume ventilation, the ventilator must adjust either the peak flow or inspiratory time to maintain the delivered tidal volume (Figure 6-11).

If peak flow is adjusted, then inspiratory time and I:E ratio are constant. For a descending ramp flow pattern, the peak flow ($\dot{V}_{pk}$) is determined by the inspiratory time (T_I) and the flow at the end of inspiration ($\dot{V}f$):

$$\dot{V}_{pk} = [V_T - (0.5)(\dot{V}f)(T_I)]/[(0.5)(T_I)]$$

For example, if V_T is 0.75 L, T_I is 1.5 s, and $\dot{V}f$ is 5 L/min (0.083 L/s), then $\dot{V}_{pk}$ will need to be 55 L/min (0.92 L/s).

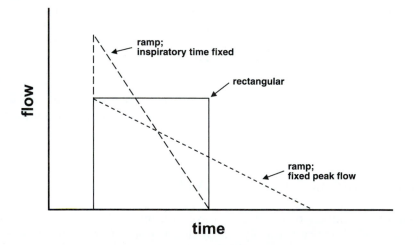

Figure 6-11 When the flow pattern is changed from a constant flow to a descending ramp flow, either the inspiratory time or the peak inspiratory flow must increase.

If inspiratory time is adjusted when the flow pattern is changed, then the peak flow set on the ventilator will be the initial flow. For a descending ramp flow pattern, the increase in inspiratory time will be determined by the peak flow and the flow at the end of inspiration:

$$T_I = (V_T)/(0.5)(\dot{V}_{pk} + \dot{V}f)$$

For example, if V_T is 0.75 L, $\dot{V}_{pk}$ is 90 L/min (1.5 L/s), and $\dot{V}f$ is 5 L/min (0.083 L/s), then T_I will be 0.95 s. For full deceleration (i.e., $\dot{V}f = 0$), either the inspiratory time or the peak flow must double.

SIGH VOLUME

The sigh breath is a deliberate increase in tidal volume for one or more breaths at regular intervals. Sighs during mechanical ventilation were commonly used in the 1970s, but then became less commonly used. There is again interest in the use of sighs during mechanical ventilation as a recruitment maneuver, but the value of this is yet to be determined. One way of producing a sigh during pressure support ventilation is to set an inspiratory pressure of 20 to 30 cm H_2O, for 1 to 3 s, 2 to 4 times/min, using Bilevel or PCV+ (BIPAP) (Figure 6-12).

I:E RATIO

The relationship between inspiratory time and expiratory time (I:E ratio) is an important consideration during mechanical ventilation. A longer inspiratory time (and a shorter expiratory time) increases the mean airway pressure, which often increases arterial oxygenation but may decrease cardiac output. A longer inspiratory time may also result in air trapping (auto-PEEP), particularly if inspiratory time is greater than the expiratory time (inverse I:E ratio). Normally, expiratory time is longer than inspiratory time. An inspiratory time of 1–2 s is usually appropriate during adult mechanical ventilation. A shorter inspiratory time is

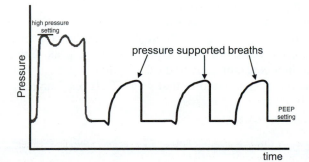

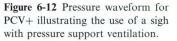

Figure 6-12 Pressure waveform for PCV+ illustrating the use of a sigh with pressure support ventilation.

desirable for patients who are spontaneously breathing (≤ 1 s), and a longer inspiratory time is desirable to increase mean airway pressure and improve oxygenation. If very long inspiratory times are used (> 2 s), hemodynamics and auto-PEEP must be monitored. Long inspiratory times are often uncomfortable, and require patient sedation and/or paralysis. Several approaches can be used by ventilators to set the I:E ratio.

- I:E ratio and rate. For example, at an I:E ratio of 1:3 and a rate of 15/min (cycle time of 4 s), the inspiratory time is 1 s and the expiratory time is 3 s.
- Flow, tidal volume, and rate. For example, suppose there is a constant inspiratory flow of 60 L/min, tidal volume of 0.7 L, and rate of 12/min. The inspiratory time is therefore 0.7 s, the expiratory time is 4.3 s, and the I:E ratio is 1:6.
- Inspiratory time and respiratory rate. With an inspiratory time of 1 s and a rate of 10/min, the expiratory time is 5 s and the I:E ratio is 1:5.
- Per cent inspiratory time and rate. At a rate of 15/min and 25% inspiratory time, the inspiratory time is 1 s (25% of the total cycle time of 4 s), the expiratory time is 3 s, and the I:E ratio is 1:3.

POINTS TO REMEMBER

- The time constant is the product of resistance and compliance.
- Inspiratory flow waveforms can be categorized as constant or descending ramp flow.
- With pressure controlled ventilation, the inspiratory flow is determined by the resistance and compliance of the respiratory system.
- With pressure support ventilation, the initial inspiratory flow is high and then decreases to a manufacturer-specific end-inspiration flow cycle.
- Rise time can be adjusted with pressure control and pressure support ventilation.
- Some current generation ventilators allow adjustment of the termination flow criteria during pressure support ventilation.
- Descending ramp flow patterns generate higher mean airway pressures, lower peak airway pressures, and improved gas distribution.
- An end-inspiratory pause increases mean airway pressure.
- When an inspiratory flow pattern other than constant flow is chosen during volume-controlled ventilation, the ventilator must adjust either the peak flow or inspiratory time to maintain a constant delivered tidal volume.
- The I:E ratio affects mean airway pressure and in that way affects oxygenation and cardiac output.

ADDITIONAL READING

BLANCH PB, JONES M, LAYON AJ, CONNER N. Pressure-preset ventilation. Part I: Physiologic and mechanical considerations. *Chest* 1993; 104:590–599.

BLANCH PB, JONES M, LAYON AJ, CONNER N. Pressure-preset ventilation. Part II: Mechanics and Safety. *Chest* 1993;104:904–912.

BRANSON RD, CAMPBELL RS. Sighs: Wasted breath or breath of fresh air? *Respir Care* 1992; 37: 462–468.

BRUCE RD, STOCK MC, TARRAS E, HANCOCK S. Does a sigh breath improve oxygenation in the intubated patient receiving CPAP? *Respir Care* 1992; 37:1409–1503.

BRUNNER JX, LAUBSCHER TP, BANNER MJ, ET AL. Simple method to measure total expiratory time constant based on the passive expiratory flow-volume curve. *Crit Care Med* 1995; 23:1117-1122.

CHATMONGKOLCHART S, WILLIAMS P, HESS DR, KACMAREK RM. Evaluation of inspiratory rise time and inspiration termination criteria in new-generation mechanical ventilators: a lung model study. *Respir Care* 2001; 46:666–677.

CHIUMELLO D, PELOSI P, CROCI M, ET AL. The effects of pressurization rate on breathing pattern, work-of-breathing, gas exchange and patient comfort in pressure support ventilation. *Eur Respir J* 2001; 18:107–114.

COHEN IL, BILEN Z, KRISHNAMURTHY S. The effects of ventilator working pressure during pressure support ventilation. *Chest* 1993; 103:588–592.

DAVIS K, BRANSON RD, CAMPBELL RS, ET AL. The addition of sighs during pressure support ventilation. Is there a benefit? *Chest* 1993; 104:867–870.

HESS DR, MEDOFF BD, FESSLER MB. Pulmonary mechanics and graphics during positive pressure ventilation. *Int Anesthesiol Clin* 1999; 37:15–34.

JUBRAN A. Inspiratory flow rate: more may not be better. *Crit Care Med* 1999; 27:670–671.

MARCY TW, MARINI JJ. Inverse ratio ventilation in ARDS. Rationale and implementation. *Chest* 1991; 100:494–504.

MARINI JJ, CAPPS JS, CULVER BH. The inspiratory work of breathing during assisted mechanical ventilation. *Chest* 1985; 87:612–618.

MARINI JJ, CROOKE PS, TRUWIT JD. Determinants and limits of pressure-preset ventilation: a mathematical model of pressure control. *J Appl Physiol* 1989; 67:1081–1092.

PATRIONITI N, FOTI G, CORTIHOVIS B, ET AL. Sigh improves gas exchange and lung volume in patients with acute respiratory distress syndrome undergoing pressure support ventilation. *Anesthesiology* 2002; 96:788–794.

PELOSI P, CADRINGHER P, BOTTINO N, ET AL. Sigh in acute respiratory distress syndrome. *Am J Respir Crit Care Med* 1999; 159:872–880.

RAU JL, SHELLEDY DC. The effect of varying inspiratory flow waveforms on peak and mean airway pressures with a time-cycled volume ventilator: A bench study. *Respir Care* 1991; 36:347–356.

RAVENSCRAFT SA, BURKE WC, MARINI JJ. Volume-cycled decelerating flow. An alternative form of mechanical ventilation. *Chest* 1992; 101:1342–1351.

UCHIYAMA A, IMANAKA H, TAENAKA N. Relationship between work of breathing provided by a ventilator and patients' inspiratory drive during pressure support ventilation; effects of inspiratory time. *Anaesth Intensive Care* 2001; 29:349–358.

SEVEN

HUMIDIFICATION AND THE VENTILATOR CIRCUIT

INTRODUCTION

Care of mechanically ventilated patients requires attention to both physiologic and technical issues. The outcome from mechanical ventilation is often affected by the patient-ventilator interface. This interface is more than simply an attachment between the machine and the patient. To deliver an adequate tidal volume, the patient-ventilator interface must be unobstructed, leak-free, and have minimal compliance and compressible volume. This chapter discusses issues related to humidification and the ventilator circuit.

HUMIDIFICATION

Physiologic Principles

Inspired gases are conditioned in the airway so that they are fully saturated with water at body temperature by the time they reach the alveoli ($37°$ C, 100% relative humidity, 44 mg/L absolute humidity, 47 mm Hg water vapor pressure). The point in the airway at which the inspired gases reach body temperature and humidity is the isothermic saturation boundary (ISB), and below this point there is no fluctuation of temperature and humidity. The ISB is normally just below the carina. Above the ISB, heat and humidity are added to the inspired gases, and heat and humidity are extracted from the expired gases. Thus, this portion of the airway acts as a heat and moisture exchanger. Much of this portion of the airway is bypassed in patients with an artificial airway (endotracheal or tracheostomy tube), necessitating the use of external humidifying apparatus in the breathing circuit. Under normal conditions, about 250 mL of water are lost from the lungs each day to humidify the inspired gases.

Problems with Inadequate and Excessive Humidity

Gases delivered from mechanical ventilators are typically dry and the upper airways of such patients are functionally bypassed by artificial airways. The physiologic effects of inadequate humidity can be due to heat loss or moisture loss. Heat loss from the respiratory tract occurs due to humidification of the inspired gases. However, heat loss due to mechanisms other than respiration is usually more important for temperature homeostasis. Moisture loss from the respiratory tract, and subsequent dehydration of the respiratory tract, results in epithelial damage, particularly of the trachea and upper bronchi. The result of this is an alteration in pulmonary function such as decreased compliance and decreased surfactant activity. Clinically, drying of secretions, atelectasis, and hypoxemia can occur.

Over-humidification is possible only if the temperature of the inspired gases is greater than $37°$ C and the absolute humidity is greater than 44 mg/L. This is unlikely with heated humidifiers, and usually will not occur in a device that does not produce an aerosol. Although it is difficult to produce excessive humidification with a heated humidifier, complete humidification of the inspired gases (during mechanical ventilation) eliminates the insensible water loss that normally occurs during breathing. Failure to consider this could result in a positive water balance (250 mL/day). With humidification systems, significant heat gain is unlikely and tracheal injury due to high temperature output of a humidifier is rare. Because the specific heat of gases is low, it is difficult to transfer significant amounts of heat without the presence of aerosol particles to cause tracheal burns. In hypothermic patients, super-warming of inspired gases has little effect in the facilitation of core rewarming. Breathing gases warmed and humidified to normal body conditions, however, complements other rewarming techniques because it prevents further heat loss from the respiratory tract.

Problems of excessive humidity are more likely when aerosols are administered. Excessive aerosol therapy may result in a positive water balance, particularly in neonates and patients with renal failure. Aerosols have also been associated with contamination of the lower respiratory tract. Cool aerosols can increase airway resistance by increasing the volume of secretions and by irritation of airways. Molecular humidity rather than aerosol therapy should be used for humidification for patients with reactive airways, and all patients requiring mechanical ventilation.

TECHNIQUES OF HUMIDIFICATION OF INSPIRED GASES

The output of any therapeutic gas delivery system should match the normal conditions at that point of entry into the respiratory system (Figure 7-1). If the temperature and humidity are less than this, a humidity deficit is produced. If the temperature and humidity are greater than this, fluid overload and patient discomfort may occur. Inspired gases that bypass the upper respiratory tract (e.g., endotracheal tubes and tracheostomy tubes) should be heated to at least 32 to 34° C at 95 to 100% relative humidity.

Heated Humidifiers

Humidifiers produce molecular water (water vapor). High flow heated humidifiers are capable of providing a relative humidity of nearly 100% at temperatures near body temperature. Specific devices include the passover, cascade, wick, and vapor

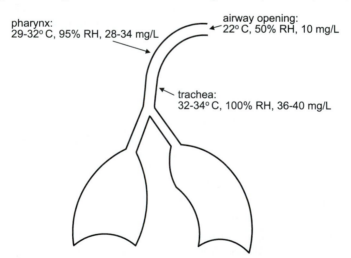

pharynx:
29-32° C, 95% RH, 28-34 mg/L

airway opening:
22° C, 50% RH, 10 mg/L

trachea:
32-34° C, 100% RH, 36-40 mg/L

Figure 7-1 Normal temperature, relative humidity, and absolute humidity levels at three sites in the respiratory tract. The output of any therapeutic gas delivery system should match the normal conditions at that point of entry into the respiratory system.

phase humidifiers. The water level in the reservoir of a humidifier can be maintained by manually adding water, adding water from a bag attached to the humidifier, or by a continuous-feed system that will keep the water level constant. Closed-feed systems avoid interruption of ventilation to fill the humidifier. Continuous feed systems avoid fluctuations in the temperature of gas delivered, and maintain a low compressible gas volume. Many heated humidifier systems are servo-controlled with a thermistor at the proximal airway to maintain the desired gas delivery temperature. Cooling of the gas between the humidifier and the patient results in condensation (rain-out), which should be collected in a water trap, and removed aseptically.

The circuit that carries gas from the humidifier to the patient can be heated. This prevents a temperature drop in the circuit, and a more precise temperature of gas can be delivered to the patient. By heating the inspiratory and expiratory limbs, a heated circuit also decreases the amount of condensation in the circuit. If the temperature of the circuit is less than the temperature of the gas leaving the humidifier, condensation will occur in the circuit. On the other hand, if the temperature of the circuit is greater than the temperature of the gas leaving the humidifier, the relative humidity of the gas will drop. This decrease in relative humidity, which can occur with heated circuits, may produce drying of secretions (Figure 7-2). Water condensation in the inspiratory limb of the ventilator circuit

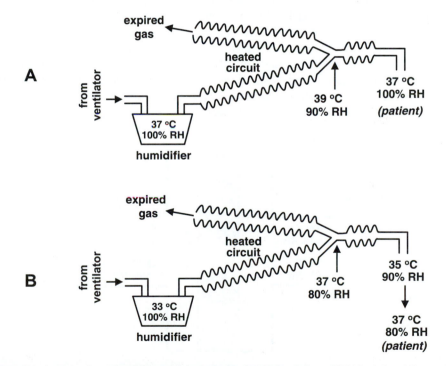

Figure 7-2 A. Properly set humidifier with heated wire circuit that delivers 100% body humidity to the patient. B. Heated wire circuit with setting too low, delivering inadequate humidity to the patient.

near the patient, or in the proximal endotracheal tube, indicates 100% relative humidity of the inspired gas.

Another issue related to the use of humidifiers in ventilator circuits relates to flow resistance. Depending on the point where the ventilator senses patient effort, this may affect the ability of the ventilator to adequately respond to patient effort during assisted modes. If the humidifier is between the patient and the point at which the ventilator is triggered, patient work-of-breathing will increase. However, the flow resistance through the humidifier may be less important if trigger pressure is measured at the proximal airway of the patient.

Artificial Noses

Artificial noses passively humidify the inspired gases by collecting the patient's expired heat and moisture and returning it during the following inspiration (Figure 7-3). These devices are attractive alternatives to active heated humidifiers because of their passive operation (they do not require electricity or heating) and their relatively low cost. A number of laboratory evaluations of artificial noses have generally found them capable of providing 22–28 mg/L of water to the airway.

The additional resistance and dead space of these devices can be problematic because it increases the imposed work-of-breathing and minute ventilation requirement. The dead space of these devices is particularly problematic when the tidal volume is low. There has recently been increasing interest in long term use of artificial noses during mechanical ventilation. Although the most efficient devices can provide nearly 30 mg/L of water, the output of artificial noses is less than that with a heated humidifier. When the artificial nose is used during pro-longed mechanical ventilation, the patient must be frequently assessed for signs of inadequate humidification (e.g., thick secretions, bronchial casts, mucus plug-

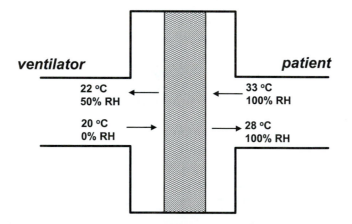

Figure 7-3 Schematic diagram of an artificial nose, showing the temperature and relative humidity on the patient and ventilator sides of the device during inhalation and exhalation.

ging). If signs of inadequate humidification are present, heated humidification should be initiated. There are several clinical conditions that contraindicate the use of an artificial nose (Table 7-1).

THE VENTILATOR CIRCUIT

A typical ventilator circuit consists of those components that deliver gas from the ventilator to the patient and return the patient's exhaled gas to the atmosphere. In addition to gas delivery, the circuit conditions the inspired gases by filtering and humidification as discussed previously. Some ventilator circuits can be sterilized and re-used, but many are disposable single-patient-use devices.

Compression Volume

Compression volume is based on the internal volume of the ventilator, the volume of the humidifier, and the characteristics of the circuit tubing. The compression volume of the system is a function of the volume of the circuit, the compliance (elasticity) of the tubing material, and the ventilation pressure. Circuit compression volume does not reach the patient, and becomes clinically important with high pressures and low tidal volumes. The volume that leaves the exhalation valve of the ventilator includes the exhaled volume from the patient as well as the volume of gas compressed in the ventilator circuit. Unless volume is measured directly at the patient's airway, the exhaled volume displayed by the ventilator may overestimate the patient's actual tidal volume by the amount of the

Table 7-1 Contraindications for the use of artificial noses

- Copious secretions. Secretions in the artificial nose will significantly increase resistance to flow. If a patient has copious amounts of secretions, the lack of therapeutic humidity may result in thickening of secretions.
- Very small or very large tidal volumes. With small tidal volumes, the dead space of the device may compromise ventilation and lead to retention of CO_2. With very large tidal volumes (> 1.0 L), the ability of the artificial nose to humidify inspired gases may be compromised.
- High spontaneous minute ventilation (> 10 L/min). The resistance through artificial noses increases with time, and this may make spontaneous breathing difficult.
- Low ventilatory reserve with spontaneous breathing. The resistance through these devices may result in decreased breathing ability for patients who have low ventilatory reserves.
- Expired tidal volume less than 70% of the inspired tidal volume. To function properly, both inspired gases and expired gases must travel through the artificial nose. Patients with a bronchopleural fistula or an incompetent airway cuff will not have an adequate expired volume through the device.
- Hypothermia. Artificial noses are contraindicated with a body temperature < 32° C.
- An artificial nose should be removed from the ventilator circuit during aerosol treatments when the nebulizer is placed in the circuit.

compressible volume. Some current generation microprocessor ventilators correct measured volume for circuit compression volume.

The compressible volume is often expressed as the compression factor, which is calculated by dividing the compression volume by the corresponding ventilation pressure. If the compression factor is known, the compressible volume can be calculated by multiplying it by the ventilating pressure. The delivered tidal volume is the volume leaving the exhalation valve minus the compression volume:

$$V_T = V_T exh - (factor \times (PIP - PEEP))$$

where $V_T exh$ is the volume leaving the exhalation valve, and V_T is the tidal volume corrected for compression volume (Figure 7-4).

Consideration of compression volume is important for several reasons. Most important, it decreases the delivered tidal volume to the patient. Failure to consider compression volume results in overestimation of lung compliance. Auto-PEEP measurements are also affected by circuit compression volume:

$$auto\text{-}PEEP = (Crs + Cpc)/Crs \times estimated\ auto\text{-}PEEP$$

where Crs is the compliance of the respiratory system, Cpc is the compliance of the patient circuit and estimated auto-PEEP is the value that is measured. Compression volume also affects the measurement of mixed exhaled P_{CO_2}, and the following correction can be used:

$$P\bar{E}_{CO_2} = Pexh_{CO_2} \times (V_T exh/V_T)$$

where $P\bar{E}_{CO_2}$ is the true mixed exhaled P_{CO_2} and $Pexh_{CO_2}$ is measured mixed exhaled P_{CO_2} (including gas compressed in the ventilator circuit). Compression volume does *not* affect measurements of oxygen consumption and carbon dioxide production.

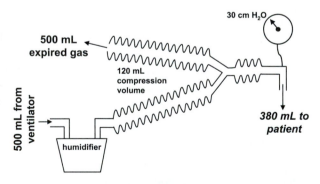

Figure 7-4 Illustration of compression volume. In this example, if airway pressure is 30 cm H_2O, set tidal volume is 500 mL, and compression factor is 4 mL/cm H_2O, then the actual tidal volume delivered to the patient is only 380 mL.

Circuit Resistance

Ventilator circuits and endotracheal tubes increase the imposed work-of-breathing for the patient. Patient-ventilator interaction is dependent upon the ability of the patient (and ventilator) to overcome these effects. During spontaneous modes of ventilation, the resistance through the ventilator circuit and endotracheal tube can contribute to patient-ventilator dys-synchrony. The inspiratory work-of-breathing due to circuit resistance is a function of the patient's peak inspiratory flow and the response of the ventilator. When this is coupled with the resistance through an endotracheal tube, the imposed work reaches a level of clinical importance at high flows for most systems. Circuit resistance, although important, may not become important until it is added to the resistance of the endotracheal tube.

The effect of inspiratory circuit resistance is only important for patient triggering. Pressure should be measured at the patient's airway, trigger sensitivity should be low, and response time should be high. Flow-triggering, rather than pressure-triggering, often reduces the imposed work during patient-initiated modes of ventilation. The effects of both circuit resistance and endotracheal tube resistance may be overcome by ventilator triggering within the trachea (rather than the proximal airway), but the clinical utility of this method is unknown.

The resistance through the expiratory limb of the circuit is primarily that due to the exhalation valve and PEEP devices. Mushroom and scissors valves have significant expiratory resistance. Current generation ventilators use an exhalation valve with a large diaphragm that is electrically controlled, and thus produces a more consistent circuit pressure regardless of flow. Excessive expiratory circuit resistance can prolong exhalation, resulting in auto-PEEP. High expiratory circuit resistance can also result in high airway pressures if the patient coughs. Some newer generation ventilators have an active exhalation valve during pressure controlled ventilation, reducing the risk of circuit over-pressurization during these events.

Circuit Dead Space

The circuit dead space is the volume of the circuit through which rebreathing occurs. It is commonly called mechanical dead space and is functionally an extension of the patient's anatomic dead space. Mechanical dead space is the volume of tubing between the Y-piece and the artificial airway. The mechanical dead space becomes particularly important when the patient is ventilated with a small tidal volume. During low tidal volume ventilation, such as is used as part of a lung protective strategy, the volume of mechanical dead space should be minimized.

Ventilator Circuits and Nosocomial Pneumonia

Intubated mechanically ventilated patients are at risk for nosocomial pneumonia. These pneumonias are associated with high morbidity and mortality, increased length of hospitalization, and increased cost of care. The ventilator circuit has been historically associated with the risk of ventilator-associated pneumonia. For example, the condensate in mechanical ventilator circuits is often contaminated, raising the question as to whether this might pose a risk for pneumonia. It is now appreciated, however, that organisms contaminating the circuit are usually organisms that originate from the patient. The patient contaminates the circuit, and ventilator-associated pneumonia (VAP) may not be ventilator-related. VAP is usually the result of aspiration of pharyngeal secretions. Ventilator-associated pneumonia might be better called endotracheal-tube associated pneumonia. Ventilator circuits do not need to be changed on a scheduled basis. Circuit changes are only necessary between patients, if the circuit malfunctions, and when the circuit is visibly soiled. It has also been reported that artificial noses can be safely used for extended intervals of three to five days. There is no strong evidence that the use of heated wire circuits or artificial noses decreases the risk of VAP. Similarly, there is little evidence that use of a filter at the proximal endotracheal tube decreases the risk of VAP.

Troubleshooting

Because mechanical ventilation is technically complex, the patient-ventilator system should be evaluated periodically by a clinician who appreciates the technical aspects of the ventilator system and the pathophysiology of the patient. In the United States, this person is a respiratory therapist who is trained in both technology and pathophysiology. Guidelines for patient-ventilator system checks have been published by the American Association for Respiratory Care (Table 7-2). The patient-ventilator system check is a documented evaluation of a ventilator and the patient's response to mechanical ventilatory support. It should be performed at regular intervals and more frequently if the patient becomes unstable or requires ventilator adjustments. A ventilator flow sheet is typically used to record these assessments.

Table 7-2 Components of a patient-ventilator system check

- All data relevant to the patient-ventilator system check must be recorded on the appropriate hospital forms at the time of performance.
- Patient-ventilator system checks must include patient information and observations indicative of the ventilator's settings at the time of the check (e.g., current ventilator settings, alarm settings, description of any instance of equipment failure).
- Documentation of a physician order for mechanical ventilator settings [this may be in the form of desired ranges for blood gases or other parameters, and ventilator variables to manipulate to achieve the desired blood gas results or other targets of interest (e.g., plateau pressure)].
- Patient-ventilator system checks must include clinical observations indicative of the patient's response to mechanical ventilation at the time of the check.

Adapted from AMERICAN ASSOCIATION FOR RESPIRATORY CARE GUIDELINE: Patient-Ventilator System Checks. *Respir Care* 1992; 37:882–886.

Perhaps the most troublesome aspect of ventilator troubleshooting is the detection and correction of circuit leaks. These must be corrected promptly to prevent patient harm due to hypoventilation. To avoid patient injury due to hypoxia (and possibly death), a disconnect alarm must be set at all times. The disconnect alarm is usually low exhaled volume or low airway pressure. A manual resuscitator should be at the bedside of all mechanically ventilated patients to allow ventilation in the event of a ventilator failure.

Between patients, all ventilators should be calibrated and an operational verification procedure (OVP) should be conducted as recommended by the manufacturer. At the bedside, an OVP can be performed by occluding the patient connection and assessing the airway pressure increase on a manometer. With current generation microprocessor ventilators, sophisticated integral computerized self-test diagnostics are available. At manufacturer-determined intervals, more complete ventilator preventive maintenance is required by a biomedical engineering technician.

ALARMS

All critical care ventilators feature a variety of alarms to warn of events. These events may be malfunctions of the ventilator (e.g., circuit leak), malfunctions of the patient-ventilator interface (e.g., disconnect), or pathologic changes affecting the patient (e.g., high airway pressure). The American Association for Respiratory Care has classified these alarms as:

- immediately life-threatening (Level 1)
- potentially life threatening (Level 2)
- those that are not life threatening but a possible source of patient harm (Level 3).

Although ventilator alarms are necessary, they contribute to noise pollution in the critical care unit. Alarms should be set sensitive enough to detect critical events without producing false alarms. If false alarms occur frequently, desensitization of the clinical staff can occur, with potentially disastrous results if a true alarm situation occurs. Newer generation ventilators incorporate smart alarms, which are less likely to produce false alarms. Some current generation critical care ventilators have so many alarms that a false positive alarm is likely at virtually any time.

POINTS TO REMEMBER

- Inadequate humidification of the inspired gases can result in drying of secretions and atelectasis.

- The temperature and humidity output of any therapeutic gas delivery device should match the normal conditions at that point of entry into the respiratory system.
- Heated humidifiers produce molecular water vapor.
- Artificial noses passively heat and humidify the inspired gases.
- Compression volume is that volume of gas compressed in the ventilator circuit during inspiration, and thus not delivered to the patient.
- Ventilator-associated pneumonia is usually not ventilator-related, and ventilator circuits do not need to be changed on a scheduled basis.
- Ventilator alarms should be set sensitive enough to detect critical events without producing false alarms.

ADDITIONAL READING

AMERICAN ASSOCIATION FOR RESPIRATORY CARE. Consensus statement on the essentials of mechanical ventilators – 1992. *Respir Care* 1992; 37:1000–1008.

AMERICAN ASSOCIATION FOR RESPIRATORY CARE GUIDELINE: Patient-ventilator system checks. *Respir Care* 1992; 37:882–886.

BRANSON RD, CAMPBELL RS. Humidification in the intensive care unit. *Respir Care Clin N Am* 1998; 4:305–320.

BRANSON RD, DAVIS K, BROWN R, ET AL. Comparison of three humidification techniques during mechanical ventilation: patient selection, cost, and infection considerations. *Respir Care* 1996; 41:809–816.

BRANSON RD, DAVIS K, CAMPBELL RS, ET AL. Humidification in the intensive care unit. Prospective study of a new protocol utilizing heated humidification and a hygroscopic condenser humidifier. *Chest* 1993; 104:1800–1805.

DREYFUSS D, DJEDAINI K, WEBER P, ET AL. Prospective study of nosocomial pneumonia and of patient and circuit colonization during mechanical ventilation with circuit changes every 48 hours versus no change. *Am Rev Respir Dis* 1991; 143:738–743.

FINK JB, KRAUSE SA, BARRETT L, ET AL. Extending ventilator circuit change interval beyond 2 days reduces the likelihood of ventilator-associated pneumonia. *Chest* 1998; 113:405–411.

HESS D. Prolonged use of heat and moisture exchangers: Why do we keep changing things? *Crit Care Med* 2000; 28:1667–1668.

HESS D, BURNS E, ROMAGNOLI D, ET AL. Weekly ventilator circuit changes: a strategy to reduce costs without affecting pneumonia rates. *Anesthesiology* 1995; 89:903–911.

HESS D, MCCURDY S, SIMMONS M. Compression volume in adult ventilator circuits: A comparison of five disposable circuits and a nondisposable circuit. *Respir Care* 1991; 36:1113–1118.

KOLLEF MH, SHAPIRO SD, FRASER VJ, ET AL. Mechanical ventilation with or without 7-day circuit changes. A randomized controlled trial. *Ann Intern Med* 1995; 123:168–174.

MACINTYRE NR, DAY S. Essentials for ventilator alarm systems. *Respir Care* 1992; 37:1108–1112.

MIYAO H, HIROKAWA T, MIYASAKA K, KAWAZOE T. Relative humidity, not absolute humidity, is of great importance when using a humidifier with a heating wire. *Crit Care Med* 1992; 20:674–679.

MIYAO H, MIYASAKA T, HIROKAWA T. Consideration of the international standard for airway humidification using simulated secretions from an artificial airway. *Respir Care* 1996; 41:43–49.

WILLIAMS R, RANKIN N, SMITH T, ET AL. Relationship between the humidity and temperature of inspired gas and the function of the airway mucosa. *Crit Care Med* 1996; 24:1920–1929.

EIGHT

PRESSURE AND VOLUME VENTILATION

OBJECTIVES

1. Discuss the gas delivery patterns of pressure and volume ventilation.
2. Describe the effect of varying rise time and inspiratory cycle criteria during pressure support and pressure control ventilation.
3. Describe how an end-inspiratory plateau can be achieved with pressure control ventilation.

4. Describe approaches to monitor gas delivery during both pressure and volume ventilation.
5. Contrast the advantages and disadvantages of pressure and volume ventilation.

INTRODUCTION

Controversy has always followed the introduction of new modes of ventilation. In the late 1970s it was assist/control versus intermittent mandatory ventilation. In the mid- to late-1980s, it was intermittent mandatory ventilation versus pressure support. A debate today is whether gas delivery should be volume controlled or pressure controlled.

VOLUME VENTILATION

Many of the first mechanical ventilators were pressure limited (e.g., Bird and Puritan-Bennett IPPB machines). However, in the 1950s a number of volume ventilators were introduced. Since that time, volume ventilation has been the norm. Volume ventilation means that the variable that is constant during each breath is tidal volume. Inherent in this approach is a variable peak inspiratory pressure (PIP). As impedance to ventilation changes (e.g., resistance, compliance), PIP must vary because tidal volume is constant. With volume ventilation, the clinician sets V_T, inspiratory time, flow pattern, peak inspiratory flow, rate, and trigger sensitivity. In some ventilators, inspiratory time, minute volume and I:E ratio are set instead of V_T and flow. In practice, most ventilators provide volume control by controlling the inspiratory flow and inspiratory time to provide a constant tidal volume delivery.

PRESSURE VENTILATION

With pressure controlled ventilation, a peak inspiratory pressure is set. In addition, inspiratory time or I:E ratio and trigger sensitivity are set. As noted in Table 8-1, the primary differences between these approaches are the fixed V_T or PIP. With pressure ventilation, PIP is constant and V_T may vary. With volume ventilation, V_T is constant and PIP may vary.

Pressure Support

Despite the fact that pressure support is pressure limited, it is different from pressure controlled ventilation. Traditionally, the only variable set by the clinician is the pressure support level and all other variables are patient controlled. On a breath-by-breath basis, rate, inspiratory time, I:E ratio, inspiratory flow,

Table 8-1 Pressure control versus volume control ventilation

	Pressure	Volume
V_T	Variable	Constant
PIP	Constant	Variable
Peak alveolar pressure	Constant	Variable
Flow pattern	Decreasing	Preset
Peak flow	Variable	Constant
Inspiratory time	Preset	Preset
Minimum rate	Preset	Preset

and V_T are patient controlled and may change. In newer generation ventilators, the clinician may also set the rise time, which is the amount of time it takes for the pressure limit to be reached. With some ventilators, the pressure limit can be achieved within 100 to 150 ms, whereas with others the pressure limit may not be achieved until the end of the inspiratory phase (Figure 8-1). Exhalation is initiated when inspiratory flow decreases to a predetermined level dependent upon the ventilator design (i.e., 5 L/min or 25% of peak flow). Although inspiratory cycle criteria are often set as a percentage of peak flow, some ventilators use an absolute terminal flow. The ability to adjust the cycle criteria is also possible in some ventilators. Although controversy exists over the most appropriate rise time and inspiratory termination criteria, both should be set to enhance patient comfort. The inspiratory termination criteria should be adjusted so that the patient does not activate expiratory muscles to terminate the inspiratory phase. Set appropriately, a pressure increase above the set level at end-inhalation is not present. When end-inspiratory pressure exceeds the set level, the patient has begun exhalation before the ventilator has reached its inspiratory termination criteria. This causes patient-ventilator dys-synchrony. Rise time should be set to satisfy patient peak inspiratory demand. An initial overshoot in pressure above the set pressure support level indicates that the rise time is too short, whereas a concave rise in initial airway pressure usually indicates the rise time is too long.

Rise time, inspiratory termination criteria, and the pressure support level are interrelated. Peak flow increases with a faster rise time or higher pressure. As a result, there will be a greater flow for inspiratory termination if the ventilator determines cycle criteria based on a percent of peak flow. Thus, if any of these three variables are changed (pressure, rise time, termination flow), the others should be re-evaluated. Airway pressure graphics are needed to properly set rise time and inspiratory termination criteria. Without graphics, it is difficult to determine whether these settings are appropriate.

A lengthy inspiratory time, beyond the patient's desired inspiratory time, may occur with pressure support whenever a leak is present. Cuff leaks, bronchopleural fistulae, or circuit leaks can all prolong inspiration since they may

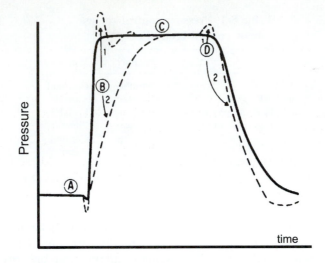

Figure 8-1 Design characteristics of a pressure supported breath. The inspiratory pressure is triggered at point A by a patient effort resulting in an airway pressure decrease. Demand valve sensitivity and responsiveness are characterized by the depth and duration of this negative pressure. The rise to pressure (line B) is provided by a fixed high initial flow delivery into the airway. Note that if flows exceed patient demand, initial pressure exceeds set level (B1), whereas if flows are less than patient demand, a very slow (concave) rise to pressure can occur (B2). The plateau of pressure support (line C) is maintained by servo control of flow. A smooth plateau reflects appropriate responsiveness to patient demand, fluctuations would reflect less responsiveness of the servo mechanisms. Termination of pressure support occurs at point D and should coincide with the end of the spontaneous inspiratory effort. If termination is delayed, the patient actively exhales (bump in pressure above plateau) (D1); if termination is premature, the patient will have continued inspiratory efforts (D2). (From McIntyre N, et al. The Nagoya conference on system design and patient-ventilator interactions during pressure support ventilation. *Chest* 1990; 97:1463–1466.)

prevent the inspiratory termination criteria from being met. That is, flow will be unable to decrease to the level required to initiate expiration. Whenever lengthy inspiratory times (> 1.5 s) are observed with pressure support, a system leak should be suspected.

Pressure Controlled CMV (Assist/Control)

Pressure support and pressure controlled CMV (assist/control) provide the same gas delivery pattern. The only difference between the two is the method of terminating inspiration. With pressure support, inspiration is normally terminated by flow. With pressure control, inspiration is terminated by a set inspiratory time. The rise time control is active during pressure control and pressure support ventilation.

FLOW RATE AND PATTERN

A difference between pressure and volume ventilation is the flow pattern. With volume ventilation, flow is set on the ventilator. With pressure ventilation, flow is determined by the pressure level, airways resistance, respiratory system compliance, and the algorithm used by the ventilator to establish the pressure target. With pressure ventilation, sufficient gas flow is provided so that the pressure limit is met within the time period of the pressure delivery algorithm. This may be 100 to 500 ms. The greater the pressure limit and the lower the resistance to gas delivery, the higher is the peak inspiratory flow rate. With some ventilators, peak inspiratory flows may approach 180 L/min during pressure ventilation.

A distinctive flow pattern occurs with pressure ventilation. Because the pressure limit is met by establishing a high initial flow rate and the pressure is constant, flow decreases exponentially as inspiratory time proceeds. The rate of decrease is dependent upon the pressure limit and the patient's resistance and compliance. When the pressure limit and compliance are low, the flow decrease occurs rapidly. When the pressure limit and resistance are high, the rate of decrease is slow.

With volume ventilation, a precise gas flow pattern is delivered per clinician selection. Various flow patterns (rectangular, ramp) can be set during volume ventilation. Most initial comparisons between pressure and volume ventilation were performed with the Servo 900C ventilator, and volume ventilation was delivered with a rectangular pattern. However, as shown in Figure 8-2, when a descending ramp flow pattern is chosen, pressure and volume ventilation cannot easily be distinguished if set to deliver gas in a similar manner.

END-INSPIRATORY PLATEAU PRESSURE

With pressure controlled ventilation, inspiratory time or I:E ratio is set and the gas flow pattern responds to the pressure limit and impedance to ventilation. For a specific pressure and lung mechanics, there is an inspiratory time beyond which an end-inspiratory plateau develops. Extending inspiratory time beyond this establishes a plateau period, whereas shortening inspiratory time below this eliminates the plateau. With volume ventilation the clinician must set an end-inspiratory pause. That is, after setting the basic gas delivery parameters, the clinician sets a specific end-inspiratory plateau time. With volume ventilation, the plateau remains constant at the set level unless changed by the clinician. With pressure ventilation the length of the end-inspiratory plateau changes with changes in lung mechanics. As compliance decreases, the end-inspiratory plateau increases. As resistance increases, the plateau decreases. A decreasing flow pattern with either volume or pressure ventilation has the advantage of delivering the majority of the tidal volume early in the inspiratory phase (Figure 8-2). This may result in better distribution in the inspired gas, a higher Pa_{O_2} and a lower Pa_{CO_2}.

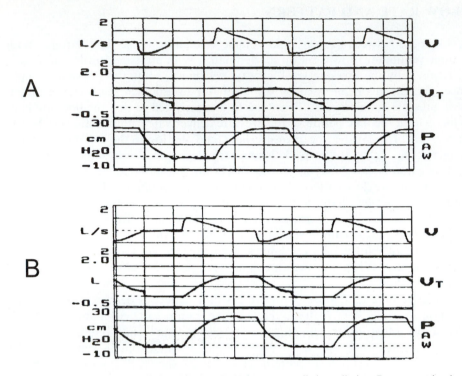

Figure 8-2 A. Pressure controlled ventilation. B. Volume controlled ventilation. Pressure and volume controlled modes generated on a lung model. Volume control was set to match pressure control gas flow delivery pattern; same peak flow, same inspiratory time, and same end inspiratory pause time. The two delivery patterns are virtually indistinguishable.

INSPIRATORY TIME AND AIR TRAPPING

Increasing inspiratory time and changing the inspiratory flow pattern are the only manipulations of the gas delivery pattern that result in an increase in mean airway pressure ($\bar{P}$aw) (Table 8-2) without increasing peak alveolar pressure or level of ventilation. Increasing inspiratory time has been used in the management of severe acute respiratory failure. However, it is important to understand the varying effects of increasing inspiratory time with volume versus pressure ventilation.

With volume ventilation, increasing inspiratory time can be accomplished by decreasing the flow, increasing the tidal volume, or adding an end-inspiratory pause. Of these, only the addition of a pause maintains constant the peak inspiratory pressure and increases the $\bar{P}$aw. Decreasing the flow increases inspiratory time without affecting the peak alveolar pressure. However, because it decreases the rate of gas delivery, the increase in $\bar{P}$aw as a result of increasing inspiratory

Table 8-2 Methods of increasing P̄aw

- Increase PEEP
- Increase V_T
- Increase rate
- Increase peak inspiratory pressure
- Select descending ramp flow pattern*
- Increase inspiratory time*

---

* Only methods that do not affect peak alveo-lar pressure, or level of ventilation (provided auto-PEEP does not occur).

time may be offset by the decrease in P̄aw associated with the slower gas delivery. Increasing V_T increases P̄aw and peak alveolar pressure.

With pressure-controlled ventilation, P̄aw is increased by increasing inspiratory time or increasing the pressure limit. Increasing the pressure limit increases V_T and peak alveolar pressures, while increasing inspiratory time may also increase V_T as P̄aw is increased. As noted in Figure 8-3, as inspiratory time increases tidal volume also increases to a point, then decreases. The specific inspiratory time where this change occurs is dependent upon resistance and compliance. If compliance is low, maximum V_T will occur at a shorter inspiratory time. If resistance is high, a longer inspiratory time is needed to maximize tidal

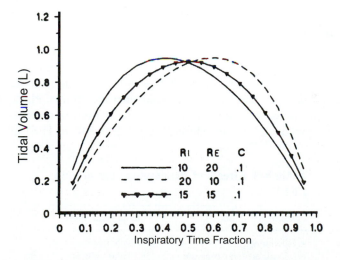

Figure 8-3 Relationship of inspiratory time fraction to tidal volume (pressure target = 20 cm H_2O). When inspiratory (R_I) and expiratory (R_E) resistance are equal, optimal duration (D) = 0.5. When $R_I > R_E$, more inspiratory time is required, and optimal D > 0.5. Conversely, when $R_E > R_I$, optimal D < 0.5. (From MARINI JJ, CROOKE PS, TRUWIT JD. Determinants and limits of pressure-preset ventilation. A mathematical model of pressure control. *J Appl Physiol* 1989; 67:1081–1092.)

volume delivery. Once an end inspiratory plateau occurs, V_T remains constant with pressure ventilation until inspiratory time is increased enough to cause air trapping and auto-PEEP (Table 8-3).

There is an inspiratory time at which expiratory time is too short to prevent air trapping. When air trapping develops, volume and pressure ventilation respond differently. With volume ventilation, since V_T is constant, the development of air trapping and auto-PEEP results in an increase in PIP and peak alveolar pressure. With pressure ventilation, air trapping and auto-PEEP result in a decrease in the delivered V_T with peak alveolar pressure remaining constant. With either approach the development of auto-PEEP compromises gas delivery.

WORK-OF-BREATHING

Generally, pressure modes result in less patient work than volume modes. With pressure ventilation, delivered flow varies with patient demand. Increased demand results in greater delivered flow. Generally, work-of-breathing is not increased with pressure ventilation unless inspiratory time is set inappropriately. With pressure control, inspiratory time should be set to avoid an end-inspiratory plateau. With volume ventilation, patient work-of-breathing is best minimized by use of a descending ramp flow pattern and the setting of flow high enough to meet patient demand. Inspiratory time in volume and pressure ventilation should be set equal to the patient's spontaneous inspiratory time (0.7 to 1.5 s).

MONITORING

With volume ventilation, monitoring should focus on airway pressures. Peak, plateau and mean airway pressures change with alterations in resistance and compliance. Of primary concern is the rapid identification of elevated pressures in the presence of a pneumothorax or airway obstruction. In patients who are not breathing spontaneously, alarms should be set 5 to 10 cm H_2O above average

Table 8-3 Effects of the development of auto-PEEP

Pressure ventilation	Volume ventilation

• No change:
  Peak alveolar pressure
  Peak inspiratory pressure
	• No change
	  Tidal volume

• Decrease:
  Tidal volume
	• Increased:
	  Peak alveolar pressure
	  Peak airway pressure

PIP. In patients breathing spontaneously, alarms should be set about 10 cm H_2O above average PIP (Table 8-4).

With pressure ventilation, monitoring should focus on V_T and $\dot{V}_E$ changes. For patients without spontaneous breathing efforts, low V_T or $\dot{V}_E$ alarms should be set about 10% lower than the average V_T or $\dot{V}_E$. For patients who are spontaneously breathing, low V_T alarms are more appropriate than low $\dot{V}_E$ alarms. Patients may compensate for the decreased V_T by increasing their respiratory rate to keep $\dot{V}_E$ constant. In this setting, low V_T alarms should be set about 20% lower than the average V_T.

Pneumothorax

Of concern with pressure ventilation is the recognition of a pneumothorax or major airway obstruction. Most clinicians are familiar with the signs of tension pneumothorax during volume ventilation (the increasing PIP). However, with pressure ventilation the signs are subtle. Since PIP is constant, V_T decreases as the pneumothorax increases, but its decrease is limited by the eventual equilibration of pressure in the thorax and in the airway. That is, the pneumothorax may not extend to the degree seen with volume ventilation. The level of hemodynamic compromise with pressure ventilation may be less than with volume ventilation. With pressure ventilation, the first indication of a problem is frequently a deterioration in blood gases. With volume ventilation the effects of a tension pneumothorax are immediate, dramatic, and usually rapidly recognized. However, with pressure ventilation the response is less dramatic, more difficult to recognize and frequently the pneumothorax goes unrecognized until a routine chest X-ray is taken or blood gases are drawn.

PRESSURE VERSUS VOLUME VENTILATION

There are advantages and disadvantages of both pressure and volume ventilation. The decision to employ one or the other approach is generally based on personal bias and which of the advantages or disadvantages are considered most important. A review of controlled studies indicates that there are no differences in physiologic effects, development of barotrauma or acute lung injury, or outcome between pressure and volume ventilation regardless of the I:E ratio used. This is

Table 8-4 Monitoring during pressure and volume ventilation

Volume ventilation – Monitor pressure	Pressure ventilation – Monitor volume

• Ventilator-triggered breaths:
  PIP alarm 5 cm H_2O above average PIP
• Patient-triggered breaths:
  PIP alarm 10 cm H_2O above average PIP
	• Ventilator-triggered breaths:
	  Low V_T or $\dot{V}_E$ alarms 10% below average volumes
	• Patient-triggered breaths:
	  Low V_T alarm 20% below average V_T

particularly true when pressure ventilation is compared to volume ventilation with a descending ramp flow waveform and an end-inspiratory plateau.

Pressure Ventilation: Advantages and Disadvantages

The major advantage of pressure ventilation is that PIP and peak alveolar pressures are maintained at a constant level. Flow also varies with patient demand, decreasing the likelihood of dys-synchrony. This may decrease the likelihood of localized over-distention with associated barotrauma and acute lung injury. The major disadvantage is that V_T varies as impedance changes, increasing the likelihood of blood gas alteration and making it more difficult to rapidly identify major alterations in impedance.

Volume Ventilation: Advantages and Disadvantages

The major advantage of volume ventilation is the delivery of a constant V_T. This insures a consistent level of alveolar ventilation and results in easily identifiable changes in PIP as impedance to ventilation changes. However, with volume ventilation peak alveolar pressure may change dramatically as impedance changes, potentially increasing the risk of lung injury. Flow pattern is also fixed, preventing response to patient demand and increasing the probability of dys-synchrony.

POINTS TO REMEMBER

- With volume ventilation, V_T is constant but PIP varies with changes in compliance and resistance.
- With pressure ventilation, PIP is constant but V_T varies with changes in compliance and resistance.
- Pressure support is a pressure mode that differs from other pressure modes because inspiratory time is not set.
- Rise time is adjustable in some ventilators during pressure control and pressure support, but inspiratory termination criteria can only be adjusted in pressure support.
- Gas delivery patterns during pressure support and pressure control are identical.
- With pressure ventilation, an exponentially decreasing flow pattern is observed, while with volume ventilation the flow pattern is set on the ventilator.
- With pressure ventilation, an end-inspiratory plateau may occur, dependent upon the pressure, inspiratory time, resistance, and compliance.
- With a descending ramp flow pattern the majority of the V_T is delivered early in inspiration.
- Pressure and volume ventilation are available in CMV (A/C) and SIMV modes.
- For a set flow pattern, the only method of increasing P̄aw that does not affect peak alveolar pressure is increasing inspiratory time.

- Increasing inspiratory time is limited by the development of auto-PEEP.
- With patient-triggered breaths, pressure ventilation unloads the work-of-breathing to a greater extent than volume ventilation.
- Careful monitoring of airway pressure is necessary with volume ventilation, while careful monitoring of V_T is necessary with pressure ventilation.
- If a leak is present (e.g., bronchopleural fistula) inspiration may be prolonged during pressure support.

ADDITIONAL READING

BONMARCHAND G, CHEVRON V, MENARD JF, ET AL. Effects of pressure ramp slope values on the work of breathing during pressure support ventilation in restrictive patients. *Crit Care Med* 1999; 27:715–722.

CINNELLA G, CORTI E, LOFASO F, ET AL. Effects of assisted ventilation on the work of breathing: volume-controlled versus pressure-controlled ventilation. *Am J Respir Crit Care Med* 1996; 153:1025–1033.

KACMAREK RM. Management of the patient mechanical ventilator system. In PIERSON DJ, KACMAREK, RM (eds.). *Foundations of respiratory care*. New York, Churchill Livingstone Inc. 1992; 973–997.

KACMAREK RM. Methods of providing mechanical ventilatory support. In PIERSON DJ, KACMAREK RM (eds). *Foundation of respiratory care*. Churchill Livingstone Inc. 1992; 953–972.

LUDWIGS U, PHILIP A. Pulmonary epithelial permeability and gas exchange: a comparison of inverse ratio ventilation and conventional ventilation in oleic acid-induced lung injury in rabbits. *Chest* 1998; 113:459–466.

MARCY TW, MARINI JJ. Inverse ratio ventilation in ARDS: Rationale and implementation. *Chest* 1991; 100:495–504.

MARINI JJ, CROOKE PS, TRUWIT JD: Determinants and limits of pressure-preset ventilation: A mathematical model of pressure control. *J Appl Physiol* 1989; 67:1081–1092.

McINTYRE N, NISHIMURA M, USADA Y, ET AL. The Nagoya conference on system design and patient-ventilator interactions during pressure support ventilation. *Chest* 1990; 97:1463–1466.

PARTHASARATHY S, JUBRAN A, TOBIN MJ: Cycling of inspiratory and expiratory muscle groups with the ventilator in airflow limitation. *Am J Respir Crit Care Med* 1998; 158:1471–1478.

ZAVALA E, FERRER M, POLESE G, ET AL. Effect of inverse I:E ratio ventilation on pulmonary gas exchange in acute respiratory distress syndrome. *Anesthesiology* 1998; 88:35–42.

F_{IO_2}, PEEP, AND MEAN AIRWAY PRESSURE: MANAGEMENT OF OXYGENATION

OBJECTIVES

1. Discuss the pathophysiology of hypoxemia.
2. Discuss the physiologic effects of PEEP.
3. Discuss the indications for the application of PEEP.
4. Discuss the application, monitoring, and withdrawal of PEEP in ARDS.
5. Discuss the overall management of oxygenation in critically ill patients.

INTRODUCTION

The principles associated with management of oxygenation are more complex than those associated with ventilation. Provided that cardiovascular function and $\dot{V}_{CO_2}$ are constant, increases in alveolar ventilation generally result in decreases in Pa_{CO_2} and vice versa. Oxygenation status, although dependent on $F_{I_{O_2}}$, is also affected by cardiopulmonary disease, PEEP and mean airway pressure ($\bar{P}$aw). In this chapter, the aspects of mechanical ventilation that affect oxygenation are discussed, as well as approaches to these techniques during patient management.

PATHOPHYSIOLOGY OF HYPOXEMIA

Normal Pa_{O_2} is 80 to 100 mm Hg when breathing room air at sea level, with hypoxemia defined as a Pa_{O_2} of < 80 mm Hg. To maintain normal tissue oxygenation it is necessary to provide an adequate inspired O_2 concentration, appropriate matching of ventilation and perfusion ($\dot{V}/\dot{Q}$), sufficient hemoglobin, adequate cardiac output, and appropriate O_2 unloading to the tissue. A breakdown at any stage in this process may result in tissue hypoxia. At sea level, hypoxemia results from one of a number of alterations in cardiopulmonary function. Specifically, hypoxemia is caused by shunt, $\dot{V}/\dot{Q}$ mismatch, diffusion defect, and hypoventilation. Hypoxemia is also worsened by cardiovascular compromise.

Shunt

Shunt is perfusion without ventilation. When present, venous blood (shunted blood) mixes with arterialized blood in the pulmonary veins or left heart causing a decrease in the Pa_{O_2} of blood leaving the left heart. Because the majority of O_2 is carried by hemoglobin, even a small shunt (Figure 9-1) can result in significant hypoxemia. Increasing $F_{I_{O_2}}$ improves oxygenation only in settings of small shunts. Large shunts are usually unresponsive to $F_{I_{O_2}}$ increases. Improvement in oxygenation in the setting of a large shunt is usually focused on resolution of the shunt (e.g., decompression of a pneumothorax, resolution of a pneumonia, re-expansion of atelectasis, diuresis). The use of PEEP, recruitment maneuvers and maneuvers to

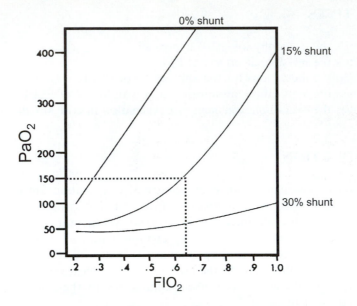

Figure 9-1 Comparison of the theoretical F_{IO_2}–Pa_{O_2} relationships with 0%, 15% and 30% true shunts. These relationships were calculated assuming normal ventilation, hemoglobin of 15 g, $C(a - v)O_2$ difference of 5 vol %, and normal cardiac output, metabolic rate, pH and P_{CO_2}. Note that as shunt increases, the Pa_{O_2} at a given F_{IO_2} decreases substantially. (From SHAPIRO BA, ET AL: *Clinical application of blood gases.* 4th ed. Chicago, Mosby-Yearbook, 1989, p 115.)

elevate $\bar{P}aw$ are often useful to improve oxygenation in this setting. A common, but often unrecognized, cause of shunt in mechanically ventilated patients is a patient foramen ovale. A functionally closed foramen ovale may open if pulmonary vascular resistance increases during mechanical ventilation.

$\dot{V}/\dot{Q}$ Mismatch

The normal $\dot{V}/\dot{Q}$ is 0.8. Hypoxemia results when this ratio is low (Figure 9-2). The most effective methods of altering Pa_{O_2} in the presence of $\dot{V}/\dot{Q}$ mismatch are to improve distribution of ventilation and increase the F_{IO_2}. This is particularly true for patients with chronic obstructive lung disease, where gross mismatching of $\dot{V}/\dot{Q}$ is present. As illustrated in Figure 9-2, in some settings minor increases in F_{IO_2} can cause marked increases in Pa_{O_2}. In many ventilated patients, hypoxemia is caused by both shunting and $\dot{V}/\dot{Q}$ mismatch. In these patients, management of oxygenation may require increasing F_{IO_2}, PEEP and Paw.

Diffusion Defect

Hypoxemia in this setting is due to the increased time for equilibration of O_2 across the alveolar capillary membrane. This is a result of thickening of the

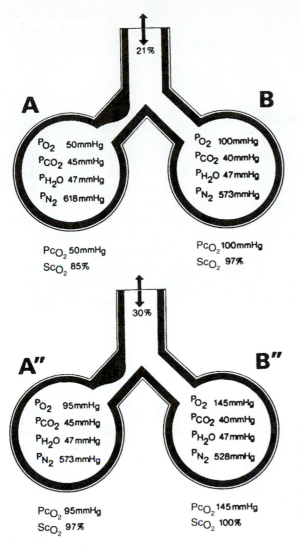

Figure 9-2 Effect of $\dot{V}/\dot{Q}$ mismatch on oxygenation. In alveolus A (A″), $\dot{V}/\dot{Q}$ is < 0.8. As a result, less O_2 reaches the lung unit than is removed by circulation causing the alveolar P$_{O_2}$ to decrease and the alveolar P$_{CO_2}$ to increase. In alveolus B (B″), the normal $\dot{V}/\dot{Q}$ is maintained. Increasing the F$_{IO_2}$ from 0.21 to 0.30 (A″ and B″) markedly diminishes the effect that the low $\dot{V}/\dot{Q}$ has on oxygenation. (From SHAPIRO BA, ET AL: *Clinical application of blood gases*, 4th ed. Chicago, Mosby-Year Book, 1989, 114.)

alveolar-capillary membrane or a decrease in surface area available for diffusion. Interstitial fluid, fibrotic changes of the alveolar-capillary membrane, and emphysematous changes of the lung parenchyma are the primary causes of a diffusion defect. Increasing F$_{IO_2}$ improves oxygenation with a diffusion defect.

Hypoventilation

Elevation of alveolar P$_{CO_2}$ decreases the alveolar P$_{O_2}$, as predicted by the alveolar gas equation. The elevated arterial P$_{CO_2}$ causes the oxyhemoglobin dissociation curve to shift to the right, decreasing Sa_{O_2} but increasing the unloading of O_2 at tissue. Improvement in ventilation is the best treatment for hypoxemia caused by hypoventilation, although this cause of hypoxemia also responds to O_2 administration.

Decreased Cardiovascular Function

In the healthy individual, decreased cardiac output does not result in hypoxemia. However, altered cardiovascular function can magnify the hypoxemic effects of either $\dot{V}/\dot{Q}$ mismatch or shunting. When cardiac output is low, tissue O_2 extraction is high and mixed venous P_{O_2} and O_2 content are low. When shunt or $\dot{V}/\dot{Q}$ mismatch is present with low cardiac output, blood with a lower O_2 content from shunted areas mixes with blood from non-shunted areas, resulting in a greater degree of hypoxemia than if the cardiac output were higher. Management of hypoxemia due to cardiovascular dysfunction must be corrected by appropriate hemodynamic management. Although increasing FI_{O_2} is an appropriate ventilator alteration in this setting, there are certain settings (e.g., cardiogenic pulmonary) where moderate levels of PEEP are useful.

FI_{O_2}

Since mechanical ventilation may cause $\dot{V}/\dot{Q}$ mismatching, even patients without marked cardiopulmonary dysfunction (e.g., postoperative, drug overdose) may require an elevated FI_{O_2} to maintain a normal Pa_{O_2}. In these settings, however, rarely is an $FI_{O_2} > 0.40$ necessary except during specific procedures (e.g., suctioning, bronchoscopy).

O_2 Toxicity

The issue of oxygen toxicity in critically ill patients is controversial. In healthy mammals, breathing 100% O_2 for 24 hours results in structural changes at the alveolar-capillary membrane, pulmonary edema, atelectasis and decreased Pa_{O_2}. In healthy humans, the same process has been observed, but requires a longer period of time. Thus, the lowest FI_{O_2} necessary to maintain the target Pa_{O_2} should always be used. However, in the severely diseased lung, antioxidants capable of minimizing the effect of high FI_{O_2} may be induced, allowing the lung to tolerate a high FI_{O_2} without further damage. For patients with acute lung injury, a $FI_{O_2} > 0.60$ is generally avoided. However, it may be less dangerous to increase the FI_{O_2} above this level than to expose the lungs to the damaging effects of high peak alveolar pressure (> 30 cm H_2O).

100% O_2

As indicated above, the continuous use of 100% O_2 should be avoided. In addition to the potential for O_2 toxicity, high F_{IO_2} may cause absorption atelectasis in poorly ventilated, unstable lung units due to denitrogenation. This does not mean that 100% O_2 should never be used. Whenever oxygenation status is in question or generalized cardiopulmonary instability occurs, 100% O_2 should always be administered. F_{IO_2} should be reduced as rapidly as possible to more appropriate levels when the acute concerns have been resolved. Use of 100% O_2 during patient transport, bronchoscopy, suctioning, and any other stressful procedures is recommended. In addition, unless the required F_{IO_2} is already established, 100% O_2 should be administered during initial ventilator setup and quickly reduced when appropriate Pa_{O_2} and Sp_{O_2} are established.

POSITIVE END-EXPIRATORY PRESSURE (PEEP)

The application of a supra-atmospheric pressure at end-expiration is referred to as PEEP. The term is generally used in reference to patients receiving mechanical ventilatory support. Continuous positive airway pressure (CPAP) is the provision of a supra-atmospheric end-expiratory pressure to the spontaneously breathing patient. The physiologic effects, indications and precautions are the same for both and the only distinction between them is the use of ventilatory support with PEEP.

Physiologic Effects

End expiratory pressure increases $\bar{P}aw$ and mean intrathoracic pressure. This has effects on many physiologic functions (Table 9-1). When applied to appropriate levels for the clinical setting, PEEP improves pulmonary mechanics and gas exchange, and may have varying effects on the cardiovascular system.

Pulmonary mechanics Since pressure and volume in the lung are directly related, the application of PEEP increases the functional residual capacity (FRC). In acute lung injury where unstable lung units have collapsed, PEEP recruits functional lung units by preventing their collapse. If recruitment of collapsed lung units occurs, lung compliance may improve. However, since compliance in ventilated patients is based on the difference between end-expiratory and end-inspiratory static airway pressures, compliance frequently decreases as PEEP is applied. This is a result of PEEP preventing derecruitment and the recruitment of lung with each tidal breath (Figure 9-3). In a given patient, an end-inspiratory pressure of 30 cm H_2O may result in the same overall lung volume regardless of PEEP level. Thus, the application of PEEP may increase, decrease or not affect compliance. An appropriate level of PEEP also decreases the work-of-breathing in spontaneously breathing patients. Excessive PEEP places the lung on the upper

Table 9-1 Potential physiological effects of appropriately and excessively applied PEEP

	Appropriate level	Excessive level
Intrapulmonary pressure	Increased	Increased
Intrathoracic pressure	Increased	Increased
FRC	Increased	Increased
Lung compliance	No change, increase, or decrease	No change, increase, or decrease
Closing volume	Decreased	Decreased
Pa_{O_2}	Increased	Increased or decreased
Pa_{CO_2}	No change or decreased	Increased
Q_S/Q_T	Decreased	Decreased or increased
$P(A-a)O_2$	Decreased	Decreased or increased
$C(a-\bar{v})O_2$	Decreased	Decreased or increased
$P\bar{v}_{O_2}$	Increased	Increased, decreased, or no change
$Pa_{CO_2} - Pet_{CO_2}$	Decreased	Increased
V_D/V_T	Decreased	Increased
Work-of-breathing	Decreased	Increased
Extravascular lung water	No change or increased	No change or increased
Pulmonary vascular resistance	No change	Increased
Pulmonary perfusion	No change	Decreased
Cardiac output	No change	Decreased
Pulmonary artery pressure	No change	Decreased, increased, or no change
Pulmonary capillary wedge	No change	Decreased, increased, or no change
Central venous pressure	No change	Decreased, increased, or no change
Left ventricular afterload	Decreased	Decreased
Arterial pressure	No change	Decreased
Intracranial pressure	No change	Increased
Urine output	No change	Decreased

Abbreviations: FRC, functional residual capacity; Q_S/Q_T, shunt fraction; $P(A-a)O_2$, alveolar-arterial O_2 pressure difference; $C(a-\bar{v})O_2$, arterial-mixed venous O_2 content difference; $P\bar{v}_{O_2}$, mixed venous O_2 pressure; Pet_{CO_2}, end-tidal P_{CO_2} pressure; V_D/V_T, dead space/tidal volume ratio.

flat portion of the pressure-volume curve, thus decreasing compliance and increasing work-of-breathing.

Gas exchange In most clinical applications, PEEP is applied to improve Pa_{O_2}. This is accomplished primarily by preventing alveolar collapse and decreasing intrapulmonary shunt. Appropriate PEEP may also improve the Pa_{CO_2}-Pet_{CO_2} (end-tidal CO_2) difference and Pa_{CO_2} by decreasing dead space. However, excessive PEEP can decrease perfusion to well ventilated areas causing an increase in Pa_{CO_2}-Pet_{CO_2} difference, Pa_{CO_2}, and dead space. For patients with unilateral lung

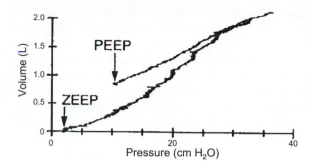

Figure 9-3 Inspiratory pressure volume curve with and without the application of 10 cm H$_2$O PEEP. Since the end inspiratory pressure-volume relationship is unchanged, compliance is decreased with PEEP. (From JONSON B, ET AL. Pressure-volume curve and compliance in acute lung injury. *Am J Respir Crit Care Med* 1999; 159:1172–1178.)

disease, PEEP may result in over-distension of healthy lung units with shunting of blood to the diseased lung units worsening hypoxemia.

Cardiovascular function The effect of PEEP on the cardiovascular system is dependent upon the level of PEEP, the compliance of the respiratory system, and cardiovascular status. Because PEEP increases P̄aw and mean intrathoracic pressure, venous return and cardiac output may decrease as PEEP is applied. PEEP has the greatest effect on cardiac output in a setting where lung compliance is high, chest wall compliance is low and cardiovascular reserve is low. High levels of PEEP decrease right ventricular preload. High levels of PEEP also increase right ventricular afterload (increased pulmonary vascular resistance), which increases end-diastolic volume, decreases ejection fraction, and shifts the inter-ventricular septa to the left. This, along with a reduction in pericardial pressure gradient, limits left ventricular distensibility, reducing left ventricular end-diastolic volume and stroke volume. Thus, both pulmonary and systemic vascular pressures are affected by PEEP. Because PEEP increases pressure outside of the heart, it decreases left ventricular afterload. If flow is maintained when PEEP is applied, vascular pressures remain unchanged or increase. However, if pulmonary perfusion is decreased, vascular pressures generally decrease as PEEP is applied. The result is decreased cardiac output, arterial blood pressure, urine output and tissue oxygenation. Thus, PEEP may increase arterial oxygenation but decrease tissue oxygenation.

Intracranial pressure Since PEEP decreases venous return, intracranial pressure increases with the application of PEEP. This is usually not an issue unless intra-cranial pressure is already increased. The effects of PEEP can generally be neu-tralized by elevating the head of the patient a distance equivalent to the amount of PEEP applied. PEEP should be used cautiously in any patient where increased intracranial pressure is a concern.

Barotrauma Three factors must be present for barotrauma to occur: lung disease, over-distention and pressure. Since the primary indication for the use of PEEP is acute lung injury, disease is present when PEEP is applied. Thus, the amount of over-distention achieved at a given PEEP level essentially determines the probability of barotrauma. Because acute lung injury is heterogeneous, over-distention of any lung unit may be achieved at any PEEP level. As a result, carefully monitoring for the presence of barotrauma must be routinely performed, and PEEP must be maintained at the minimal level required to achieve the therapeutic endpoints of PEEP therapy. However, barotrauma usually occurs because of high end-inspiratory pressure. The higher the PEEP, generally the higher will be the end-inspiratory pressure.

Indications

General indications for the use of PEEP (Table 9-2) are associated with prevention of de-recruitment of unstable lung units, stabilization of the chest wall, counteracting auto-PEEP, and improving left ventricular performance by decreasing preload and afterload.

Acute respiratory distress syndrome (ARDS) The traditional indication for PEEP is ARDS, with restoration of FRC as the overall goal. In early ARDS, the pressure-volume curve of the respiratory system is characterized by a lower inflection point and marked hysteresis. Application of 10–20 cm H_2O PEEP eliminates the lower inflection point and decreases the hysteresis. In later stages of ARDS, marked fibroproliferation is observed with the loss of the lower inflection point, decreased lung volumes, and 8 to 10 cm H_2O PEEP required to maintain oxygenation. In general, 10 to 20 cm H_2O PEEP is needed in early ARDS to prevent derecruitment.

Chest trauma PEEP in this setting is used to stabilize the chest wall and prevent paradoxical movement in the area of trauma. If ARDS is not present, 5 to 10 cm H_2O PEEP is indicated, provided no pulmonary air leak is present and the patient is hemodynamically stable. However, this is an area of controversy and PEEP may not be necessary if oxygenation is satisfactory.

Postoperative atelectasis The use of end-expiratory pressure in this setting is usually by CPAP to improve gas distribution to areas with low $\dot{V}/\dot{Q}$. CPAP

Table 9-2 Indications for PEEP

- Acute respiratory distress syndrome
- Chest trauma
- Postoperative atelectasis
- Cardiopulmonary edema
- Acute artificial airway
- Auto-PEEP

(i.e., spontaneous breathing) has been applied in this setting, usually for 15 to 30 min every 2 to 6 hr at levels of 5 to 10 cm H_2O.

Cardiogenic pulmonary edema Pulmonary edema in this setting is the result of increased left ventricular performance. The application of PEEP (CPAP for spontaneously breathing patients) decreases preload and afterload. The use of PEEP or CPAP at 10 cm H_2O improves oxygenation, decreases work-of-breathing, increases left-ventricular ejection fraction, decreases left ventricular end-diastolic pressure, and improves cardiac output.

Artificial airways The insertion of an artificial airway decreases FRC and may compromise gas exchange. The use of 3 to 5 cm H_2O PEEP or CPAP in infants with an endotracheal tube is standard practice. Application of 5 cm H_2O PEEP is typically used with intubated patients unless otherwise contraindicated. However, most patients with long-term tracheostomies adapt to a bypassed glottis without the need for PEEP or CPAP.

Auto-PEEP Auto-PEEP is end-expiratory pressure caused by airflow limitation (increased time constant), increased tidal volume or an inadequate expiratory time. Since auto-PEEP results from an alteration in the normal intrinsic function of the lung, it is not observed on the ventilator pressure manometer unless an end-expiratory hold is used. The magnitude of auto-PEEP developed in individual lung units is dependent upon the lung unit's time constant, expiratory time, and volume. If auto-PEEP is created for patients with airflow limitation breathing spontaneously, work-of-breathing is elevated. It is difficult to identify auto-PEEP in a spontaneously breathing patient, and the first indication of auto-PEEP may be an inability to trigger the ventilator. Applying PEEP in this setting, up to 80% of the actual auto-PEEP level, counter-balances auto-PEEP, decreases the effort needed to trigger, and may not affect total PEEP (applied PEEP plus auto-PEEP). For the patient who is having difficulty triggering the ventilator, the PEEP can be slowly increasing until patient rate and ventilator rate are equal. At the appropriate level of applied PEEP, patient rate generally decreases and signs of cardiopulmonary stress subside. Note that PEEP balances auto-PEEP with flow limitation (dynamic airway closure). However, PEEP does not affect auto-PEEP with fixed airway obstruction or when the auto-PEEP is due to high minute ventilation. In volume ventilation, if the applied PEEP increases total PEEP, PIP and plateau pressure increase. In pressure ventilation, V_T decreases if applied PEEP increases the total PEEP level. If changes in applied PEEP do not affect peak airway pressure (volume ventilation) or tidal volume (pressure ventilation), then auto-PEEP is present.

PEEP in ARDS

The primary indication for PEEP is ARDS. The goal of PEEP in this setting is prevention of derecruitment and maintenance of tissue oxygenation. More specifically, PEEP is applied to improve shunt, reverse hypoxemia, decrease the work-of-breathing, and decrease the work of the myocardium. Further, this should be accomplished without adversely affecting cardiac output.

In adults, setting PEEP at a level that prevents derecruitment is recommended. Arterial blood pressure and pulse oximetry are monitored whenever PEEP is applied. A given PEEP level after a large V_T or recruitment maneuver maintains a greater lung volume than before the maneuver. Ideally, PEEP should be set above the lower inflection point on the pressure-volume curve. However, identifying this point is difficult in the clinical setting. For patients with ARDS and hemodynamic stability, PEEP should be set at a level likely to maintain alveolar recruitment and then slowly decreased until the lowest PEEP maintaining a Sp_{O_2} of 90 to 95% is identified. PEEP in ARDS is generally set between 10 and 20 cm H_2O. PEEP should not be arbitrarily decreased. PEEP should be maintained at the best level identified until the F_{IO_2} is < 0.50. Once the F_{IO_2} is < 0.5, PEEP may be slowly decreased with appropriate monitoring.

Since PEEP has a marked potential of adversely affecting the cardiovascular system, careful monitoring of this system should be performed (Table 9-1). Pulse oximetry before and after each increase in PEEP should be evaluated. Of particular concern is O_2 delivery. If PEEP increases Sp_{O_2} but decreases cardiac output (i.e., with a net decrease in O_2 delivery), the overall effect of PEEP may be to decrease tissue oxygenation. Since improved oxygenation reduces cardiovascular stress, the benefit provided by PEEP may be to improve Sp_{O_2}, decrease myocardial work and return of cardiac output to a more acceptable level, without markedly altering O_2 delivery. Generally, oxygenation status can be adequately assessed with Sp_{O_2}. Arterial blood gases are not necessarily required with each PEEP or F_{IO_2} change.

PEEP should not be abruptly withdrawn. If PEEP is re-evaluated on a regular basis, the need to make large changes in PEEP rarely exists. Of concern is alveolar derecruitment with the withdrawal of PEEP. Also of concern is the development of hemodynamic instability if patients are fluid positive at the time PEEP is withdrawn. The level of PEEP may be maintaining a delicate pulmonary vascular fluid balance in association with a compromised left ventricle. PEEP reduction in this setting can cause alteration in left ventricular preload and afterload with subsequent pulmonary edema. If arterial oxygenation is satisfactory with an $F_{IO_2} \leq 0.5$, PEEP is slowly decreased (Table 9-3). If the Sp_{O_2} decreases when PEEP is decreased, the prior level should be re-established rather than increasing the F_{IO_2}.

MEAN AIRWAY PRESSURE

$\bar{P}aw$ is the pressure applied to the lung over the entire ventilatory cycle. $\bar{P}aw$ is dependent upon all of the factors that effect ventilation (Table 9-4). Increasing the inspiratory time increases $\bar{P}aw$ without elevating peak alveolar pressure and maintains a constant level of ventilation, provided no auto-PEEP is developed. If auto-

Table 9-3 Withdrawal of oxgenation support

1st: Reduce F$_{I_{O_2}}$ to ≤ 0.50
2nd: Return I:E ratio to 1:2 (if prolonged inspiratory time is used)
3rd: Reduce PEEP to 5 cm H$_2$O
4th: Reduce F$_{I_{O_2}}$ to 0.40
Discontinue mechanical ventilation at this level.

PEEP develops, either peak alveolar pressure or tidal volume is compromised. With volume ventilation, auto-PEEP increases peak alveolar pressure because V$_T$ is constant. With pressure ventilation, tidal volume is decreased as auto-PEEP develops. Because peak airway pressure and peak alveolar pressure are constant with pressure ventilation, the pressure gradient establishing V$_T$ decreases when auto-PEEP occurs. If inspiratory time is increased, it should be limited to the level that does not create auto-PEEP. Auto-PEEP causes a less uniform distribution of PEEP and FRC than applied PEEP. That is, as a result of heterogeneous lung disease, pulmonary time constants can vary considerably from one lung unit to another. With auto-PEEP, FRC and total PEEP will be largest in the most compliant lung unit (longest expiratory time constant) and lowest in the least compliant lung unit (shortest expiratory time constant). Auto-PEEP measured in the ventilator circuit is the mean auto-PEEP.

MANAGEMENT OF OXYGENATION

Assuming appropriate treatment of the underlying condition, optimization of oxygenation requires the use of PEEP, administration of O$_2$, and the assurance of adequate cardiovascular function. With high PEEP (> 15 cm H$_2$O), a higher cardiac filling pressure may be required. Management of oxygenation should always be based on the presenting pathophysiology. In ARDS, high levels of PEEP may be indicated, whereas in localized severe pneumonia high PEEP may compromise oxygenation. In addition, some ARDS patients may benefit from prone positioning or lateral positioning (good lung down) with unilateral lung disease.

Table 9-4 Factors affecting mean airway pressure

- Inspiratory pressure
- PEEP
- I:E ratio (inspiratory time and rate)
- Inspiratory pressure pattern

POINTS TO REMEMBER

- To maintain normal tissue oxygenation, an adequate Pa_{O_2} must be available, sufficient hemoglobin must be present, and adequate cardiac output must be available.
- Hypoxemia often results from shunt, $\dot{V}/\dot{Q}$ mismatch, and cardiovascular compromise.
- Always use the lowest $F_{I_{O_2}}$ to maintain the target Pa_{O_2}.
- Use 100% O_2 during ventilator setup, cardiopulmonary instability and whenever stressful procedures are performed.
- PEEP increases FRC and prevents derecruitment of unstable lung units.
- Prevention of derecruitment of unstable lung units with PEEP decreases intrapulmonary shunt and improves oxygenation.
- The effect of PEEP on the cardiovascular system is dependent upon the level of PEEP, the compliance of the respiratory system, and cardiovascular status.
- If pulmonary blood flow is maintained as PEEP is applied, pulmonary vascular pressures remain unchanged or increase.
- Indications for PEEP are ARDS, chest trauma, postoperative atelectasis, cardiogenic pulmonary edema, and counterbalancing auto-PEEP.
- Monitoring of blood gases, pulse oximetry and hemodynamics must be performed during the application of PEEP.
- In ARDS, apply PEEP at the lowest level that prevents derecruitment (10 to 20 cm H_2O).

ADDITIONAL READING

AMATO MBP, BARBAS CSV, MEDEIROS DM, ET AL. Effect of a protective-ventilation strategy on mortality in the acute respiratory distress syndrome. *N Engl J Med* 1998; 338:347–354.

HICKLING KG. The pressure-volume curve is greatly modified by recruitment: A mathematical model of ARDS lung. *Am J Respir Crit Care Med* 1998; 158:194–202.

HUDSON LD, WEAVER LJ, HIRSCH CE, CARRICO CJ. Positive end-expiratory pressure: reduction and withdrawal. *Respir Care* 1988; 33:613–619.

JONSON B, RICHARD JC, STRAUS C, MANCEBO J, LEMAIRE F, BROCHARD L. Pressure-volume curve and compliance in acute lung injury. *Am J Respir Crit Care Med* 1999; 159:1172–1178.

KACMAREK RM. Positive end-expiratory pressure. In PIERSON DJ, KACMAREK RM (eds) *Foundations of respiratory care*. New York, Churchill Livingstone Inc. 1993, 891–920.

MARINI JJ, RAVENSCROFT SA. Mean airway pressure: Physiologic determinants and clinical importance - Part 1: Physiologic determinants and measurements. *Crit Care Med* 1992; 20:1461–1472.

MARINI JJ, RAVENSCROFT SA. Mean airway pressure: Physiologic determinants and clinical importance - Part 2: Clinical implications. *Crit Care Med* 1992; 20:1604–1616.

CHAPTER TEN

DETERMINING APPROPRIATE PHYSIOLOGIC GOALS

OBJECTIVES

1. Define permission hypercapnia, discuss when it should be employed, and discuss problems with its use.
2. Discuss concerns regarding the use of high oxygen concentrations in critically ill patients.
3. Discuss the pressure and volume targets to be used when ventilating patients.
4. List the gas exchange and acid-base targets for critically ill patients.

INTRODUCTION

The concept of normal has been ingrained in all students as they progress through their basic science and clinical education. Many clinical management decisions are designed to return abnormal physiologic function to normal or to return abnormal laboratory data to normal. However, during the course of mechanical ventilation, it may not be advisable to strictly adhere to normal blood gas values irrespective of the tidal volume delivered, pressure applied, or F_{IO_2} used. The inappropriate use of the ventilator may cause severe lung injury, activate inflammatory mediators, and potentially cause or extend multisystem organ failure. Physiologic goals of mechanical ventilation vary considerably over the ventilatory course of a given patient, dependent upon their specific pathophysiologic state. Of particular concern are patients with ARDS, asthma, or COPD whose lungs have high resistance or low compliance.

PERMISSIVE HYPERCAPNIA

Permissive hypercapnia is the deliberate limitation of ventilatory support to avoid alveolar over-distension, allowing Pa_{CO_2} to rise to levels greater than normal (50–100 mm Hg). Allowing the Pa_{CO_2} to rise to these levels should be considered when the only alternative is a potentially dangerous increase in peak alveolar pressure. The potential adverse effects of an elevated Pa_{CO_2} are listed in Table 10-1. Most of the more important clinical problems occur at Pa_{CO_2} levels above 150 mm Hg. However, even small increases in Pa_{CO_2} increase cerebral blood flow and permissive hypercapnia is generally contraindicated when intracranial pressure is increased (e.g., acute head injury). Elevated Pa_{CO_2} also stimulates ventilation, but patients are usually sedated in the settings where permissive hypercapnia is considered.

Permissive hypercapnia may adversely affect the oxygenation of some patients. Elevated Pa_{CO_2} and low pH shift the oxyhemoglobin dissociation

Table 10-1 Physiological effects of permissive hypercapnia

- Shift in the oxyhemoglobin dissociation curve to the right
- Decreased alveolar P_{O_2}
- Both stimulation and depression of the cardiovascular system
- Central nervous system depression
- Stimulation of ventilation
- Dilation of vascular bed
- Increased intracranial pressure
- Anesthesia ($Pa_{CO_2} > 200$ mm Hg)
- Decreased renal blood flow ($Pa_{CO_2} > 150$ mm Hg)
- Leakage of intracellular potassium ($Pa_{CO_2} > 150$ mm Hg)
- Alteration of the action of pharmacologic agents (a result of intracellular acidosis)

curve to right. This decreases the affinity of hemoglobin for oxygen, decreasing oxygen loading in the lungs but facilitating the unloading of oxygen at the tissues. As illustrated by the alveolar gas equation, an increase in the alveolar P_{CO_2} results in a decrease in alveolar P_{O_2}. For each Pa_{CO_2} rise of one mm Hg, the Pa_{O_2} decreases by about one mm Hg. When permissive hypercapnia is allowed, optimal efforts to maximize oxygenation should be used.

The effect of carbon dioxide on the cardiovascular system is difficult to predict. As illustrated in Figure 10-1, carbon dioxide elicits competing responses from the cardiovascular system. Carbon dioxide directly stimulates or depresses some parts of the cardiovascular system, but opposite effects can occur via stimulation of the autonomic nervous system. It is thus difficult to predict the precise response of the cardiovascular system to permissive hypercapnia. In our experience, an increase in P_{CO_2} most frequently causes pulmonary hypertension and an increase in cardiac output. Dosages of pharmaceutical agents affecting the cardiovascular and autonomic nervous systems may need to be adjusted in the

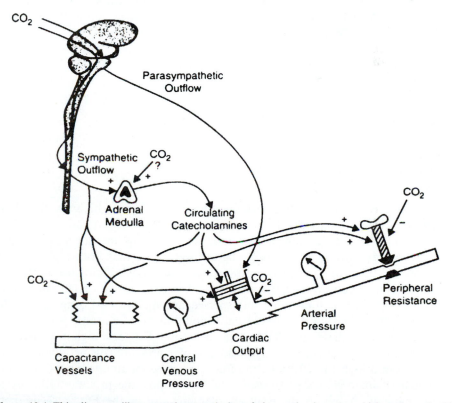

Figure 10-1 This diagram illustrates the complexity of the mechanisms by which carbon dioxide influences the circulatory system. See text for details. (From NUNN JF. Carbon Dioxide. In: NUNN JF, ed. *Applied Respiratory Physiology*, 2nd edition. London, Butterworth and Co., 1977, 334–374.)

presence of permissive hypercapnia, but this is a result of the acidosis and not the elevated P_{CO_2}.

The primary factor limiting permissive hypercapnia is the pH produced. Patients without primary cardiovascular disease or renal failure usually tolerate a pH of 7.20 to 7.25, and younger patients may tolerate an even lower pH. The specific minimal pH acceptable needs to be determined on an individual patient basis. If necessary, Pa_{CO_2} is allowed to gradually increase from the onset of ventilation, which allows a gradual renal compensation. Abrupt changes in ventilator strategies that result in rapid and marked elevation of Pa_{CO_2} are more poorly tolerated.

Whether buffers should be administered to manage the acidosis induced by permissive hypercapnia is debatable. In the setting of cardiac arrest, sodium bicarbonate is contraindicated because of the resulting increased intracellular acidosis. Its use in permissive hypercapnia, however, has not been extensively studied. One can expect a short-term increase in carbon dioxide load when sodium bicarbonate is administered, which is exhaled over time if the level of ventilation is held constant. However, whether the use of buffers has any effect on an overall tolerance of permissive hypercapnia is not known. An alternative buffer is THAM, which does not generate CO_2 and produces intracellular as well as extracellular buffering of pH.

Cautious use of permissive hypercapnia is recommended only when the airway pressure target has been met and increases in respiratory rate maximized. There does not seem to be any significant short-term adverse effect in the majority of patients. However, what is not known is if there are any long-term effects of permissive hypercapnia on the central nervous system.

OXYGEN TOXICITY

Debate has occurred over the years regarding the effect of high F_{IO_2} on lung injury in critically ill patients. In normal lungs of experimental animals, an F_{IO_2} of 1.0 results in the development of non-cardiogenic pulmonary edema (i.e., ARDS) within 24 to 48 hours. It is interesting to note that both high alveolar pressures and high oxygen concentrations can cause ARDS changes in normal alveoli. This is of concern because acute lung diseases such as ARDS are heterogeneous, with normal lung units interspersed among diseased lung units. The lowest F_{IO_2} that achieves the desired Pa_{O_2} should always be used.

The concern with severe ARDS is whether a high F_{IO_2} or a high peak alveolar pressure is more detrimental. A high peak alveolar pressure is generally a greater concern than a high F_{IO_2}. Ideally, the F_{IO_2} should be maintained ≤ 0.6 to avoid the potential toxic effects of oxygen. This is not possible in some critically ill ARDS patients. As either the peak alveolar pressure or the F_{IO_2} exceeds these potentially injurious targets, consideration should be given to accepting a lower Pa_{O_2}. When some chemotherapeutic agents are used (e.g., bleomycin), the effects of oxygen toxicity are exaggerated. In this case, the $F_{I_{O_2}}$ should be kept as low as possible without producing tissue hypoxia.

VOLUME AND PRESSURE TARGETS

Volume

Historically, conventional approaches to mechanical ventilation suggested tidal volumes of 10 to 15 mL/kg of ideal body weight. Today these volumes are only acceptable for patients who require mechanical ventilation and have normal lung function (e.g., post-operative, drug overdose, neuromuscular disease) where the set V_T results in low peak alveolar pressure. However, the presence of chronic or acute pulmonary disease requires that these volumes be lowered to prevent localized over inflation. Since it is clinically impossible to detect localized over-distention, an acceptable tidal volume in a given patient must be judged by measuring the peak alveolar pressure.

Peak Alveolar Pressure

The pressure most reflective of peak alveolar pressure is the end-inspiratory plateau pressure, which actually reflects the mean peak alveolar pressure. To most appropriately determine an end-inspiratory plateau pressure, a 0.5 to 1 s end-inspiratory breath-hold must be established. A maximum plateau pressure of 30 cm H_2O is recommended provided chest wall compliance is normal. This is generally achieved by using a V_T of 4 to 8 mL/kg for ARDS patients. There are cases in which an unacceptable level of ventilation is established with a plateau pressure of 30 cm H_2O. However, exceeding this target should not occur without careful consideration of the potential adverse effects or the presence of a stiff chest wall.

PEEP

The recommended PEEP in early ARDS is 10 to 20 cm H_2O, which is needed to maintain lung recruitment. If PEEP is set at 10 to 20 cm H_2O and peak alveolar pressure is limited to 30 cm H_2O, then only 10 to 20 cm H_2O ventilating pressure is available. This may result in tidal volumes as low as 4 to 5 mL/kg with non-compliant lungs. Ventilation can be increased with the respiratory rate provided that air trapping does not develop.

For patients who do not have ARDS, a PEEP of 5 cm H_2O is reasonable to maintain functional residual capacity and prevent atelectasis. This level of PEEP will usually have no adverse affects. However, PEEP levels as low as zero may be necessary for patients who are hemodynamically unstable, who have elevated intracranial pressure, or who have a large bronchopleural fistula. For patients with dynamic airway closure (e.g., COPD) who have auto-PEEP, applied PEEP may be useful to improve triggering.

GAS EXCHANGE TARGETS

Oxygenation

The normal Pa_{O_2} is 80 to 100 mm Hg breathing room air at sea level. This is the ideal target in all patients requiring ventilatory assistance. However, the cost with respect to oxygen and pressure injury requires adjustment of this target in many critically ill patients. Table 10-2 lists target Pa_{O_2} associated with severity of pulmonary disease. The Pa_{O_2} target may be 50 mm Hg in some patients whose cardiovascular function is adequate, who have no metabolic acidosis (i.e., lactate is not elevated), and who have their metabolic rate controlled by sedation/paralysis and have a normal body temperature. Although maintaining Pa_{O_2} at these levels is not recommended, the potential detrimental effects of high pressure and $F_{I_{O_2}}$ may outweigh the potential benefits of a Pa_{O_2} above 50 mm Hg in some patients.

Ventilation

Normal Pa_{CO_2} is 35–45 mm Hg, and should be the target in all mechanically ventilated patients unless the risks of ventilator-induced lung injury due to high peak alveolar pressure outweigh the benefit of a normal Pa_{CO_2}. In the case of high peak alveolar pressures, the Pa_{CO_2} can be allowed to rise to as high as 80 to 100 mm Hg if necessary, provided increased intracranial pressure is not of concern and marked metabolic acidosis is not present. Pa_{CO_2} levels higher than 100 mm Hg are almost never required, and have been associated with reduced renal and splanchnic blood flow, hyperkalemia, and convulsions (Pa_{CO_2} > 150 mm Hg).

Table 10-2 Gas exchange targets

Condition	Target value
Pa_{O_2}	
Normal lung	$\geq$ 80 mm Hg
Mild lung injury	$\geq$ 70 mm Hg
Moderate lung injury	$\geq$ 60 mm Hg
Severe lung injury	$\geq$ 50 mm Hg
Pa_{CO_2}	
Normal lung	35–45 mm Hg
Lung injury	< 80 mm Hg
pH	
Normal lung	7.35–7.45
Lung injury	$\geq$ 7.20

Acid-Base

In most mechanically ventilated patients, the target pH is 7.35 to 7.45. However, when a maximum peak alveolar pressure is set and Pa_{CO_2} is allowed to rise, the potential for respiratory acidosis exists. If the rise in Pa_{CO_2} is gradual and renal and cardiovascular function are adequate, a pH of 7.20 to 7.30 is usually not a problem, although a rapid rise in Pa_{CO_2} will cause a marked decrease in pH. Most patients without significant cardiovascular disease or sepsis tolerate a pH as low as 7.25. Allowing the pH to fall below 7.20 may be tolerated in some patients, but cardiovascular and renal function must be closely followed.

With the exception of an acutely elevated intracranial pressure, respiratory alkalosis should be avoided. Many clinicians have traditionally regarded respiratory alkalosis as benign. However, respiratory alkalosis is associated with a variety of potential problems including electrolyte disturbances (e.g., hypokalemia, decreased ionized calcium), decreased oxygen unloading from hemoglobin (i.e., left-shifted oxyhemoglobin dissociation curve), and decreased cerebral blood flow.

POINTS TO REMEMBER

- Because mechanical ventilation may itself induce lung injury, the concept of physiologic normal must be reconsidered during mechanical ventilation.
- To reduce the risk of ventilator-induced lung injury, end-inspiratory plateau pressure (peak alveolar pressure) should be maintained ≤ 30 cm H_2O.
- Tidal volumes in patients with acute or chronic lung disease should be ≤ 10 mL/kg.
- In early ARDS, PEEP is set to maintain lung recruitment (10 to 20 cm H_2O).
- Permissive hypercapnia is the deliberate adjustment of mechanical ventilation to allow the Pa_{CO_2} to rise above 40 mm Hg (50 to 100 mm Hg).
- Most patients tolerate a pH as low as 7.20 if no significant cardiovascular, renal, or neurologic disease is present.
- The $F_{I_{O_2}}$ should be kept as low as possible, with a target of ≤ 0.6.
- A high $F_{I_{O_2}}$ causes less lung injury than a high end-inspiratory plateau pressure.
- The Pa_{O_2} target should be decreased as the severity of acute lung disease increases; this may result in a Pa_{O_2} as low as 50 mm Hg in some patients.

ADDITIONAL READING

AMATO MBP, BARBAS CS, MEDEIROS DM, ET AL. Effects of a protective-ventilatory strategy on mortality in the acute respiratory distress syndrome. *New Engl J Med* 1998; 338:347–354.
DURBIN CG, WALLACE KK. Oxygen toxicity in the critically ill patient. *Respir Care* 1993; 38:739–753.
FEIHL F, PERRET C. Permissive hypercapnia, how permissive should we be? *Am J Respir Crit Care Med* 1994; 150:1722–1737.

HICKLING KG, HENDERSON SJ, JACKSON R. Low mortality associated with low volume, pressure limited ventilation with permissive hypercapnia in severe adult respiratory distress syndrome. *Intensive Care Med* 1990; 16:372–377.

HICKLING KG, WALSH J, HENDERSON S, JACKSON R. Low mortality rate in adult respiratory distress syndrome using low-volume, pressure-limited ventilation with permissive hypercapnia: A prospective study. *Crit Care Med* 1994; 22:1568–1578.

KACMAREK RM. Management of the patient-mechanical ventilator system. In PIERSON DJ, KACMAREK RM (eds) *Foundations of Respiratory Care*. New York, Churchill Livingstone 1992, 995–996.

KACMAREK RM, HICKLING KG. Permissive hypercapnia. *Respir Care* 1993; 38:373–387.

MARINI JJ, SLUTSKY AS. Physiological basis of ventilatory support. New York, Marcel Dekker Inc., 1998.

MUSCEDERE JG, MULLEN JBM, GAN K, SLUTSKY AS. Tidal ventilation at low airway pressures can augment lung injury. *Am J Respir Crit Care Med* 1994; 149:1327–1334.

TUXEN DV. Permissive hypercapnia ventilation. *Am J Respir Crit Care Med* 1994; 150:870–874.

ELEVEN

INDICATIONS AND INITIAL SETTINGS FOR MECHANICAL VENTILATION

OBJECTIVES

1. Discuss the difference between hypoxemic and hypercapnic respiratory failure and list the causes of each.
2. Describe the indications for mechanical ventilation.
3. Discuss concerns and approaches to the initiation of mechanical ventilation.
4. Discuss the criteria used to initially set the mechanical ventilator for patients with normal lungs, and with obstructive and restrictive diseases.

5. Discuss the ethical considerations related to initiation of mechanical ventilation.

INTRODUCTION

Mechanical ventilatory support should be instituted when a patient's ability to maintain gas exchange has failed to the level that death is imminent if support is not provided. Generally, failure of the respiratory system is categorized as either hypoxemic or hypercapnic. Although there are times when ventilatory support is indicated for primary hypoxemic respiratory failure, mechanical ventilation is usually indicated only in the presence of hypercapnic respiratory failure. Once the decision is made to initiate mechanical ventilation, careful selection of the initial ventilator settings based on the patient's physiologic status should be made. Whenever mechanical ventilation is considered, the ethical consequences of the decision must be addressed.

HYPOXEMIC VS. HYPERCAPNIC RESPIRATORY FAILURE

Hypoxemic respiratory failure is characterized by a failure of gas exchange – principally a failure to oxygenate. Hypercapnic respiratory failure is a failure of the ventilatory pump or ventilatory muscles. Frequently, respiratory failure is a result of both hypoxemic and hypercapnic failure, and can be classified as compensated or uncompensated. Mechanical ventilation is most commonly instituted to treat uncompensated hypercapnic respiratory failure.

Hypercapnic Respiratory Failure

The ventilatory pump comprises all of the bones and muscles of the chest wall as well as the neural network controlling their function. This total apparatus is responsible for insuring adequate alveolar ventilation. Four aspects of the ventilatory pump, either alone or in combination, can result in pump failure: inadequate ventilatory muscle function, excessive ventilatory load, impaired neuromuscular transmission or compromised central ventilatory drive (Table 11-1). Hypercapnic respiratory failure is associated with an elevated Pa_{CO_2}.

Inadequate ventilatory muscle function may occur as a result of malnutrition, inadequate electrolyte balance, inadequate peripheral nerve function, or compromised delivery of substrates to muscles. Drugs of various categories can also compromise muscle function. Long term use of corticosteroids and the administration of aminoglycoside antibiotics or calcium channel blockers can impair neuromuscular transmission. Chronic pulmonary disease as well as neuromuscular disease may precipitate pump failure because of a decrease in the force-velocity relationship of the muscle, decreasing maximal muscular contraction.

Table 11-1 Causes of hypercapnic respiratory failure

Inadequate ventilatory muscle function
- Electrolyte imbalance
  - Magnesium
  - Potassium
  - Phosphate
- Malnutrition
- Pharmacologic agents
  - Long-term corticosteroids
  - Aminoglycoside antibiotics
  - Calcium channel blocking agents
- Diminished contractility
- Mechanical disadvantage
  - Flattened diaphragm
  - Thoracic deformity
- Atrophy
- Fatigue

Impaired neural transmission
- Spinal cord injury
- Peripheral neuropathies
- Neuromuscular blockade

Excessive ventilatory load
- Secretions
- Mucosal edema
- Bronchospasm
- Increased dead space
- Increased carbon dioxide production
- Dynamic hyperinflation (auto-PEEP)

Decreased central ventilatory drive
- Pharmacologic agents (sedatives and narcotics)
- Hypothyroidism
- Idiopathic central alveolar hyperventilation
- Severe medullary brainstem injury

Ventilatory muscle force may also be decreased by the mechanical disadvantage caused by a flattening of the diaphragm as in severe COPD or a deformed thoracic cage as in kyphoscoliosis. Patients in the ICU who are mechanically ventilated, especially those paralyzed and receiving steroids, may develop critical illness myopathies. In addition, chronic pulmonary disease or neuromuscular disease may lead to detraining, atrophy, or fatigue of ventilatory muscles, all leading to a reduced efficiency of ventilation and carbon dioxide retention.

Excessive ventilatory load may cause failure but is usually associated with other factors that compromise pump function. For patients with chronic pulmonary or neuromuscular disease, the increased load resulting from secretion accumulation, mucosal edema or bronchospasm may be sufficient to precipitate failure. For patients with thoracic deformities, increased ventilatory load is a chronic problem. Any factor that elevates minute ventilation requirements increasing ventilatory load may precipitate failure when associated with reduced neuromuscular capability.

Depressed central ventilatory drive may be caused by drugs, hypothyroidism, idiopathic central alveolar hypoventilation syndrome or severe brainstem injury at the level of the medulla. Increased ventilatory drive may also precipitate acute ventilatory failure, especially when coupled with compromised pump function and increased ventilatory load. For example, metabolic acidosis, increased carbon dioxide production, and dyspnea-related anxiety may result in an intolerable increase in ventilatory drive.

Table 11-2 Causes of hypoxemic ventilatory failure

- Ventilation–perfusion imbalance
- Right to left shunt
- Alveolar hypoventilation
- Diffusion deficit
- Inadequate F_{IO_2}

Hypoxemic Respiratory Failure

Failure of the lung to maintain arterial oxygenation is referred to as hypoxemic respiratory failure (Table 11-2). Hypoxemic respiratory failure usually does not result in carbon dioxide retention unless acute or chronic pump failure is also present. The five basic mechanisms associated with hypoxemic respiratory failure are:

1. Ventilation-perfusion mismatch.
2. Right-to-left shunt.
3. Alveolar hypoventilation.
4. Diffusion defect.
5. Inadequate F_{IO_2}.

- overventilating with good lung up - gets ventil but not perfusion

Hypoxemic respiratory failure can usually be treated with oxygen and CPAP. However, mechanical ventilation may also be necessary in severe cases of ARDS, heart failure, or pneumonia.

INDICATIONS FOR MECHANICAL VENTILATION

From a physiologic perspective, indications for mechanical ventilation are

1. Apnea.
2. Acute ventilatory failure.
3. Impending acute ventilatory failure.
4. Severe oxygenation deficit (Table 11-3).

Acute ventilatory failure requires ventilatory support when the Pa_{CO_2} is elevated sufficiently to cause an acute acidosis (pH < 7.30), although the precise limits on pH and Pa_{CO_2} cannot be defined and must be individually evaluated in each patient.

Impending acute ventilatory failure is an indication for mechanical ventilation when the patient's clinical course shows progress towards failure despite maximal treatment. Examples include the neuromuscular diseased patient or the patient with asthma who demonstrates increasingly compromised ventilatory

Table 11-3 Indications for mechanical ventilation

- Apnea
- Acute ventilatory failure
- Impending acute ventilatory failure
- Severe oxygenation deficit

function in the presence of maximal therapy. The decision to ventilate may actually occur before acute ventilatory failure occurs.

Oxygenation deficit is the least likely indication for mechanical ventilation. However, the severe hypoxemia caused by ARDS or pneumonia may drive the ventilatory pump to failure if not corrected. Whenever high F_{IO_2} (> 0.80) and CPAP (≤ 10 cm H_2O) are required, mechanical ventilation should be considered. Unloading the work of the ventilatory pump with mechanical support frequently improves oxygenation status because of the reduced oxygen cost of breathing.

INITIATION OF MECHANICAL VENTILATION

Hemodynamic compromise to some level is common when mechanical ventilation is started. Mean intrathoracic pressure swings go from negative to positive when ventilation is begun. Adequate ventilation and oxygenation may result in decreased autonomic tone. Sedation is frequently provided, further altering autonomic and vascular tone. This coupled with an inadequate vascular volume leads to hypotension. Normally, the hemodynamic compromise associated with the initiation of mechanical ventilation can be controlled with fluid administration, although vasoactive pharmacology may also be necessary for patients with a compromised cardiovascular system.

INITIAL VENTILATOR SETTINGS

A precise definition of how to set the mechanical ventilator for each patient is impossible. Actual settings depend on the level of patient interaction with the ventilator, the underlying pathophysiology, and the presenting pulmonary mechanics. Two patients of similar size and age, one presenting with a drug overdose and the other with severe asthma, should not be ventilated in the same manner.

Mode

Much controversy over the best mode exists and little scientific evidence is available to direct the choice of mode. More importantly, during the initial phases of ventilatory support, full ventilatory support should be provided. The patient's total ventilatory drive should be satisfied and sedation should be provided to insure that the patient is breathing in synchrony with the ventilator. This may be accomplished with continuous mandatory ventilation (assist/control) applied as either volume control or pressure control. The key is to set the backup rate high enough to insure little if any spontaneous effort is required by the patient.

Volume and Pressure Levels

Because of concern regarding ventilator-induced lung injury, plateau pressure ideally should not exceed 30 cm H_2O unless chest wall compliance is reduced. Volume and pressure levels should always be adjusted with this in mind. However, the specific V_T delivered may vary from 4 mL/kg to 12 mL/kg based on compliance, resistance and presenting pathophysiology. Those individuals with normal lungs requiring ventilation (e.g., overdose, post-operative) may have V_T set in the 10 to 12 mL/kg range, while others with either chronic or acute restrictive lung disease may require a V_T of 4 to 8 mL/kg (Table 11-4). Another consideration for V_T setting is type of ventilator. Ventilators that automatically compensate for compressible circuit volume require a smaller V_T setting than ventilators that do not because the set V_T is the actual delivered V_T.

Setting of pressure control level is determined by the tidal volume delivered. Pressure levels should be set to achieve a tidal volume consistent with that described above. Regardless of approach used to deliver V_T, the actual volume delivered to a patient's lungs should be small (4 to 8 mL/kg) in patients with restrictive lung disease, moderate (8 to 10 mL/kg) in patients with obstructive lung diseases (to minimize air trapping), and large (10 to 12 mL/kg) in patients with normal lung mechanics.

Flow Pattern, Peak Flow, and Inspiratory Time

With volume ventilation, a peak flow and flow pattern are set on the ventilator. Although a descending ramp flow pattern may potentially improve V_T distribu-

Table 11-4 Initial V_T and rate

- Normal pulmonary mechanics
  - V_T 10 to 12 mL/kg
  - Rate 8 to 12/min
- Restrictive lung disease
  - V_T 4 to 8 mL/kg
  - Rate 15 to 25/min
- Obstructive lung disease
  - V_T 8 to 10 mL/kg
  - Rate 8 to 12/min

Always maintain peak alveolar pressure < 30 cm H_2O unless chest wall compliance is decreased

tion, a rectangular flow pattern may be equally acceptable during the initiation of mechanical ventilation. Peak flow should be set to insure an inspiratory time of about one second. This is especially important if patients are triggering the ventilator, since inspiratory flow and time should be consistent with spontaneous inspiratory demand. Actively breathing patients rarely need an inspiratory time of one second, and some may require an inspiratory time of 0.7 to one second.

Rate

The rate chosen depends on tidal volume, pulmonary mechanics and Pa_{CO_2} target (Table 11-4). For patients with obstructive lung disease, lower set rates in the range of 8 to 12/min are normally well tolerated. With obstructive lung disease, rate and minute volume are set low to avoid the development of auto-PEEP and ventilation beyond the patient's usual Pa_{CO_2}. For patients with either acute or chronic restrictive lung disease, an initial rate of about 15 to 25/min is generally adequate to meet ventilatory demand. Patients with normal pulmonary mechanics usually tolerate an initial rate of 8 to 12/min. As with all settings, adjustment should be made after monitoring the effect of mechanical ventilation.

F_{IO_2} and PEEP

At initiation of mechanical ventilation, a F_{IO_2} of 1.0 is recommended. This is to insure that hypoxemia does not complicate the initial acclimation to the ventilator. Pulse oximetry can be used to adjust F_{IO_2} once the patient has stabilized. An initial PEEP of 5 cm H_2O is often set to maintain functional residual capacity and prevent atelectasis unless marked cardiovascular instability is present, in which case PEEP is withheld until cardiovascular status is stabilized.

ETHICAL CONSIDERATIONS

Before committing a patient to mechanical ventilatory support, consideration should be given to the reversibility of the disease process. If there is no likelihood of reversing the acute disease process that necessitated mechanical ventilation, the potential for long-term ventilation must be weighed against the result of not providing ventilatory support. However, the recent increased emphasis on noninvasive positive pressure ventilation has made it easier to avoid ethical conflicts. Noninvasive support can be provided as an interim measure while discussions regarding the advisability of intubation and long-term support can be evaluated.

POINTS TO REMEMBER

- Ventilatory muscle failure may occur as a result of inadequate ventilatory muscle function, excessive ventilatory load, a compromised central ventilatory drive or a combination of the above.
- Ventilatory drive may be depressed by drugs, hypothyroidism, congenital abnormalities, or neurologic lesions.
- Physiologic indications for mechanical ventilation are apnea, acute ventilatory failure, impeding acute ventilatory failure, and severe oxygenation deficit.
- During initial selection of ventilatory mode, CMV (A/C) with either pressure or volume ventilation is recommended, provided that rate is set to insure full ventilatory support.
- Tidal volume and pressure level should always be set based on pulmonary mechanics, pathophysiology and a maximum end-inspiratory plateau pressure of 30 cm H_2O.
- Set V_T at 10 to 12 mL/kg in patients with normal lungs, 8 to 10 mL/kg in patients with obstructive lung disease, and 4 to 8 mL/kg in patients with restrictive lung disease.
- Initial inspiratory flow pattern with volume ventilation may be descending ramp or rectangular; peak flow or inspiratory time should be set to insure an inspiratory time of one second.
- Rate is set based on V_T, pulmonary mechanics and targeted Pa_{CO_2}. For restrictive lung disease, set rate at 15 to 25/min; for obstructive lung disease, set rate at 8 to 12/min; and for patients with normal lungs, set rate at 8 to 12/min.
- Initial $F_{I_{O_2}}$ should be set at 1 and then adjusted based on pulse oximetry.
- Ventilatory support should not be initiated unless the acute process necessitating ventilation is reversible.

ADDITIONAL READING

ALDRICK TK, PREZANT DJ. Indications for mechanical ventilation. In TOBIN M (ed) *Textbook of Mechanical Ventilation*. New York, McGraw-Hill, 1994; 155–952.

HUDSON LD, PIERSON DJ. Ventilatory failure. In PIERSON DJ, KACMAREK RM (eds) *Foundations of Respiratory Care*. New York, Churchill Livingstone, 1992; 303–310.

PIERSON DJ. Respiratory failure: introduction and overview. In PIERSON DJ, KACMAREK RM (eds) *Foundations of Respiratory Care*. New York, Churchill Livingstone, 1992; 295–302.

ROCHESTER DF. The diaphragm in COPD: better than expected but not good enough. *N Engl J Med* 1991; 325:961–962.

STOLLER JK. Determining the need for mechanical ventilation. In PIERSON DJ, KACMAREK RM (eds) *Foundations of Respiratory Care*. New York, Churchill Livingstone, 1992; 945–952.

TOBIN MJ. Respiratory muscle involvement in chronic obstructive pulmonary disease and asthma. *Prob Respir Care* 1990; 3:375–395.

CHAPTER TWELVE

WEANING FROM MECHANICAL VENTILATION

OBJECTIVES

1. Discuss those physiologic variables that are used to indicate readiness to wean from ventilatory support.
2. Contrast the approaches used to wean patients from ventilatory support.
3. Discuss the use of protocols to wean patients from ventilatory support.
4. Discuss the criteria used to indicate readiness for extubation.
5. Describe the most common reasons why patients fail to wean from mechanical ventilation.

INTRODUCTION

The ultimate goal of mechanical ventilatory support is ventilator discontinuation and in the vast majority of patients this is a simple process. About 75% of mechanically ventilated patients can be liberated from the ventilator when the physiologic reason for ventilatory support is reversed. The others may require weaning before ventilator discontinuation is possible. A small percentage of patients may never be physiologically ready for ventilator discontinuation and become chronically ventilator-dependent. This chapter addresses issues defining readiness for weaning, assessments of pulmonary mechanics that predict weaning outcome, the various approaches used to wean patients from ventilatory support, and the use of protocols to wean patients.

READINESS TO WEAN

Before a patient is considered a candidate for discontinuation of ventilatory support, a basic level of physiologic readiness must be established (Table 12-1).

Table 12.1 Readiness to wean

- Improvement of respiratory failure
- $Pa_{O_2} \geq 60$ mm Hg with $F_{I_{O_2}} \leq 0.40$ and PEEP ≤ 5 cm H_2O
- Intact ventilatory drive
- Cardiovascular stability
- Electrolytes normal
- Normal body temperature
- Adequate nutritional status
- Absence of major organ system failure

Reversal of Indication for Ventilatory Support

The most important indicator of readiness for discontinuation of ventilatory support is the reversal of the specific indication for ventilatory support. Although this seems obvious, it is frequently forgotten when management of a given patient focuses on discontinuing ventilatory support. If a patient developed ventilatory failure because of pneumonia superimposed on chronic pulmonary disease, or because anesthesia was not reversed, consideration for weaning should not be made until the pneumonia has been effectively treated or the anesthetic has been completely reversed.

Gas Exchange

In the broadest sense, weaning occurs each time the $F_{I_{O_2}}$ or PEEP is decreased. However, before attempts to discontinue ventilatory support are made, the patient should be able to maintain gas exchange with minimal support. From an oxygenation perspective, this means a $Pa_{O_2} \geq 60$ mm Hg with an $F_{I_{O_2}} \leq 0.40$ and PEEP ≤ 5 cm H_2O. If higher levels of oxygenation support are required during mechanical ventilation, the likelihood of discontinuation is markedly decreased. A high minute ventilation during ventilatory support should not be required to maintain the Pa_{CO_2} in the patient's normal range. Generally, a dead space to tidal volume ratio $(V_D/V_T) < 60\%$ during ventilatory support or a minute ventilation < 12 L/min is optimal. In addition, patients must be able to spontaneously ventilate, they should be capable of controlling their own level of ventilation (no central ventilatory drive issues), and they should not be tachypneic (rate < 30/min).

Function of Other Organ Systems

For weaning to be successful, all major organ systems must be functioning appropriately. Cardiovascular function must be optimized. Arrhythmias, fluid overload, and myocardial contractility should all be properly managed before weaning. Body temperature should ideally be normal before weaning is initiated. Each degree centigrade increase in body temperature increases CO_2 production and O_2 consumption by about 5%. Electrolyte levels should be normal. Imbalances in potassium, calcium, magnesium, and phosphate result in muscle weakness. Nutritional status should be addressed, because both under- and over-feeding can compromise ventilatory muscle function. Renal, liver or gastrointestinal dysfunction may all adversely impact ventilatory capabilities.

Psychologic Factors

The need for mechanical ventilatory support is a very terrifying experience, but also may be a welcome change from dyspnea. It is possible, though rare, that patients develop a psychological dependence on ventilatory support. Thus, the weaning process should always be conducted in a supportive manner. Assurance of assistance when needed should be discussed and a supportive clinician should be present throughout the weaning trial. For patients who are physiologically ready for weaning and in whom no reason for failure to wean is identified, psychologic dependence should be considered before the patient is labeled chronically ventilator-dependent.

PREDICTORS OF WEANING OUTCOME

Most predictors of weaning outcome focus on the ability to achieve or sustain a specific ventilatory parameter. Unfortunately, no predictive parameter is 100% accurate in identifying individuals who will successfully wean. In fact, the best predictor of weaning success may be patient response to a spontaneous breathing trial. Some patients who never meet standard weaning criteria eventually wean, whereas others do not wean in spite of acceptable weaning parameters. Generally, failure to wean indicates the need to reinstate ventilatory support within 48 hr after discontinuation.

The most commonly used predictors of weaning success are listed in Table 12-2. Note that they are subdivided into indices that evaluate ventilatory drive, ventilatory muscle capability and ventilatory performance. The primary index of ventilatory drive is $P_{0.1}$ or the airway pressure change generated in the first 100 ms (0.1 s) of inspiration with an occluded airway. Failure to wean is associated with a high ventilatory drive. Since greater effort is required to ventilate when ventilator drive is high, exhaustion is more likely.

The two historically used indices of ventilatory muscle strength are vital capacity and maximum inspiratory pressure ($P_{I max}$). Of these, vital capacity is the least precise since it requires patient cooperation. $P_{I max}$ inaccurately predicts weaning success but is the best predictor of weaning failure (≥ -15 cm H_2O). Reproducibility of $P_{I max}$ is not dependent upon patient cooperation but upon

Table 12-2 Predictors of weaning outcome

Predictor	Value
• Evaluation of ventilatory drive	
$\quad P_{0.1}$	< 6 cm H_2O
• Ventilatory muscle capabilities	
$\quad$ Vital capacity	> 10 mL/kg
$\quad$ Maximum inspiratory pressure	< −30 cm H_2O
• Ventilatory performance	
$\quad$ Minute ventilation	< 10 L/min
$\quad$ Maximum voluntary ventilation	> 3 times $\dot{V}_E$
$\quad$ Rapid shallow breathing index	< 100
$\quad$ Repiratory rate	< 30/ min

measurement technique. To insure maximum effort, measurement of P_{Imax} should be performed at residual volume (RV). To insure lung volume is at residual volume, a one-way valve as illustrated in Figure 12-1 is employed. This allows exhalation but not inspiration. Thus the lung volume at which P_{Imax} is evaluated decreases with each attempt to breathe. P_{Imax} measurements should be performed for about 20 s provided no arrhythmias or desaturation occurs.

Another group of indices evaluates ventilatory performance. The most accurate predictor of weaning success of all indices is the rapid-shallow breathing index. This index is determined by dividing the respiratory rate by the tidal volume in liters, determined one minute after discontinuation of ventilatory and oxygenation support. If this parameter is ≤ 100, the probability of successful weaning is high and if it is > 100, the probability of failure is high.

Another index of ventilatory performance is work-of-breathing. However, as with most of the other weaning parameters, no specific level has been consistently identified with weaning success or failure. In addition, work-of-breathing is a poor indicator of patient effort because no work is performed even if large intrathoracic pressure changes develop but no volume is moved. The assessment of work-of-breathing is also invasive, costly, and requires significant expertise. Thus, assessment of work-of-breathing for evaluation for weaning readiness is not recommended.

Observation of ventilatory pattern provides insight into the level of stress experienced by patients during weaning. Paradoxical abdominal and chest wall

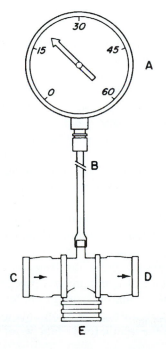

Figure 12-1 Apparatus used to determine P_{Imax} for patients with artificial airways. (A) manometer; (B) connecting tubing; (C) inspiratory one-way valve with port for thumb occlusion; (D) expiratory one-way valve with port; (E) 22-mm ID port for attachment to artificial airway. (From KACMAREK RM, ET AL. Determination of maximal inspiratory pressure: a clinical study and literature review. *Respir Care* 1989; 34:868–878.)

movement, use of accessory muscles, nasal flaring and retractions, and respiratory alternans are all indicators of ventilatory stress and are associated with a high probability of weaning failure.

APPROACHES TO WEANING

In general, approaches to weaning can be grouped into four categories:

1. Spontaneous breathing trials.
2. Pressure support ventilation (PSV).
3. SIMV.
4. Newer weaning modes.

Regardless of the approach used, our underlying rule is "DO NOT WEAN TO EXHAUSTION." The stress associated with a weaning trial should not result in fatigue of ventilatory muscles or in the compromise of a patient's ventilatory ability during subsequent weaning trials. In addition, in those patients requiring a lengthy period of weaning (more than a day), it is important to adjust ventilatory support at night to insure ventilatory muscle rest and sleep. Approaches that appropriately alternate work and rest periods with proper nutrition and sleep are recommended.

Spontaneous Breathing Trials

The classic approach to weaning is the spontaneous breathing trial (T-piece or CPAP). There are two uses of the spontaneous breathing trial (SBT). In the first case, the SBT is used to assess extubation readiness. Patients who tolerate spontaneous breathing for 30 to 120 min should be considered liberated from ventilatory support and candidates for extubation. In the second case, weaning is achieved by increasing periods of unsupported spontaneous breathing interspersed with periods of full ventilatory support. The length of the trials is increased as the patient's tolerance improves, allowing periods of rest between trials and during the night. For patients with tracheotomy tubes, spontaneous breathing trials may continue for as long as 24 hours to insure ventilator discontinuation is complete.

The approach to a spontaneous breathing trial can vary greatly. Original trials were conducted with a T-piece. However, the newest generation of ventilators impose little work when set to CPAP and many clinicians use the ventilator for spontaneous breathing trials. Performing spontaneous breathing trials with the patient attached to the ventilator has the advantage of maintaining a precise F_{IO_2}, as well as the patient monitoring activities of the ventilator. In addition, low levels of CPAP and pressure support can be applied during the spontaneous breathing trial. The primary disadvantage of using the ventilator is that work-of-breathing may be imposed or low-level ventilatory support may be provided during the trial.

Most patients do equally well on T-piece trials or CPAP trials on the mechanical ventilator with CPAP set at zero. Due to auto-PEEP, many patients with COPD may benefit from the application of 5 cm H_2O CPAP during the spontaneous breathing trial. Patients with high airway resistance, small endotracheal tubes, and nasal intubation may benefit from the application of low levels of pressure support (5 to 10 cm H_2O). Others may benefit from spontaneous breathing trials with low levels of CPAP and low levels of pressure support. During all spontaneous breathing trials, $F_{I_{O_2}}$ should be maintained at the level previously applied during mechanical ventilation.

Pressure Support

Many clinicians use gradual reductions in the level of PSV for weaning, provided the patient can maintain a target respiratory rate and V_T. The process is begun by setting the PSV at a level where the tidal volume and respiratory rate are consistent with the level expected upon discontinuation of ventilatory support. A PSV level that prevents activation of accessory muscles is the most appropriate. PSV is then decreased on a regular basis (hours or days) to a minimum level (5 to 8 cm H_2O) that unloads the work-of-breathing imposed by the ventilator/endotracheal tube system, provided the desired ventilatory pattern is maintained. Once the patient is capable of maintaining the target ventilatory pattern and gas exchange at this minimal level, mechanical ventilation is discontinued.

Although this approach works well with most patients requiring short-term weaning (8 to 24 hrs), it can be problematic for patients who require longer periods to wean. First, it may not allow the patient to rest. If the level of ventilatory support is maintained at the minimal level necessary, this may not be appropriate for patients requiring lengthy weaning periods. In addition, because of the lack of ability to modify the terminal flow criteria used to cycle PSV from inspiration to expiration in some ventilators, a high level of PSV ($\geq$ 15 cm H_2O) may increase expiratory muscle activity.

SIMV

SIMV was introduced as a ventilator mode to facilitate weaning. A gradual reduction in SIMV rate has been a commonly used approach for weaning. However, in contrast to PSV, with SIMV two different breath types are applied – a mandatory breath and a spontaneous breath. Many patients experience dyssynchrony with low SIMV rates. Weaning with SIMV also results in significant work of the respiratory muscles during both the mandatory and spontaneous breaths. SIMV is commonly used with PSV to unload spontaneous breaths. Because SIMV has the worst weaning outcomes in clinical trials, its use is not recommended.

New Weaning Modes

A number of ventilator manufacturers have introduced new modes of ventilation that they claim increases the rate of weaning from mechanical ventilation. Volume support, automode, and automatic tube compensation have been introduced for this purpose. Although there may be benefits from some of these new modes, there is no data to support more rapid weaning from ventilatory support with these modes.

PROTOCOLS

A successful approach to weaning patients from ventilatory support is the use of protocols implemented by respiratory therapists and nurses. These protocols result in shorter weaning times and shorter lengths of mechanical ventilation than physician-directed weaning. The primary reason for the success of protocols is that they are developed by multidisciplinary teams and are implemented by respiratory therapists and nurses empowered to make clinical decisions. In the United States, weaning protocols are most commonly implemented by respiratory therapists.

Although protocols can be developed for any approach to weaning, the approach that has been most commonly used is based on spontaneous breathing trials. Mechanically ventilated patients are regularly screened for weaning readiness according to specific criteria (Table 12-3). Patients meeting these criteria are evaluated during a short trial of spontaneous breathing using the rapid-shallow breathing index (RSBI). If the RSBI is ≤ 100, a spontaneous breathing trial is conducted.

Patients successfully completing a spontaneous breathing trial of 30 to 120 min are considered for extubation (Table 12-4). Many clinicians conduct the spontaneous breathing trial while the patient is attached to the ventilator. This allows use of the monitoring available on the ventilator and rapid reinstitution of ventilatory support if necessary. For patients who successfully complete the spontaneous breathing trial, extubation is performed unless there is a reason to delay extubation.

Table 12-3 Evaluation for readiness for spontaneous breathing trial

- $Pa_{O_2}/F_{I_{O_2}} \geq 200$ mm Hg
- PEEP ≤ 5 cm H_2O
- Intact airway reflexes
- No need for continuous infusions of vasopressors or inotropes

Table 12-4 Criteria for failure of a spontaneous breathing trial

---

- Respiratory rate > 35/min
- Sp_{O_2} < 90%
- Heart rate > 140/min or sustained 20% increase in heart rate
- Systolic BP > 180 mm Hg, diastolic > 90 mm Hg
- Anxiety
- Diaphoresis

EXTUBATION

Extubation is a process separate from weaning. Successful extubation requires that patients are able to protect their airway, mobilize secretions, and do not have a level of airway obstruction requiring an artificial airway. In most mechanically ventilated patients, ventilator discontinuation and extubation occur simultaneously. However, there are some patients who may require an endotracheal tube for airway protection or secretion mobilization after they are able to breathe on their own. Generally, patients who can sustain spontaneous ventilation can mobilize secretions provided that the secretions are not large in quantity, thick and tenacious. Airway obstruction is usually the primary concern following extubation. After suction of the trachea and the oropharynx, the cuff may be deflated and air leak around the tube should be evaluated. Auscultating the lateral neck can determine gas flow around the endotracheal tube. If no air movement around the tube is identified, the probability of airway obstruction after removal of the tube is higher. A short course of steroid therapy may be indicated prior to extubation and personnel trained to re-intubate should be at the bedside at the time of extubation.

NONINVASIVE VENTILATION

It may be useful to provide noninvasive positive pressure ventilation (NPPV) post-extubation in those patients with limited ventilatory reserve or chronic pulmonary disease. NPPV may be necessary for several days and makes the transition from invasive ventilatory support to spontaneous breathing easier in some patients. In those patients who have failed weaning attempts but are progressing, a trial of NPPV may be appropriate before tracheostomy is considered.

FAILURE TO WEAN

Patients fail to wean from ventilatory support for physiologic reasons (Table 12-5), some that are simple to correct, and others that may be impossible to correct.

Table 12-5 Common reasons for failure to wean

- Weaning to exhaustion
- Auto-PEEP
- Excessive work-of-breathing
- Poor nutritional status
- Overfeeding
- Left heart failure
- Decreased magnesium and phosphate levels
- Infection/fever
- Major organ system failure
- Technical limitations

Weaning to Exhaustion

One of the biggest mistakes made when weaning patients is to push them to the point of exhaustion. Whether fatigue actually develops during weaning is controversial, but the exhaustion observed in some patients results in a delay in weaning progression. As indicated above, care must be exercised to prevent exhaustion. The guidelines outlined in Table 12-4 determine when weaning should be terminated. A respiratory rate, V_T, heart rate, and blood pressure that signal excess stress should be identified. Rest is always a key component to any lengthy weaning program.

Work-of-Breathing

Although work-of-breathing is not a good predictor, an excessive workload may be the primary reason why a patient fails a weaning trial. High airways resistance and low compliance contribute to the increased effort necessary to breathe. Aerosolized bronchodilators, bronchial hygiene and normalized fluid balance assist in normalizing compliance, resistance, and work-of-breathing.

Auto-PEEP

Auto-PEEP is a problem in many patients with chronic lung disease during lengthy weaning periods. Auto-PEEP increases the pressure gradient needed to inspire, whether triggering the ventilator or spontaneously breathing. Use of CPAP is important in these patients to balance alveolar pressure with ventilator circuit pressure. Generally, 5 to 10 cm H_2O CPAP is needed. This is titrated based on clinical observation of patient effort. When the CPAP or PEEP level adequately balances auto-PEEP, a decrease in indicators of patient stress (e.g., retractions, respiratory rate, heart rate) occurs. For patients triggering the ventilator, patient and ventilator rate become equal. Inspiratory changes in esophageal pressure can be used to titrate CPAP, but few patients have an esophageal balloon in place.

Nutritional Status/Electrolyte Balance

Imbalance of electrolytes causes muscular weakness. Specifically, decreased potassium, magnesium, phosphate, and calcium levels impair ventilatory muscle function. Nutritional support frequently improves outcome. However, care should be exercised to avoid overfeeding since excessive carbohydrate ingestion elevates CO_2 production.

Infection/Fever/Organ System Failure

Failure of any major organ system can precipitate weaning failure. Fever and infection are of particular concern, since both O_2 consumption and CO_2 production are increased, resulting in increased ventilatory drive.

Left Heart Failure

Of particular concern for patients with cardiopulmonary disease is poorly managed left heart failure. A delicate balance between mean airway pressure and hemodynamics may exist, that is easily disrupted by the decrease of mean airway pressure during weaning trials (Figure 12-2). These patients may rapidly develop pulmonary edema during weaning. Some patients develop myocardial ischemia during weaning. Appropriate management of cardiovascular status is necessary before weaning will be successful.

Technical Limitations

Particularly with older generation mechanical ventilators, the imposed work-of-breathing during CPAP trials may be excessive or the work imposed by a small endotracheal tube may prevent weaning. If a newer generation ventilator is not available, continuous flow CPAP may be more appropriate than CPAP on the ventilator. If a small endotracheal tube is in place, use of PSV may be useful.

CHRONIC VENTILATOR DEPENDENCY

In spite of doing everything correctly, some patients will not be able to wean from ventilatory support. Their level of chronic pulmonary or neuromuscular/neurologic disease may make it impossible for them to wean. However, before declaring a patient ventilator-dependent, all of those factors affecting weaning failure should be addressed. Some patients in this category can be transitioned to noninvasive nocturnal positive pressure ventilation while others will require continued invasive ventilatory support.

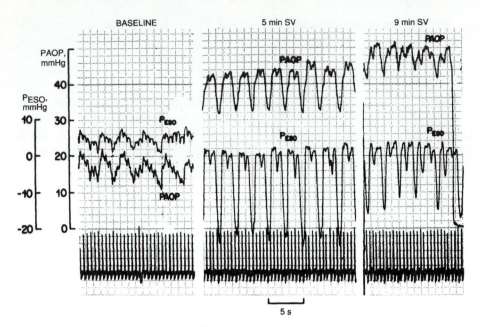

Figure 12-2 Weaning of a patient from mechanical ventilation (baseline) to spontaneous ventilation (SV). There is a progressive increase of pulmonary artery occlusion pressure (PAOP) from 14 mm Hg (baseline) to 50 mm Hg (9 min SV). The esophageal pressure is reduced during SV with marked negative inspiratory excursions. (From LEMAIRE F, TEBOUL JL, CINOTTI L, ET AL. Acute left ventricular dysfunction during unsuccessful weaning from mechanical ventilation. *Anesthesiology* 1988; 69:171–179.)

ACCP-SCCM-AARC EVIDENCE-BASED VENTILATOR WEANING/DISCONTINUATION GUIDELINES

1. In patients requiring mechanical ventilation for more than 24 hours, a search for all causes that may be contributing to ventilator dependence should be undertaken. This is particularly true in the patient who has failed attempts at withdrawing the mechanical ventilator. Reversing all possible ventilatory and non-ventilatory issues should be an integral part of the ventilator discontinuation process.

2. Patients receiving mechanical ventilation for respiratory failure should undergo a formal assessment of discontinuation potential if the following criteria are satisfied: evidence for some reversal of the underlying cause for respiratory failure, adequate oxygenation (e.g., $Pa_{O_2}/FI_{O_2} \leq 150$–$200$; requiring PEEP ≤ 5–8 cm H_2O; $FI_{O_2} \leq 0.4$–0.5) and pH (e.g., ≥ 7.25), hemodynamic stability as defined by absence of active myocardial ischemia and absence of clinically significant hypotension (i.e., requiring no or only low dose vasopressors such as dopamine or dobutamine < 5 mcg/kg/min), capability to initiate an inspiratory effort. The decision to use these criteria must

be individualized. Some patients not satisfying all of the above criteria (e.g., patients with chronic hypoxemia below these thresholds) may be ready for attempts at discontinuation of mechanical ventilation.

3. Formal discontinuation assessments for patients receiving mechanical ventilation for respiratory failure should be done during spontaneous breathing rather than while the patient is still receiving substantial ventilatory support. An initial brief period of spontaneous breathing can be used to assess the capability of continuing onto a formal spontaneous breathing trial (SBT). Criteria to assess patient tolerance during SBTs are the respiratory pattern, adequacy of gas exchange, hemodynamic stability, and subjective comfort. Tolerance of SBTs lasting 30 to 120 min should prompt consideration for permanent ventilator discontinuation/liberation.

4. Removal of the artificial airway from a patient who has successfully been discontinued from ventilatory support should be based upon assessments of airway patency and the ability of the patient to protect the airway.

5. Patients receiving mechanical ventilation for respiratory failure who fail an SBT should have the cause for the failed SBT determined. Once reversible causes for failure are corrected, subsequent SBTs should be performed every 24 hrs.

6. Patients receiving mechanical ventilation for respiratory failure who fail an SBT should receive a stable, non-fatiguing, comfortable form of ventilatory support.

7. Anesthesia/sedation strategies and ventilator management aimed at early extubation should be used in post-surgical patients.

8. Weaning/discontinuation protocols designed for non-physician health care professionals should be developed and implemented by intensive care units. Protocols aimed at optimizing sedation should also be developed and implemented.

9. Tracheostomy should be considered after an initial period of stabilization on the ventilator when it becomes apparent that the patient will require prolonged ventilator assistance. Tracheostomy should then be performed when the patient appears likely to gain one or more of the benefits ascribed to the procedure. Patients who may derive particular benefit from early tracheostomy are: those requiring high levels of sedation to tolerate translaryngeal tubes; those with marginal respiratory mechanics (often manifested as tachypnea) in whom a lower resistance tracheostomy tube might reduce the risk of muscle overload; those who may derive psychological benefit from the ability to eat orally, communicate by articulated speech, and experience enhanced mobility; those in whom enhanced mobility may assist physical therapy efforts.

10. Unless there is evidence for clearly irreversible disease (e.g., high spinal cord injury, advanced amyotrophic lateral sclerosis), a patient requiring prolonged mechanical ventilatory support for respiratory failure should not be considered permanently ventilator dependent until three months' of weaning attempts have failed.

11. Critical care practitioners should familiarize themselves with facilities in their communities, or units in hospitals they staff, that specialize in managing patients with prolonged dependence on mechanical ventilation. Such familiarization should include reviewing published peer-reviewed data from those units, if available. When medically stable for transfer, patients who have failed ventilator discontinuation attempts in the ICU should be transferred to those facilities that have demonstrated success and safety in accomplishing ventilator discontinuation.
12. Weaning strategy in the prolonged mechanically ventilated patient should be slow-paced, and should include gradually lengthening self-breathing trials.

POINTS TO REMEMBER

- The primary prerequisite for weaning is reversal of the indication for mechanical ventilation.
- Adequate gas exchange should be present, with minimal oxygenation and ventilatory support, before weaning is attempted.
- The most successful predictor of weaning is the rapid-shallow breathing index; ≤ 100 indicates high likelihood of weaning and > 100 indicates a high likelihood of failure.
- Regardless of the approach used to wean, an appropriate mix of work and rest periods, and the assurance of proper sleep and nutrition are essential.
- The poorest weaning outcomes are with the use of SIMV.
- The use of protocols results in the most rapid weaning from ventilatory support.
- Extubation should be considered separately from weaning.
- The primary reason that patients fail weaning trials is that the process stresses them to exhaustion.
- The presence of auto-PEEP, increased work-of-breathing, left heart failure, electrolyte imbalance, fever, poor nutritional status, and technical limitations are frequent causes of weaning failure.
- Post-extubation NPPV is useful in some patients to allow a smooth transition to spontaneous breathing.

ADDITIONAL READING

BROCHARD L, KAUSS A, SALVADOR B, ET AL. Comparison of three methods of gradual withdrawal from mechanical support during weaning from mechanical ventilation. *Am J Respir Crit Care Med* 1994; 150:896–903.

BUTLER R, KEENAN SP, INMAN KJ, ET AL. Is there a preferred technique for weaning the difficult-to-wean patient? A systematic review of the literature. *Crit Care Med* 1999; 27:2331–2336.

ELY EW. The utility of weaning protocols to expedite liberation from mechanical ventilation. *Respir Care Clin N Am* 2000; 6:303–319.

ELY EW, BAKER AM, DUNAGAN DP ET AL. Effect on the duration of mechanical ventilation of identifying patients capable of breathing spontaneously. *N Engl J Med* 1996; 335:1864–1869.

ELY EW, BENNETT PA, BOWTON DL, ET AL. Large scale implementation of a respiratory therapist-driven protocol for ventilator weaning. *Am J Respir Crit Care Med* 1999; 159:439–446.

EPSTEIN SK. Weaning parameters. *Respir Care Clin N Am* 2000; 6:253–301.

ESTEBAN A, FRUTOS F, TOBIN MJ ET AL. A comparison of four methods of weaning patients from mechanical ventilation. *N Engl J Med* 1995; 332:345–350.

HESS D, BRANSON RD. Ventilators and weaning modes. *Respir Care Clin N Am* 2000; 6:407–435.

HORST HM, MOURO D, HALL-JENSSENS RA, PAMUKOU N. Decrease in ventilation time with a standardized weaning protocol. *Arch Surg* 1998; 133:483–489.

HURFORD WE, FAVORITO F. Myocardial ischemia during weaning of mechanical ventilator-dependent patients. *Crit Care Med* 1995; 23:1475–1480.

KHAMIEES M, RAJU P, DEGIROLAMO A, ET AL. Predictors of extubation and outcome in patients who have successfully completed a spontaneous breathing trial. *Chest* 2001; 120:1262–1270.

KOLLEF MH, SHAPIRO SD, SILVER P, ET AL. A randomized, controlled trial of protocol-directed versus physician-directed weaning from mechanical ventilation. *Crit Care Med* 1997; 25:567–574.

LEMAIRE F, TEBOUL J-L, CINOTTI L, ET AL. Acute left ventricular dysfunction during unsuccessful weaning from mechanical ventilation. *Anesthesiology* 1988; 69:171–179.

MACINTYRE NR, COOK DJ, ELY EW, ET AL. Evidence-based guidelines for weaning and discontinuing ventilator support. *Chest* 2001; 120:375S–395S.

MARELICH GP, MURIN S, BATTISTELLA F, ET AL. Protocol weaning of mechanical ventilation in medical and surgical patients by respiratory care practitioners and nurses. Effect on weaning time and incidence of ventilator-associated pneumonia. *Chest* 2000; 118:459–467.

MEADE MO, GUYATT GH, COOK DJ. Weaning from mechanical ventilation: The evidence from clinical research. *Respir Care* 2001; 46:1408–1415.

SASSOON CSH, TE TT, MAHUTTE CK, LIGHT RW. Airway occlusion pressure: an important indicator for successful weaning in patients with chronic obstructive pulmonary disease. *Am Rev Respir Dis* 1987; 135:107–113.

TOBIN MJ, ALEX CG. Discontinuation of mechanical ventilation. In TOBIN MJ (ed): *Mechanical Ventilation*. New York, McGraw Hill Publishers, 1994, 1117–1124.

YANG KL, TOBIN MJ. A prospective study of indexes predicting the outcome of trials of weaning from mechanical ventilation. *N Engl J Med* 1991; 324:1445–1450.

VENTILATOR MANAGEMENT

THIRTEEN

ACUTE LUNG INJURY AND ACUTE RESPIRATORY DISTRESS SYNDROME

INTRODUCTION

OVERVIEW
  Clinical Presentation
  Ventilator-Induced Lung Injury

MECHANICAL VENTILATION
  Indications
  Ventilator Settings
  Monitoring
  Weaning

POINTS TO REMEMBER

ADDITIONAL READING

OBJECTIVES

1. Describe the clinical presentation of patients with acute lung injury (ALI) and ARDS.
2. Discuss the potential of ventilator induced lung injury with ALI and ARDS patients.
3. List the indications for mechanical ventilation for patients with ALI and ARDS.
4. Discuss approaches used to set the ventilator for patients with ALI and ARDS.
5. Describe the approach used to monitor and wean patients with ALI and ARDS.

INTRODUCTION

Acute respiratory distress syndrome (ARDS) is used to represent the pulmonary symptoms associated with severe lung injury of diverse etiology. ARDS frequently develops in the presence of sepsis and multi-organ failure, and is associated with high mortality. ARDS results in diffuse alveolar damage, pulmonary microvascular thrombosis, aggregation of inflammatory cells, and stagnation of pulmonary blood flow. Because thousands of individuals per year develop ARDS in the United States, it consumes much of the time, energy and resources of ICU clinicians.

OVERVIEW

Clinical Presentation

ARDS is characterized by hypoxemia and decreased pulmonary compliance. Specifically, bilateral infiltrates are present on the chest X-ray, the Pa_{O_2}/F_{IO_2} ratio is ≤ 200, and there is no evidence of left heart failure. The definition of acute lung injury (ALI) is similar to ARDS, except that the Pa_{O_2}/F_{IO_2} is ≤ 300. Evaluation of ARDS by chest computed tomography (CT) reveals a very heterogeneous disease with areas of consolidation, areas of lung collapse that are recruitable, and areas of normal lung tissue. Rather than considering ARDS lungs stiff, they should be considered small when compared with normal lungs.

The pathology of ARDS progresses through two phases, although the process may resolve at any point in either phase. The first phase is characterized by an intense inflammatory response resulting in alveolar and endothelial damage, increased vascular permeability, and increased lung water. This phase lasts about 7 to 10 days and then progresses to extensive fibrosis (Phase 2). ARDS has been categorized as pulmonary and extrapulmonary ARDS. With pulmonary ARDS, there is direct injury to the lungs as occurs with aspiration, infectious pneumonia, trauma (lung contusion and penetrating chest injury), near drowning, and fat embolism. With extrapulmonary ARDS, the initial injury is to an organ system distant from the lungs including sepsis syndrome, multiple trauma, burns, shock, hypoperfusion, and acute pancreatitis.

Ventilator-induced Lung Injury

As a result of the areas of low lung compliance and the heterogeneous nature of this disease, ARDS is one of the most likely pathologies to develop ventilator-induced injury. To avoid ventilator-induced lung injury, a peak alveolar pressure (end-inspiratory plateau pressure) < 30 cm H_2O and PEEP that maintains alveolar recruitment is recommended. Peak alveolar pressure is limited to prevent overdistention, whereas an appropriate level of PEEP is maintained to avoid the shear stresses of repeatedly opening and closing unstable lung units.

MECHANICAL VENTILATION

Indications

Patients with ARDS initially present with hypoxemia and increased work-of-breathing. Ventilatory support is indicated to reverse hypoxemia with the application of PEEP, delivery of a high F_{IO_2}, and reduction of the work-of-breathing (Table 13-1). The ability to ventilate may become compromised with CO_2 retention. At this stage, mechanical ventilation is indicated because of acute ventilatory failure. The use of mask CPAP and noninvasive ventilation is generally not recommended for patients with ARDS.

Ventilator Settings

Two approaches have been advocated for the ventilation of patients with ARDS. The open lung approach uses pressure-controlled ventilation, focuses on maintaining a low plateau pressure while monitoring tidal volume, and uses recruitment maneuvers and high levels of PEEP to maximize alveolar recruitment. The ARDSnet approach focuses on maintaining a low tidal volume while monitoring plateau pressure and sets PEEP based upon the F_{IO_2} requirement.

Patients should ideally be allowed to trigger the ventilator. This may promote alveolar recruitment in dorsal lung regions, it may facilitate venous return, and it may decrease the requirement for sedation. Ventilator modes that allow spontaneous breathing in patients with ARDS have been advocated by some clinicians, but further study is needed of this approach. In the early phase of ARDS, as well as during the recovery phase, pressure support is a useful mode. As the disease worsens, however, patient-triggered ventilation may result in compromised gas exchange and hemodynamics – particularly if patient-ventilator dys-synchrony occurs. As a result, pharmacologic control of ventilation is usually necessary at some stage in the ventilatory course of these patients. However, paralysis should be avoided except for the most severe cases.

The open lung approach targets a specific pressure with pressure-controlled ventilation (Table 13-2 and Figure 13-1). A V_T of 4 to 8 mL/kg while maintaining peak alveolar pressure 25 to 30 cm H_2O is selected. Permissive hypercapnia may become necessary. Respiratory rates as high as 35/min are selected. PEEP of 10 to

Table 13-1 Indications for mechanical ventilation in patients with ARDS

- Increased work-of-breathing
- Oxygenation impairment
- Impending ventilatory failure
- Acute ventilatory failure

Table 13-2 Ventilator settings for ARDS using the open lung approach

Setting	Recommendation
Mode	A/C (CMV) in most acute stages; pressure support in early stages and during recovery
Rate	As high as 35/min; avoid auto-PEEP
Volume/pressure control	Pressure
Tidal volume	4 to 8 mL/kg and plateau pressure < 30 cm H_2O
Inspiratory time	Set to insure synchrony in patient-triggered ventilation, incorporate a short end-inspiratory pause in passive ventilation (0.1–0.3 s)
PEEP	10 to 20 cm H_2O
F_{IO_2}	As needed to achieve Sp_{O_2}/Pa_{O_2} target
Mean airway pressure	Lowest level to achieve Sp_{O_2}/Pa_{O_2} target (20 to 25 cm H_2O may be required)

20 cm H_2O is set to maintain alveolar recruitment, although a lower level of PEEP is needed when the fibrotic phase of ARDS develops. A recruitment maneuver is applied before setting PEEP. PEEP is initially set higher than required and then decreased to the minimal level maintaining recruitment. F_{IO_2} is set before the titration of PEEP to insure Sp_{O_2} and Pa_{O_2} at or above the targeted level (Table 13-3). A high alveolar pressure is of greater concern than a high F_{IO_2}, and a F_{IO_2} up to 0.60 is usually used without concern. In patients experiencing persistent severe hypoxemia in spite of the use of recruitment maneuvers and the application of PEEP, prone positioning may be considered. Prone positioning results in short term improvement in oxygenation, although the long-term effect is unclear. Table 13-4 lists the sequence of adjustments used in managing oxygenation with the open lung approach.

The principle focus of the ARDSnet approach is limitation of tidal volume delivery using volume controlled ventilation. Compared to a tidal volume of 12 mL/kg, this approach – which uses a tidal volume target of 6 mL/kg – has demonstrated a 22% improvement in survival with a number-needed-to-treat of 12 patients. In other words, for every 12 patients managed with this strategy, one life will be saved. The ARDSnet approach is applicable to patients with ALI and ARDS. For the acute phase (Table 13-5 and Figure 13-2), volume-controlled CMV (assist/control) is used. The target tidal volume is 6 mL/kg and is maintained between 4 and 8 mL/kg. Tidal volume is set based upon predicted body weight, which is determined by measuring the height of the patient (heel to crown with the patient in supine position). The target plateau pressure is 25 to 30 cm H_2O. The oxygenation target is a Pa_{O_2} of 55 to 80 mm Hg (Sp_{O_2} 88 to 95%). PEEP is set according to the F_{IO_2}/PEEP combination required to maintain the Pa_{O_2} or F_{IO_2} within the target range. The arterial pH target range is 7.30 to 7.45, and respiratory rates as high as 35/min are used to maintain pH within this range.

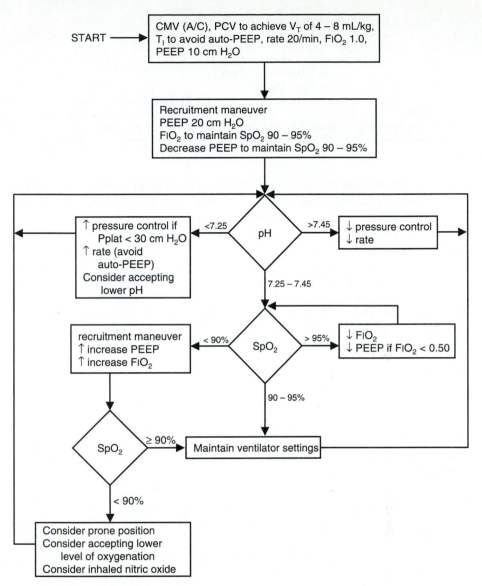

Figure 13-1 Algorithm for ventilator management of ARDS using the open lung approach.

Monitoring

With the high PEEP levels and mean airway pressures required during ARDS, pulmonary artery catheters were frequently used in the past to monitor hemodynamic status and to properly titrate fluid therapy and other hemodynamic support. However, pulmonary artery catheters are generally not necessary unless

Table 13-3 Gas exchange and pressure targets

Pa_{O_2}	ALI	> 70 mm Hg
	Moderate ARDS	> 60 mm Hg
	Severe ARDS	> 50 mm Hg
Pa_{CO_2}	40 mm Hg if possible	
	Permissive hypercapnia to avoid high peak alveolar pressure	
PEEP:	As necessary to maintain alveolar recruitment (10 to 20 cm H_2O)	
Plateau pressure:	< 30 cm H_2O, provided normal chest wall compliance	

left ventricular dysfunction is present. Monitoring of central venous pressure is usually adequate to assess fluid status. As with any patient requiring high airway pressure, pneumothorax is a concern necessitating daily chest X-rays. Continuous monitoring of Sp_{O_2} is required, since oxygenation may be difficult to maintain in these patients. Blood gases are indicated when the patient's clinical status changes. Since it is difficult to maintain ventilation and targeted peak alveolar pressure, the development of auto-PEEP is always a concern and should be carefully monitored with each ventilator setting change. Re-evaluation of the F_{IO_2}, level of PEEP, plateau pressure and mean airway pressure that results in the best gas exchange should occur frequently (Table 13-6).

Weaning

Return to spontaneous ventilation following ARDS may be a protracted process. Fibrosis may leave lung function compromised for weeks. Prolonged ventilatory muscle disuse and the use of paralyzing agents may result in prolonged ventilatory muscle weakness. In the recovery phase (i.e., when the F_{IO_2} is 0.40 and the PEEP is 8 cm H_2O with the Pa_{O_2} within the target range), the patient is liberated from

Table 13-4 Guidelines for the management of oxygenation with ARDS using the open lung approach

Initial adjustments:
- Set F_{IO_2} to 1
- Set PEEP to 10 cm H_2O
- Apply recruitment maneuver
- Set PEEP at 20 cm H_2O
- Decrease F_{IO_2} until Sp_{O_2} 90–95%
- Decrease PEEP to lowest level maintaining Sp_{O_2} 90–95%

Subsequent adjustments:
- Adjust PEEP as needed to maintain alveolar recruitment
- Adjust F_{IO_2} as necessary
- Consider prone positioning
- Evaluate plateau pressure on a regular basis

Table 13-5 The ARDSnet protocol for ventilation of patients with ALI and ARDS

INITIAL VENTILATOR TIDAL VOLUME AND RATE ADJUSTMENTS
A. Calculate predicted body weight (PBW)
   Male $= 50 + 2.3$ [ht (in) $- 60$] kg
   Female $= 45.5 + 2.3$ [ht (in) $- 60$] kg
B. Mode: Volume Assist-Control
C. Set initial tidal volume to 8 mL/kg PBW
D. Reduce tidal volume to 7 mL/kg PBW after 1–2 hrs and then to 6 mL/kg PBW
   after a further 1–2 hrs
E. Set initial ventilator rate to maintain baseline minute ventilation (not > 35/min)

SUBSEQUENT TIDAL VOLUME ADJUSTMENTS
Plateau Pressure Goal: ≤ 30 cm H_2O
Check inspiratory plateau pressure (Pplat) with 0.5 s pause at least every 4 hrs and
   after each change in PEEP or tidal volume.

- If Pplat > 30 cm H_2O, decrease tidal volume by 1 mL/kg PBW steps to 5 or if
  necessary to 4 mL/kg PBW.
- If Pplat < 25 cm H_2O and tidal volume < 6 mL/kg, increase tidal volume by 1 mL/kg
  PBW until Pplat > 25 cm H_2O or tidal volume $= 6$ mL/kg.
- If breath stacking or severe dyspnea occurs, tidal volume may be increased (not
  required) to 7 or 8 mL/kg PBW if Pplat remains ≤ 30 cm H_2O.

ARTERIAL OXYGENATION
GOAL: Pa_{O_2} 55–80 mm Hg or Sp_{O_2} 88–95%
Use these Fi_{O_2}/PEEP combinations to achieve oxygenation goal

Fi_{O_2}	0.3	0.4	0.4	0.5	0.5	0.6	0.7	0.7	0.7	0.8	0.9	0.9	0.9	1.0
PEEP	5	5	8	8	10	10	10	12	14	14	14	16	18	20–24

RESPIRATORY RATE AND ARTERIAL pH

ARTERIAL pH GOAL: 7.30–7.45
A. Acidosis Management:
If pH 7.15–7.30:

- Increase set rate until pH > 7.30 or $Pa_{CO_2} < 25$ (max set rate $= 35$/min)
- If set rate $= 35$/min and pH < 7.30, $NaHCO_3$ may be given (not required)

If pH < 7.15:

- Increase set respiratory rate to 35/min
- If set rate $= 35$/min and pH < 7.15 and $NaHCO_3$ has been considered, tidal volume
  may be increased in 1 mL/kg PBW steps until pH > 7.15 (Pplat target may be exceeded)

B. Alkalosis Management: (pH > 7.45):
Decrease set rate until patient rate $>$ set rate. Minimum set rate $= 6$/min
C. I:E Ratio Goal: 1:1–1:3
Adjust flow and inspiratory flow waveform to achieve goal.

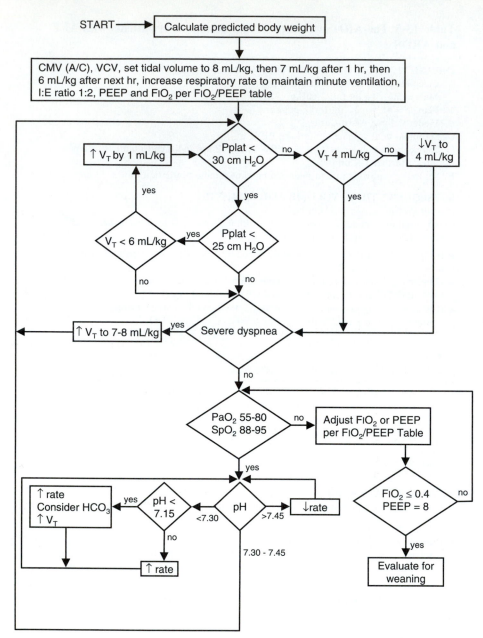

Figure 13-2 Algorithm for ventilator management of ARDS using the ARDSnet protocol.

Table 13-6 Monitoring during mechanical ventilation of patients with ARDS

- Pulse oximetry, periodic blood gases
- Central venous catheter or pulmonary artery catheter
- Presence of pneumothorax
- Auto-PEEP
- Tidal volume and plateau pressure
- Mean airway pressure

ventilatory support using pressure support ventilation and spontaneous breathing trials. Patients recovering from ARDS frequently have a high ventilatory drive and low lung compliance. Because weaning in ARDS may take weeks, care to insure rest and sleep is necessary.

POINTS TO REMEMBER

- ARDS is a heterogeneous disease with areas of consolidation, areas of collapse that are recruitable, and areas of normal tissue.
- The gas exchange area of the lung in ARDS is small compared to normal (rather than noncompliant).
- ARDS progresses through two distinct phases; the first phase is an intense inflammatory response resulting in alveolar and endothelial damage, increased vascular permeability, and increased lung water and lung protein; the second phase is characterized by extensive fibrosis.
- With ARDS, peak alveolar pressure < 30 cm H_2O and PEEP to maintain lung recruitment minimize the risk of ventilator induced lung injury.
- Mechanical ventilation is indicated in ARDS to reverse shunting and severe hypoxemia, reduce the work-of-breathing, and treat acute ventilatory failure.
- Pharmacologic support should be used to prevent patient-ventilator dyssynchrony.
- Low tidal volumes (4 to 8 mL/kg) are used to maintain a peak alveolar pressure < 30 cm H_2O. Respiratory rate is limited by the development of auto-PEEP.
- With the open lung approach, lung recruitment maneuvers should be performed before PEEP is set, and PEEP is decreased from a level higher than needed rather than from a level less than required.
- PEEP in early ARDS should be set to maintain alveolar recruitment (10 to 20 cm H_2O).

ADDITIONAL READING

AMATO MBP, BARBOS CSV, MEDEIROS DM, ET AL. Effect of protective ventilation strategy on mortality in the acute respiratory distress syndrome. *N Engl J Med* 1998; 338:347–354.

ARDS NETWORK. Ventilation with lower tidal volumes as compared with traditional tidal volumes for acute lung injury and the acute respiratory distress syndrome patients. *N Engl J Med* 2000; 342:1301–1308.

BROWER RG, WARE LB, BERTHIAUME Y, MATTHAY MA. Treatment of ARDS. *Chest* 2001; 120:1347–1367.

KACMAREK RM, HICKLING K. Permissive hypercapnia. *Respir Care* 1993; 38:373–387.

KALLET RH, CORRAL W, SILVERMAN HJ, LUCE JM. Implementation of a low tidal volume protocol for patients with acute lung injury or acute respiratory distress syndrome. *Respir Care* 2001; 46:1024–1037.

MARINI JJ. Pressure control ventilation. In TOBIN MJ (ed.) *Principles and Practice of Mechanical Ventilation*. New York, McGraw-Hill Publishers, 1994, 305–318.

WARE LB, MATTHAY MA. The acute respiratory distress syndrome. *N Engl J Med* 2000; 342:1334–1349.

FOURTEEN

CHRONIC PULMONARY DISEASE

OBJECTIVES

1. Discuss the impact of respiratory muscle dysfunction on the need for ventilatory support in patients with chronic pulmonary disease.
2. Describe how auto-PEEP develops in patients with chronic obstructive lung disease.
3. List indications for mechanical ventilation in patients with chronic pulmonary disease.
4. List the initial ventilator settings in obstructive and restrictive lung disease patients requiring acute application of mechanical ventilation.
5. Discuss the monitoring and weaning of chronic pulmonary disease patients from mechanical ventilation.

INTRODUCTION

Chronic pulmonary diseases can be divided into two general categories; obstructive and restrictive. Chronic obstructive pulmonary diseases (COPD) are characterized by airflow limitation. Specific diseases include emphysema, chronic bronchitis, asthma, bronchiectasis and cystic fibrosis. Chronic restrictive lung disease is characterized by reduced lung volume, with pulmonary fibrosis being the primary example. Other causes of chronic restrictive pulmonary disease are those affecting neuromuscular function and chest wall compliance. As a group, chronic pulmonary diseases are a leading cause of death in the United States and are an important percentage of the patients in medical intensive care units across the country. Most importantly, they present a significant management challenge when mechanical ventilation is required, since their underlying disease frequently makes weaning difficult if not impossible. They also represent a significant percentage of the patients requiring chronic ventilatory support.

OVERVIEW

In patients with COPD, chronic airflow limitation from inflammation, airway hyperreactivity, secretions and loss of the structural integrity of the lung parenchyma leads to air trapping with increased work-of-breathing and ventilatory muscle dysfunction. With chronic restrictive disease, fibrotic changes at the lung parenchyma result in a decreased lung compliance and increased work-of-breathing. In addition, the increased work-of-breathing along with life style issues in patients with chronic pulmonary disease commonly results in nutritional deficiency.

Respiratory Muscle Dysfunction

The diaphragm normally moves downward during contraction, decreasing the zone of apposition between the diaphragm and the rib cage (Figure 14-1). This causes the abdominal wall to move outward and the lateral rib cage to expand, increasing the cephalad to caudal and lateral dimensions of the thoracic cage, causing intrathoracic pressure to decrease facilitating inspiration. Because of the hyperinflation with COPD, the normal domed shape of the diaphragm is flattened and the zone of apposition is decreased. This results in less efficient diaphragmatic function. If the diaphragm is sufficiently flattened, during contraction the anterior abdominal wall is not distended and the lateral rib cage moves inward instead of outward. These changes compromise the diaphragm's function as an inspiratory muscle, leading to paradoxical breathing (Table 14-1). Accessory muscles of inspiration (intercostals, scalenes, sternomastoid, pectoralis and parasternal) become the primary muscle groups for normal breathing. Due to this chronic ventilatory muscle dysfunction, muscular reserve is limited and the probability of fatigue with even minor increases in stress is markedly increased.

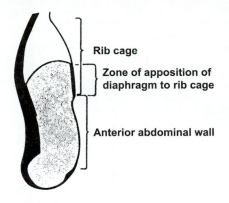

Figure 14-1 Schematic diagram of the diaphragm in relation to the rib cage and anterior abdominal wall. The zone of apposition is the area of contact between the diaphragm and the chest wall at end exhalation. With COPD, the diaphragm is flattened, the zone of apposition decreased and the ability of the diaphragm to expand the lung decreased. (From MEAD J, SMITH JC, LORING SH: Volume displacement of the chest wall and its mechanical significance. In ROUSSOS C, MAKLEM PT (eds), *The Thorax,* Part A. New York, Marcel Dekker, 1985, pp 260–281.)

Auto-PEEP

The establishment of an intrapulmonary positive end-expiratory pressure as a result of an alteration of lung mechanics and airflow limitation is termed auto-PEEP. Since no lung disease is completely homogeneous, the level of air trapping and auto-PEEP varies with each lung unit. As a result, the auto-PEEP level measured during mechanical ventilation is an average auto-PEEP of individual lung units. The longer local time constants (Table 14-2) as a result of increased airway resistance and increased lung compliance in COPD necessitate a longer expiratory time to prevent air trapping and auto-PEEP. Since end-expiratory pressure is greater than atmospheric with auto-PEEP, a pressure gradient sufficient to overcome auto-PEEP must be established for gas to move into the lungs. The presence of auto-PEEP is a primary factor associated with the increased work-of-breathing in COPD patients with acute respiratory failure.

Nutrition

It is common that patients presenting with an acute exacerbation of chronic pulmonary disease are nutritionally depleted. Because much energy is consumed in breathing, many of these patients cannot afford the added energy cost associated with the preparation and consumption of a proper diet. These patients present with caloric and protein deficiencies and electrolyte imbalances, that extend the limited function of ventilatory muscles and increase the likelihood of

Table 14-1 Characteristics of normal breathing pattern and paradoxical breathing

Normal breathing	Paradoxical breathing
• Protrusion of the anterior abdominal wall	• Anterior abdominal wall moves inward
• Expansion of the lateral rib cage	• Lateral rib cage moves inward
• Expansion of the upper chest wall	• Expansion of the upper chest wall

Table 14-2 Pulmonary time constant (τ)

- τ = compliance × resistance
- Complete passive exhalation requires 3 to 4 τ
- Normally τ is about 0.5 s
- With COPD, τ is increased due to high lung compliance and a high airway resistance
- With chronic restrictive lung disease, τ is decreased because of low lung compliance

fatigue. During acute management, nutritional supplementation is essential. Care during weaning must be exercised in these patients to insure that the proper balance between fats and carbohydrates is maintained and overfeeding is avoided to prevent excessive carbon dioxide production.

MECHANICAL VENTILATION

Invasive mechanical ventilation, although often lifesaving, should be avoided if possible in these patients. Morbidity (aspiration, barotrauma, nosocomial infection, cardiovascular dysfunction) in chronic pulmonary disease patients is high during invasive mechanical ventilation and many of these patients become ventilator dependent once intubated. As a result, non-invasive positive pressure ventilation has become a primary alternative during acute exacerbation – particularly for patients with COPD.

Indications

Most patients presenting with an acute exacerbation are hypoxemic and exhausted, with elevated Pa_{CO_2} and marked ventilatory muscle dysfunction (Table 14-3). Mechanical ventilation is indicated primarily to unload the work-of-breathing, rest ventilatory muscles, decrease Pa_{CO_2} to the patient's baseline, and treat hypoxemia.

Table 14-3 Indications for ventilation in patients with chronic pulmonary disease

- Acute on chronic ventilatory failure
- Unloading work-of-breathing
- Resting ventilatory muscles
- Improving bronchial hygiene

Noninvasive Positive Pressure Ventilation (NPPV)

All patients who present with an acute exacerbation of COPD should be considered candidates for NPPV. Many patients avoid endotracheal intubation and its associated morbidity by the use of NPPV. Provided the patient is alert and cooperative, has a stable cardiovascular status, and can clear secretions, NPPV should be attempted before the decision is made to intubate.

Ventilator Settings

Obstructive lung disease Of all the patient groups requiring ventilatory support, those with COPD can be challenging. At best, they can be returned to their baseline that is characterized by dyspnea, increased work-of-breathing, and heightened ventilatory drive. Of primary concern during ventilatory assistance is patient-ventilator synchrony to avoid unnecessary work and anxiety. Since these patients rarely require heavy sedation or paralysis unless their clinical presentation extends beyond a basic exacerbation of COPD, selecting ventilator settings that satisfy ventilatory demand is critical (Table 14-4 and Figure 14-2).

Although either may be used effectively, pressure ventilation is recommended over volume ventilation in these patients. With pressure ventilation, the peak inspiratory flow varies with the patient's ventilatory demand. This does not, however, imply that pressure support is the mode of choice. During initial ventilator setup, pressure control is recommended because of its rate and inspiratory time settings. Termination of inspiration with pressure support is flow cycled (e.g., 5 L/min, or a fixed fraction of its peak level such as 25%, or adjustable). Termination of inspiration may be either prolonged or premature, increasing ventilatory demand and activating accessory muscles of exhalation to terminate flow if patient and ventilator termination of inspiration is not synchronous. In the early phase of ventilatory support, a fixed inspiratory time may be better tolerated. Inspiratory time is set per patient comfort (0.6–1.2 s).

If volume ventilation is used, it is critical to set the peak inspiratory flow high enough to satisfy inspiratory demand and minimize patient work. Peak flow should be set $\geq$ 60 L/min to produce an inspiratory time of 0.6–1.2 s. Because

Table 14-4 Initial ventilator settings for COPD

Setting	Recommendation
Mode	A/C (CMV)
Rate	8–12/min
Volume/pressure control	Pressure or volume
Tidal volume	8–10 mL/kg provided plateau pressure < 30 cm H_2O
Inspiratory time	0.6–1.25 s (peak flow $\geq$ 60 L/min with volume ventilation)
PEEP	$\leq$ 5 cm H_2O or as necessary to counterbalance auto-PEEP
F_{IO_2}	Usually $\leq$ 0.50
Flow waveform	Descending ramp

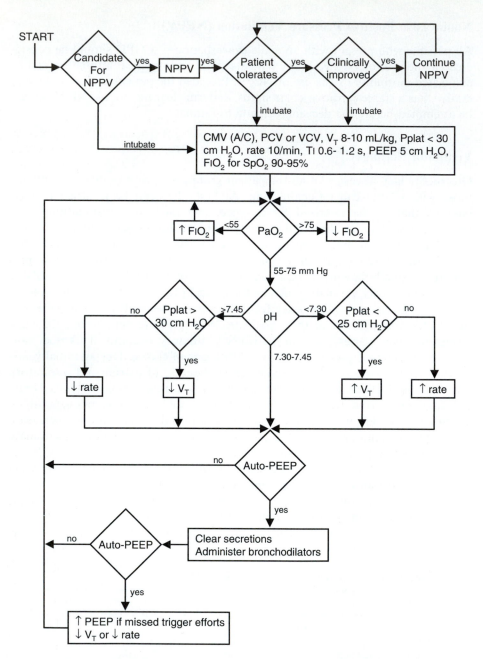

Figure 14-2 Algorithm for the ventilator management of the patient with COPD.

these patients' ventilatory demands are usually greatest at the beginning of inspiration, a descending ramp flow pattern is recommended. Further, the lower end-inspiratory flow improves gas distribution to long time constant regions. Rate should be set high enough to insure that spontaneous ventilation is not necessary during sleep. Generally, this requires a rate of 8 to 12/min, depending on patient demand and the development of auto-PEEP.

High peak alveolar pressures are usually not a problem in COPD patients unless the disease is complicated by auto-PEEP or an acute restrictive process (e.g., pneumonia). As a result, V_T in the 8 to 10 mL/kg range generally should be used (as a result of the pressure control setting or directly set with volume control). Since the goal is a slower rate to minimize air trapping and auto-PEEP, a moderate V_T is recommended. However, because chronic parenchymal damage is already present, peak alveolar pressure should be kept as low as possible (< 30 cm H_2O) to minimize the development of volutrauma.

Auto-PEEP is always a concern when ventilating patients with COPD. As a result, efforts to both minimize the auto-PEEP level and its effects on work-of-breathing should be maximized. Adequate therapy to reverse airflow limitation (e.g., steroids) and mobilize secretions (e.g., bronchoscopy, suctioning) should be used. In addition, as noted above, minute ventilation and respiratory rate should be minimized. Since auto-PEEP increases the pressure gradient required to inspire during spontaneous breathing, it also increases the pressure gradient to trigger the ventilator. This is frequently observed as accessory muscle recruitment, retractions, increased ventilatory drive, and dyspnea. However, the best sign of auto-PEEP is the difference between the patient's respiratory rate and the ventilator response. Provided the sensitivity is set properly (-1 cm H_2O or flow triggering), the only reason that the patient's rate exceeds the ventilator response rate is auto-PEEP. Many patients with COPD are unable to generate sufficient effort to overcome auto-PEEP and trigger the ventilator. In this setting, applied PEEP counterbalances auto-PEEP and improves triggering. PEEP is increased by 1 or 2 cm H_2O increments until patient rate and the ventilator rate are equal. The use of 5 cm H_2O PEEP is usually beneficial in COPD patients, and > 10 cm H_2O is seldom necessary to counterbalance auto-PEEP.

FI_{O_2} requirements in patients with COPD is rarely > 0.50 unless the exacerbation is complicated. Usually, unloading the work-of-breathing and increasing the efficiency of ventilation by improving $\dot{V}/\dot{Q}$ matching results in an acceptable Pa_{O_2} with only moderate increases in FI_{O_2}. Generally, a Pa_{O_2} of 55–75 mm Hg is adequate for these patients.

It is important to avoid hyperventilation in COPD patients. Pa_{CO_2} should only be decreased to the level maintained at baseline. In many patients, this is a Pa_{CO_2} of 50 to 60 mm Hg or that required for a near-normal pH (> 7.30). With initial ventilator settings to satisfy ventilatory drive and minimal sedation, these patients usually rest during assisted ventilation. Many of these patients are exhausted after several days of increased ventilatory demand. Complete rest is recommended for the first 24 to 48 hrs of ventilation, after which evaluation for weaning should be considered.

Restrictive lung disease Most of the discussion regarding ventilator settings for chronic obstructive pulmonary disease also apply for chronic restrictive lung disease. Exceptions are rate and V_T settings. Since lung compliance is reduced in these patients, V_T must also be reduced to decrease peak alveolar pressure. Usually V_T is set ≤ 8 mL/kg and some patients require V_T as low as 4 mL/kg. Rate, however, can be increased to maintain minute ventilation. Auto-PEEP is not a concern in these patients, allowing rate to be increased (15 to 30/min) without the development of air trapping. Because of the rapid rates, inspiratory time should be < 1 s (Table 14-5).

Monitoring

There are numerous issues that must be considered during the ventilatory assistance of patients with chronic pulmonary disease. Careful monitoring of patient-ventilator synchrony is required (Table 14-6) and the cause should be corrected or the ventilator adjusted. Monitoring auto-PEEP should occur regularly in patients with COPD. Evaluation of the expiratory flow waveform or observation of the patient's ventilatory pattern is useful to identify the presence of auto-PEEP, but not its magnitude. During passive ventilation, auto-PEEP can be quantified using an end-expiratory hold. Since cor pulmonale is a common complicating problem with chronic pulmonary disease, a pulmonary artery catheter may be indicated to monitor pulmonary artery pressure. However, a pulmonary artery catheter is generally not necessary unless concomitant left heart failure is present. It is most useful to monitor clinical findings – respiratory rate, use of accessory muscles, breath sounds, heart rate, and blood pressure. The patient comfortably ventilated without tachypnea, hypertension or tachycardia and a $Sp_{O_2} > 90\%$ usually does not require further monitoring. However, it should be remembered that Sp_{O_2} provides little indication of ventilation or acid-base balance. End-tidal CO_2 is not useful because these patients have high V_D/V_T.

Table 14-5 Initial ventilator settings for chronic restrictive pulmonary disease

Setting	Recommendation
Mode	A/C (CMV)
Rate	15–30/min
Volume/pressure control	Pressure or volume
Tidal volume	4–8 mL/kg and plateau pressure < 30 cm H_2O
Inspiratory time	< 1 s (peak flow ≥ 60 L/min with volume ventilation)
PEEP	5 cm H_2O
$F_{I_{O_2}}$	Usually ≤ 0.50
Flow waveform	Descending ramp

Table 14-6 Monitoring of the mechanically ventilated patient with pulmonary disease

- Patient-ventilator synchrony
- Auto-PEEP, peak alveolar pressure
- Hemodynamics
- Pulse oximetry and arterial blood gases
- Clinical signs of cardiopulmonary distress

Weaning

One of the most difficult questions to answer regarding respiratory intensive care is, what is the best approach to wean patients with chronic pulmonary disease? First, insure that the acute process that necessitated mechanical ventilation is reversed and that no other acute pulmonary process (i.e., infection) is present. Second, insure cardiovascular function is optimized. Many patients with chronic pulmonary disease also have cardiovascular disease that may itself require ventilatory support. Third, optimize electrolyte balance and nutritional status. Since diet can affect CO_2 load, do not try to wean until nutritional support is adequate. Since most electrolyte imbalances affect respiratory muscle function, it is critical that magnesium, phosphate and potassium be normalized. Fourth, use spontaneous breathing trials, insure that work periods are interspersed with rest periods, and that adequate sleep occurs.

As a general rule, weaning patients with chronic pulmonary disease can be divided into the categories of those that can be fully weaned (clearly the largest group) and those who will require long-term support (a very difficult subgroup). In those patients who are tracheostomized and the potential for long-term support appears possible, spontaneous breathing trials are used of increasing time interspersed with periods of near complete rest. Many of these patients slowly progress to increasing periods of ventilator independence, but periods of nocturnal ventilation are required in some.

Some patients do not wean even though they meet all traditional weaning criteria. In this group, NPPV can be used as a bridge to ventilator independence. Before committing these patients to tracheostomy, a trial of NPPV can be provided until the patient can breathe independently or requires reintubation. Weaning of the chronic pulmonary disease patient always requires assurance that overall medical status is optimized and requires patience and understanding on the part of all practitioners involved in their care.

POINTS TO REMEMBER

- Respiratory muscle dysfunction and auto-PEEP are common problems leading to increased work-of-breathing in COPD patients.

- Decreased compliance and increased work-of-breathing are common in restrictive lung disease patients.
- Ventilatory muscle dysfunction and hypoxemia lead to acute ventilatory failure in patients with chronic pulmonary disease.
- Patients with an acute exacerbation of COPD are candidates for NPPV.
- Patient-ventilator synchrony is better with pressure ventilation than with volume ventilation.
- With volume ventilation, peak inspiratory flow should be high (≥ 60 L/min) with a descending ramp flow.
- With COPD, ventilator rate should be low with moderate V_T.
- With chronic restrictive disease, a small V_T with a rapid rate is set.
- Balance the effects of auto-PEEP by applying low levels of PEEP.
- Target Pa_{CO_2} at the patient's baseline level and $Pa_{O_2} > 60$ mm Hg.
- Before weaning, insure all acute pulmonary processes are reversed, cardiovascular function is optimized, electrolytes are normalized, and nutritional support is acceptable.
- Some patients with chronic disease benefit from NPPV as a bridge from invasive ventilation to spontaneous breathing.

ADDITIONAL READING

FUMEAUX T, ROTHMEIER C, JOLLIET P. Outcome of mechanical ventilation for acute respiratory failure in patients with pulmonary fibrosis. *Intensive Care Med* 2001; 27:1868–1874.

GLADWIN MT, PIERSON DJ. Mechanical ventilation of the patient with severe chronic obstructive pulmonary disease. *Intensive Care Med* 1998; 24:898–910.

HESS DR, MEDOFF BD. Mechanical ventilation of the patient with chronic obstructive pulmonary disease. *Respir Care Clin N Am* 1998; 4:429–437.

JUBRAN A, TOBIN MJ. Pathophysiologic basic of acute respiratory distress in patients who fail a trial of weaning from mechanical ventilation. *Am J Respir Crit Care Med* 1997; 155:906–915.

JUBRAN A, TOBIN MJ. Passive mechanics of lung and chest wall in patients who failed or succeeded in trials of weaning. *Am J Respir Crit Care Med* 1997; 155:916–921.

LAGHI F, D'ALFONSO N, TOBIN MJ. Pattern of recovery from diaphragmatic failure. *J Appl Physiol* 1995; 79:539–546.

NAVA S, AMBROSINO N, CLINIE, ET AL. Noninvasive mechanical ventilation in the weaning of patients with respiratory failure due to chronic obstructive pulmonary disease: a randomized controlled trial. *Ann Intern Med* 1998; 128:721–728.

SETHI JM. Mechanical ventilation in chronic obstructive pulmonary disease. *Clin Chest Med* 2000; 21:799–818.

CHEST TRAUMA

OBJECTIVES

1. Discuss the clinical presentation of patients with both blunt and penetrating chest trauma.
2. Discuss the initial ventilator settings for patients with chest trauma.
3. Describe the monitoring of mechanically ventilated patients with chest trauma.
4. Discuss the weaning of chest trauma patients from ventilatory support.

INTRODUCTION

Particularly in developed countries, chest trauma is common. Although the chest wall can absorb significant amounts of trauma without serious injury to the patient, chest trauma is a frequent indication for critical care and mechanical ventilation. Unlike other disease states requiring mechanical ventilation (e.g.,

COPD), patients suffering chest trauma are typically young and previously healthy.

OVERVIEW

Blunt Chest Trauma

With blunt chest trauma, there are often no exterior signs or symptoms of injury to the chest. Clinical entities associated with blunt chest trauma include fractures, pulmonary contusion, tracheobronchial injury, myocardial and vascular injury, esophageal perforation, and diaphragmatic injury. Fractures can involve the ribs, sternum, vertebrae, clavicles, or scapulae. Of these, rib fractures are the most common. Rib fractures without flailing can be painful, resulting in splinting, atelectasis, and hypoxemia due to $\dot{V}/\dot{Q}$ mismatching. Isolated rib fractures almost never necessitate mechanical ventilation unless they are associated with other injuries such as pulmonary contusion. Flail chest is a loss of stability of the rib cage caused by multiple rib fractures, which frequently results in significant ventilatory disturbances due to underlying damage to the lung parenchyma, inefficient expansion of the thorax due to paradoxical movement of the chest wall, and pain leading to hypoventilation. Until recently, it was common practice to internally stabilize the rib cage in patients with flail chest by use of positive pressure ventilation and PEEP. Many patients with flail chest are now adequately managed without intubation and mechanical ventilation. This is particularly the case with appropriate pain control and aggressive pulmonary toilet. It is now generally accepted that mechanical ventilation is only required for patients with flail chest if one of the following is present: shock, closed head injury, need for immediate operation, severe pulmonary dysfunction, or deteriorating respiratory status.

Pulmonary contusion results from high impact blunt chest trauma, which produces leakage of blood and protein from the vascular to the interstitial and alveolar space of the lungs. Clinically, pulmonary contusion is similar in presentation and treatment to ARDS. Unlike other causes of ARDS, pulmonary contusion may be localized. If the contusion is localized, therapy that increases mean airway pressure (e.g., PEEP) may produce a paradoxical decrease in arterial oxygenation because blood may be diverted from normal to the injured lung increasing shunt fraction. Mild to moderate forms of pulmonary contusion may not require intubation, and hypoxemia can be adequately treated with oxygen and mask CPAP.

Tracheobronchial injuries most often occur near the trachea or near the origin of the mainstem bronchi. If they are small and do not result in pneumothorax, these may heal spontaneously. Tracheobronchial injuries that result in large air leaks and pneumothorax require surgical repair. Patients with tracheobronchial injuries may require mechanical ventilation following thoracotomy, particularly if other injuries compromising pulmonary function are present.

Myocardial injuries associated with blunt chest trauma are most often in the form of myocardial contusion. Myocardial contusion can result in arrhythmias, but rarely results in cardiac failure. The need for mechanical ventilation is rare in patients with myocardial contusion who do not have other associated injuries such as rib fractures and pulmonary contusion. Injuries to the thoracic vasculature can result in significant hypotension and the need for emergent thoracotomy. Patients with these injuries typically have multiple chest trauma and require mechanical ventilation.

Diaphragm injury secondary to blunt chest injury is very rare. This injury almost always requires operative repair. Patients with diaphragmatic injury may require post-operative mechanical ventilation and may be difficult to wean due to diaphragmatic weakness.

Penetrating Chest Trauma

Penetrating injuries can affect the lungs, the heart, and/or the vasculature, and almost always require surgical intervention. When associated with tension pneumothorax and/or significant blood loss, penetrating injuries can be immediately life-threatening. A tension pneumothorax can be rapidly corrected by insertion of a chest tube, and mechanical ventilation may not be required. Many penetrating chest injuries require extensive surgical repair, and mechanical ventilation is frequently required post-operatively.

MECHANICAL VENTILATION

Indications

Indications for mechanical ventilation in patients with chest trauma are listed in Table 15-1. None of these indications are absolute, and each is dependent upon the corresponding level of respiratory failure. Flail chest with paradoxical chest movement was once considered an absolute indication for positive pressure ventilation. However, many cases of flail chest are now managed effectively without intubation and mechanical ventilation. ARDS is a common complication of chest trauma, and may occur without associated chest contusion. When ARDS occurs in association with chest trauma, its management is similar to that with other causes of ARDS. Pain control is an issue in many patients with chest trauma. If large doses of narcotic pain control are required, respiratory depression may occur and mechanical ventilation may be necessary. Epidural narcotics, patient-controlled analgesia, and intercostal nerve blocks are commonly used to control pain without associated respiratory depression.

Table 15-1 Indications for mechanical ventilation in patients with chest trauma

- Flail chest with paradoxical chest movement, tachypnea, hypoxemia, hypercarbia
- Pulmonary contusion with tachypnea and severe hypoxemia ($Pa_{O_2} < 60$ mm Hg) breathing 100% O_2
- Rib fractures with chest pain requiring large doses of narcotics for pain control
- Post-operative thoracotomy
- Hemodynamic instability, particularly with marginal respiratory reserve (e.g., hypoxemia and tachypnea)
- Severe associated injuries (e.g., head trauma)

Ventilator Settings

Recommendations for initial ventilator settings in patients with chest trauma are listed in Table 15-2. Initially, full ventilatory support using volume control or pressure control is used (Figure 15-1). Pressure support ventilation is usually not appropriate during initial ventilatory support. Many patients require sedation, and a few may require paralysis, during the initiation of ventilation.

Oxygenation is dependant upon $F_{I_{O_2}}$, PEEP and the extent of pulmonary dysfunction. The initial $F_{I_{O_2}}$ should be set at 1, and then titrated to the desired level of arterial oxygenation using pulse oximetry. Generally, the initial PEEP level should be set at 5 cm H_2O. If the patient has significant barotrauma (e.g., subcutaneous emphysema, pneumothorax, air leaks from chest tubes), it may be desirable to set the initial PEEP level at 0 cm H_2O. If the patient has significant pulmonary shunt, a trial of higher PEEP levels is appropriate. In patients with chest trauma, however, caution must be exercised when increasing airway pressure because barotrauma is common. As the result of blood loss, hemodynamic instability may result when PEEP is increased, and increasing PEEP may increase intracranial pressure in patients with associated head trauma. If a unilateral

Table 15-2 Initial mechanical ventilation settings in patients with chest trauma

Setting	Recommendation
Mode	A/C (CMV)
Rate	10 to 20/min
Volume/pressure control	Pressure or volume
Tidal volume	8–10 mL/kg predicted body weight provided that plateau pressure < 30 cm H_2O; 4 to 8 mL/kg with ARDS
Inspiratory time	1 second
PEEP	5 cm H_2O; none with severe air leaks
$F_{I_{O_2}}$	1.0
Flow waveform	Descending ramp

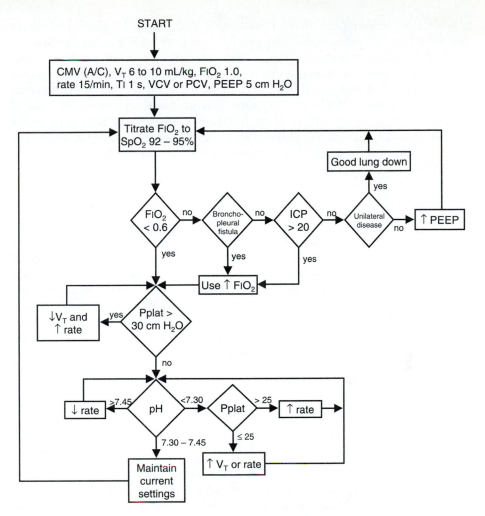

Figure 15-1 An algorithm for mechanical ventilation of the patient with chest trauma.

pulmonary contusion is present, care must also be exercised when increasing PEEP. With unilateral lung disease, PEEP may result in shunting of blood from higher compliance lung units to low-compliance non-ventilated areas, which will result in increasing shunt and hypoxemia. With unilateral pulmonary contusion, lateral positioning with the contused lung up may be more beneficial than increasing levels of PEEP.

With either volume ventilation or pressure ventilation, the plateau pressure should be kept below 30 cm H_2O. In trauma patients with satisfactory lung compliance (e.g., post-operative thoracotomy), tidal volumes of 8–10 mL/kg ideal body weight can be used with peak alveolar pressure less than 30 cm H_2O. Patients with pulmonary contusion and ARDS may require tidal volumes of 4–8 mL/kg to keep peak alveolar pressure < 30 cm H_2O. An initial respiratory rate of 10 to 20/min is often adequate. Respiratory rate can be increased if required to establish a desired Pa_{CO_2}, but care must be taken not to produce auto-PEEP. Permissive hypercapnia is generally well tolerated in chest trauma patients, provided that there is no accompanying head trauma with increased intracranial pressure. An inspiratory flow that produces an inspiratory time of one second (volume control) or a set inspiratory time of one second (pressure control) is usually adequate in patients with chest trauma. If available, a descending ramp waveform is desirable to improve distribution of ventilation.

Monitoring

Monitoring the mechanically ventilated chest trauma patient is similar in many aspects to that with any mechanically ventilated patient (Table 15-3). Air leak is more likely in patients with chest trauma, and signs of air leak must be assessed frequently. Pneumothorax should be considered following any rapid deterioration of the mechanically ventilated chest trauma patient. Chest trauma patients should be ventilated at the lowest peak alveolar pressure and PEEP level that produces adequate arterial oxygenation. Auto-PEEP must be avoided. Pulmonary embolism is also common in these patients, and should be considered if clinical status rapidly deteriorates. As is the case with many surgical patients, fluid overload frequently occurs and is associated with shunting and decreased lung compliance. With prolonged mechanical ventilation, nutritional support is necessary to facilitate healing and weaning from mechanical ventilation.

Weaning

Discontinuation of mechanical ventilation can occur early and quickly in many chest trauma patients, such as those ventilated post-operatively following repair of a penetrating chest injury. Many of these patients have no prior cardiopulmonary disease and recover rapidly if there are no associated problems (e.g., head trauma, ARDS). Those who have severe pulmonary contusion and ARDS may have a long mechanical ventilation course that may be complicated with pulmon-

Table 15-3 Monitoring of the mechanically ventilated patient with chest trauma

- Pneumothorax and extra-alveolar air
- Auto-PEEP, mean airway pressure
- Peak alveolar pressure
- Pulmonary embolism
- Fluid volume status
- Nutritional status

ary infection, empyema, sepsis, and pulmonary embolism. Some of these patients will be difficult to wean, particularly if they develop multi-system failure and malnutrition. These patients may require prolonged weaning with spontaneous breathing trials. Weaning may also be difficult in patients with severe chest wall injury and diaphragmatic injury. For patients who are difficult to wean, the goals should be treatment of injuries and pre-existing medical conditions, bronchial hygiene (e.g., secretion removal), nutritional support, and strengthening and conditioning of respiratory muscles (i.e., periods of spontaneous breathing at sub-fatiguing loads).

POINTS TO REMEMBER

- Chest trauma may be either blunt or penetrating.
- Indications for mechanical ventilation with chest trauma include flail chest, chest pain requiring large doses of respiratory depressant pain medications, pulmonary contusion, post-operative thoracotomy, hemodynamic instability, severe associated injuries.
- Flail chest is not an absolute indication for mechanical ventilation.
- Chest trauma is commonly associated with severe lung injury.
- Air leak is a common complication of mechanical ventilation in chest trauma patients.
- The ventilator course of many chest trauma patients is short and weaning occurs rapidly.
- In chest trauma patients who develop ARDS, the mechanical ventilation course can be difficult, with prolonged and difficult weaning.

ADDITIONAL READING

ALLEN GS, COATES NE. Pulmonary contusion: a collective review. *Am Surg* 1996; 62:895–900.
CALHOON JH, TRINKLE JK. Pathophysiology of chest trauma. *Chest Surg Clin N Am* 1997; 7:199–211.
COHN SM. Pulmonary contusion: a review of the clinical entity. *J Trauma* 1997; 42:973–979.
FERGUSON M, LUCHETTE FA. Management of blunt chest injury. *Respir Care Clin N Am* 1996; 2:449–466.
GENTILELLO LM, PIERSON DJ. Trauma critical care. *Am J Respir Crit Care Med* 2001; 163:604–607.
HAENEL JB, MOORE FA, MOORE EE. Pulmonary consequences of severe chest trauma. *Respir Care Clin N Am* 1996; 2:401–424.
JACKIMCZYK K. Blunt chest trauma. *Emerg Med Clin N Am* 1993; 11:81–97.
JORDEN RC. Penetrating chest trauma. *Emerg Med Clin N Am* 1993; 11:97–106.
SCHRADER KA. Penetrating chest trauma. *Crit Care Nursing Clin N Am* 1993; 5:687–696.

SIXTEEN

HEAD INJURY

OBJECTIVES

1. Describe the interactions between mechanical ventilation and head injury.
2. Define neurogenic pulmonary edema.
3. Discuss the indications, initial ventilator settings, monitoring, and ventilator weaning for the head injured patient.
4. Describe how an apnea test is performed.

INTRODUCTION

Head injury and its associated neurologic dysfunction are common in the United States and other developed countries. The morbidity and mortality associated with this problem are related to acute cerebral edema and other space occupying lesions that increase intracranial pressure. Head injury is usually traumatic in origin. However, similar effects may be seen with surgical (e.g., post craniotomy for tumor resection) and medical (e.g., cerebral vascular accident, post-resuscitation hypoxia, hepatic failure) problems.

OVERVIEW

Physiology

Because the skull is rigid, intracranial volume increases result in an increase in intracranial pressure. The relationship between intracranial volume and intracranial pressure (ICP) is described by the cerebral compliance curve (Figure 16-1). Although small increases in intracranial volume are tolerated without an increase in ICP, larger increases in volume result in large increases in ICP. This increase in ICP decreases cerebral blood flow, resulting in cerebral hypoxia. With large increases in ICP, the swelling brain herniates through the tentorium, resulting in compression of the brain stem. Much of the management of head injury relates to efforts to control ICP.

Cerebral perfusion pressure (CPP) is defined as the difference between mean arterial pressure (MAP) and ICP:

$$CPP = MAP - ICP.$$

Normally, ICP is < 10 mm Hg and MAP is about 90 mm Hg, resulting in a normal CPP > 80 mm Hg. CPP < 60 mm Hg is associated with a poor outcome. In patients with acute head injury, the ICP is frequently measured. CPP is decreased by either a decrease in MAP or an increase in ICP. Thus, treatments that decrease MAP (e.g., positive pressure ventilation, diuresis, vasodilator therapy) decrease CPP, whereas treatments that decrease ICP (hyperventilation,

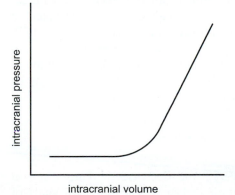

Figure 16-1 Cerebral compliance curve showing the relationship between intracranial pressure and intracranial volume. Normally (low intracranial volume), some cerebral swelling can occur without increasing intracranial pressure. However, a point is reached after which further increases in cerebral swelling result in a large increase in intracranial pressure.

mannitol) increase CPP. A normal physiologic response to an acute increase in ICP is hypertension with bradycardia, which is called the Cushing response.

Clinical Findings

Increases in ICP can result in abnormal ventilatory patterns such as Cheyne-Stokes breathing, central neurogenic hyperventilation, and apnea with severe injury. Compression of the brainstem (i.e., trans-tentorial herniation) results in dilated nonreactive pupils, posturing (decerebrate and decorticate), and cardiovascular collapse.

Neurogenic Pulmonary Edema

Acute head injury and elevated ICP can result in neurogenic pulmonary edema (NPE). NPE is a noncardiogenic pulmonary edema, and is clinically indistinguishable from ARDS. It results in a decreased functional residual capacity, decreased lung compliance, increased intrapulmonary shunt, and hypoxemia. Treatment of NPE is similar to that of other causes of ARDS, including oxygen therapy and PEEP.

Management

Management of acute head injury involves both hemodynamic and respiratory management. Techniques to control ICP are briefly summarized in Table 16-1. Hemodynamic control of arterial blood pressure is important to maintain CPP. Respiratory management involves maintenance of an adequate Pa_{CO_2} and Pa_{O_2}. Care must be taken to avoid high mean airway pressures, which can adversely affect CPP by decreasing venous return (resulting in an increase in ICP) and decreasing cardiac output (resulting in a decrease in MAP).

In the past, respiratory care of the patient with head injury has included the use of iatrogenic hyperventilation. However, this therapy has not been shown to increase survival and is no longer recommended. For an acute increase in ICP, the patient may be temporarily hyperventilated until definitive therapy is instituted, after which the Pa_{CO_2} is gradually restored to normal. Care must be taken to avoid rapid increases in Pa_{CO_2}, which may produce dangerous increases in ICP. During hyperventilation therapy, the brain quickly equilibrates to changes in Pa_{CO_2} and a new steady state is established within four to six hours. Although iatrogenic hyperventilation is not recommended, permissive hypercapnia may be associated with unacceptable elevations in ICP.

MECHANICAL VENTILATION

As shown in Figure 16-2, increases in Pa_{CO_2} and decreases in Pa_{O_2} result in increases in ICP. Thus, normal oxygenation and acid-base state are goals of

Table 16-1 Management of ICP

Technique	Comments
Hyperventilation	Pa_{CO_2} of 25 to 30 mm Hg is useful to lower ICP; Pa_{CO_2} should be normalized as soon as possible provided that ICP does not increase
Mean airway pressure	Mean airway pressure should be kept as low as possible to avoid increases in ICP and decreases in arterial blood pressure
Positioning	30 degree elevation of the head is useful to lower ICP; Trendelenburg's position should be avoided; the head should be kept in a neutral position to facilitate venous outflow from the brain
Dehydration and osmotherapy	Mannitol is useful to treat acute increases in ICP; furosemide and acetazolamide commonly used to promote clearance of fluid from the brain
Sedation and paralysis	ICP increases with agitation, Valsalva maneuvers, coughing and pain; therapy directed at suppressing these actions often lowers ICP
Corticosteroids	Steroids have been widely used in the past for treatment of cerebral edema, but no benefit has been shown to result from this treatment, and steroids should not be routinely administered for head injury
Barbiturate therapy	High dose barbiturate therapy reduces cerebral oxygen demands and lowers ICP; high dose barbiturate therapy may be a useful treatment in patients with high ICP that does not respond to conventional management
Temperature control	Hyperthermia increases cerebral injury and must be avoided; the role of hypothermia is investigational
Decompressive craniectomy	Removal of part of the skull bone can allow mass expansion without increasing pressure; the role of this therapy is unclear for diffuse edema
Ventriculostomy	Draining a small amount of cerebral spinal fluid can be used to reduce ICP

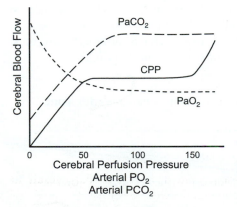

Figure 16-2 The effects of Pa_{CO_2}, Pa_{O_2}, and cerebral perfusion pressure on cerebral blood flow. Note that hypercarbia and hypoxemia increase cerebral blood flow, and thus intracranial pressure. Normally, cerebral blood flow remains relatively constant over a wide range of cerebral perfusion pressures (autoregulation), but this relationship is lost with acute head injury (loss of autoregulation).

ventilation in patients with an increased ICP. Increases in mean airway pressure can adversely affect cerebral perfusion in patients with cerebral edema. Increases in alveolar pressure may result in an increase in ICP due to a decrease in venous return and a decrease in cardiac output.

Indications

Indications for mechanical ventilation in patients with head injury are listed in Table 16-2. The most common reason to ventilate these patients is central respiratory depression due to the primary injury. In such patients, lung function may be near normal, and mechanical ventilation is straightforward. In patients with traumatic injury, associated injuries to the spine, chest, and abdomen may also require the initiation of mechanical ventilation. Positive pressure ventilation may also be necessary due to neurogenic pulmonary edema. Finally, some therapies for acute head injury (e.g., barbiturates, sedation, and paralysis) result in central respiratory depression, necessitating mechanical ventilation.

Ventilator Settings

Recommendations for initial ventilator settings for patients with head injury are shown in Table 16-3 and Figure 16-3. Full ventilator support is almost always initially required for these patients, and can be provided by CMV (A/C). Because of the depressed neurologic status of these patients and the need to control Pa_{CO_2}, pressure support ventilation as the initial mode in these patients is usually not appropriate.

Because patients with head injury often have relatively normal lung function, oxygenation is usually not a problem. With these patients, 100% oxygen is initially administered and can be rapidly weaned using pulse oximetry. A Pa_{O_2} of 70 to 100 mm Hg is often used because this minimizes the potential for periodic episodes of hypoxemia and associated rises in ICP. An initial PEEP level of 5 cm H_2O is usually appropriate and adequate. Although there is concern related to the effects of PEEP on ICP, PEEP usually does not adversely affect ICP at levels ≤ 10 cm H_2O. With neurogenic pulmonary edema, the management of oxygenation is similar to that with other causes of ARDS, although care must be taken to avoid the effects of high mean airway pressures on ICP.

Table 16-2 Indications for mechanical ventilation in patients with acute head injury

- Depression due to primary neurologic injury
- Associated injuries to the spine, chest, and abdomen
- Neurogenic pulmonary edema
- Treatment with respiratory suppressant medications (barbiturates, sedatives, paralytics)

Table 16-3 Initial mechanical ventilator settings with head injury

Setting	Recommendation
Mode	CMV (A/C)
Rate	15 to 20 breaths/min (20 to 30 breaths/min if necessary to control ICP, provided that auto-PEEP not present)
Volume/pressure control	Volume or pressure
Tidal volume	8–12 mL/kg predicted body weight provided that plateau pressure < 30 cm H_2O
Inspiratory time	1 s
PEEP	5 cm H_2O provided that PEEP does not increase ICP
FI_{O_2}	1.0
Flow waveform	Rectangular or descending ramp

Volume-controlled ventilation is usually appropriate in patients with head injury, although the choice of volume controlled or pressure controlled ventilation is usually based on clinician bias. A tidal volume in the range of 8 to 12 mL/kg ideal weight can be used provided that plateau pressure is kept below 30 cm H_2O. This is usually not a problem, because these patients typically have a nearly normal lung and chest wall compliance. If the patient has concomitant acute or chronic respiratory disease, a lower tidal volume is selected. A respiratory rate appropriate to achieve normal acid-base balance should be chosen. This can often be achieved at a rate of 15 to 20 breaths/min. An inspiratory time of one second is usually adequate.

Monitoring

Monitoring of mechanically ventilated head injured patients is similar to that of any mechanically ventilated patient (Table 16-4). If minute ventilation is increased to produce iatrogenic hyperventilation, the presence of auto-PEEP must be evaluated. Capnography may be useful to monitor the level of ventilation in these patients, who often have normal lung function and do not tolerate well an increase in Pa_{CO_2}. Close observation of ICP should be used when ventilator settings are manipulated. If an ICP monitor is not present, clinical signs of an increased ICP (e.g., pupillary response, posturing, changes in level of consciousness) should be evaluated when ventilator changes occur. Jugular venous bulb oxygen saturation (Sjv_{O_2}) may be used as an index of the adequacy of cerebral blood flow and oxygenation. Although pulmonary toilet is important in these patients, care must be taken to avoid deleterious increases in ICP during suctioning. Nutritional support is necessary to facilitate healing and weaning from mechanical ventilation. Pulmonary embolism can occur in patients with prolonged immobility, and pulmonary infection is also common in these patients.

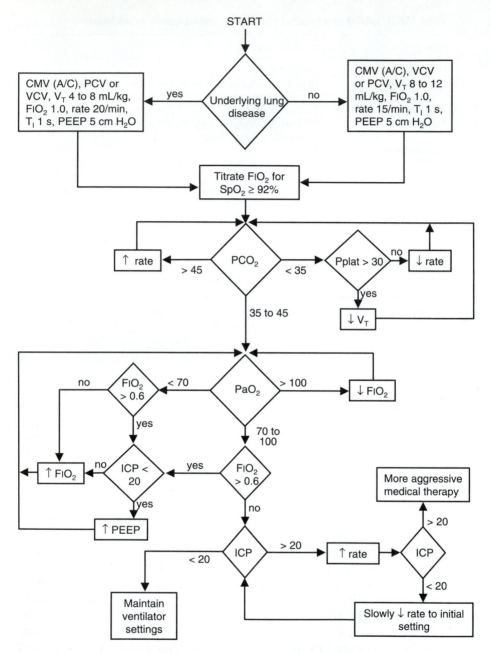

Figure 16-3 An algorithm for mechanical ventilation of the patient with head injury.

Table 16-4 Monitoring of the mechanically ventilated patient with head injury

- Peak alveolar pressure, mean airway pressure, auto-PEEP
- Pa_{CO_2} end-tidal P_{CO_2}
- Intracranial pressure, jugular venous oxygen saturation
- Pulse oximetry
- Heart rate and systemic blood pressure

Weaning

Weaning should not be considered until respiratory depressant therapy is no longer required. Weaning can often be initiated before the patient's neurologic function is maximally restored if the ventilatory drive is intact. For some patients, maintenance of a stable airway is required for a longer time than ventilatory support (i.e., tracheostomy). However, extubation should not be delayed solely on the basis of depressed neurologic status. Due to central neurologic dysfunction, weaning, extubation, and decannulation of some of these patients can be prolonged and difficult. Weaning approaches should incorporate spontaneous breathing trials and appropriate rest following a failed trial of spontaneous breathing.

Apnea Test

An apnea test is commonly conducted as part of the diagnosis of brain death. Before conducting the apnea test, the following prerequisites should be met: core temperature $\geq 36.5\,°C$, systolic blood pressure ≥ 90 mm Hg, euvolemia, normoxemia (or $Pa_{O_2} > 200$ mm Hg), and eucapnia (or $Pa_{CO_2} > 40$ mm Hg in the patient with chronic hypercapnia). The following procedure is used:

- Disconnect the ventilator.
- Administer 6 L/min O_2, either by T-piece or by a catheter passed into the trachea.
- Observe the patient closely for signs of respiratory movements. If respiratory movements occur, the apnea test is negative (i.e., does not support the clinical diagnosis of brain death), and mechanical ventilation is resumed.
- If respiratory movements do not occur, measure arterial blood gases after eight minutes and reconnect the ventilator.
- If respiratory movements are absent and Pa_{CO_2} is 60 mm Hg (or 20 mm Hg greater than baseline), the apnea test result is positive and consistent with the clinical diagnosis of brain death.
- If hypotension or desaturation occur during the apnea test, the ventilator is reconnected and the test is resumed at a later time.
- If no respiratory movements are observed, Pa_{CO_2} is < 60 mm Hg, and no adverse effects occur, the test may be repeated with 10 minutes of apnea.

POINTS TO REMEMBER

- The requirement for mechanical ventilation in head injured patients is usually due to central respiratory depression.
- Cerebral perfusion pressure is the difference between mean arterial pressure and intracranial pressure.
- Positive pressure ventilation can adversely affect cerebral perfusion pressure.
- Some head injured patients develop a form of ARDS called neurogenic pulmonary edema.
- Iatrogenic hyperventilation is used to control acute increases in ICP, but prolonged hyperventilation therapy is not recommended.
- Because many head injured patients have relatively normal lung function, mechanical ventilation is usually straightforward.
- The effects of mechanical ventilation on ICP and Sjv_{O_2} must be closely evaluated.
- The neurologic effects of respiratory care procedures such as suctioning must be closely monitored.
- Extubation should not be delayed solely on the basis of depressed neurologic function.
- The apnea test is used to confirm brain death.

ADDITIONAL READING

BERROUSCHOT J, ROOSSLER A, KOSTER J, SCHNEIDER D. Mechanical ventilation in patients with hemispheric ischemic stroke. *Crit Care Med* 2000; 28:2956–2961.

CAMPBELL RS, HURST JM. Respiratory support of the head-injured patient. *Respir Care Clin N Am* 1997; 3:51–68.

COPLIN WM, PIERSON DJ, COOLEY KD, ET AL. Implications of extubation delay in brain-injured patients meeting standard weaning criteria. *Am J Respir Crit Care Med* 2000; 161:1530–1536.

DE DEYNE C. Jugular bulb oximetry: the link between cerebral and systematic management of severe head injury. *Intensive Care Med* 1999; 25:430–431.

MCGUIRE G, CROSSLEY D, RICHARDS J, WONG, D. Effects of varying levels of positive end-expiratory pressure on intracranial pressure and cerebral perfusion pressure. *Crit Care Med* 1997; 25:1059–1062.

SKIPPEN P, SEEAR M, POSKITT K, ET AL. Effect of hyperventilation on regional cerebral blood flow in head injured children. *Crit Care Med* 1997; 25:1402–1409.

SUAZO JAC, MAAS AIR, VAN DEN BRINK WA, ET AL. CO_2 reactivity and brain oxygen pressure monitoring in severe head injury. *Crit Care Med* 2000; 28:3268–3274.

THIAGARAJAN A, GOVERDHAN PD, CHARI P, SOMASUNDERAM K. The effect of hyperventilation and hyperoxia on cerebral venous oxygen saturation in patient with traumatic brain injury. *Anesth Analg* 1998; 87:850–853.

VIGUE B, RACT C, BENAYED M, ET AL. Early Sjv_{O_2} monitoring in patients with severe brain trauma. *Intensive Care Med* 1999; 25:445–451.

WIJDICKS EFM. The diagnosis of brain death. *N Engl J Med* 2001; 344:1215–1221.

SEVENTEEN

POSTOPERATIVE PATIENTS

OBJECTIVES

1. List indications for mechanical ventilation of postoperative patients.
2. Describe the initial ventilator settings for postoperative patients without prior pulmonary disease, with prior pulmonary disease and patients with single lung transplantation.
3. Describe monitoring of the ventilated postoperative patient.
4. Discuss weaning of patients requiring postoperative ventilatory support.

INTRODUCTION

A frequently encountered category of patients requiring ventilatory support are those in the immediate postoperative period. This is particularly true of patients following thoracic or cardiac surgery, although changes in surgical and anesthesia techniques have decreased the requirement for mechanical ventilation. Generally, these patients do not present complex ventilatory management problems and many are extubated within 24 hrs.

OVERVIEW

It has been well established that surgical procedures that include general anesthesia, especially those affecting the thoracic or abdominal cavities, result in impairment of ventilatory function. The reasons for these impairments include the effects of general inhalation anesthetics on hypoxic pulmonary vaso-constriction and a blunting of hypoxemic and hypercapnic ventilatory drive when intravenous narcotics are used. As a result of alteration in the shape and motion of the diaphragm and chest wall, thoracic or cardiac surgery can decrease lung volume by 20 to 30% and upper abdominal surgery can reduce the vital capacity by up to 60%. As many as 60 to 80% of thoracic surgical and cardiac surgical patients have radiographic evidence of atelectasis. In the patient with normal pre-operative pulmonary function, this may not present significant postoperative problems. Cardiac surgical patients are at risk of diaphragmatic dysfunction due to phrenic nerve injury. In patients with pre-existing pulmonary disease, however, postoperative management can be complex. With the increased use of lung resection surgery, reduction pneumoplasty, heart and lung transplantation, and complex cardiac surgery performed on older patients, postoperative ventilatory failure is likely to remain a common reason for venti-latory support.

MECHANICAL VENTILATION

Indications

The primary reason for mechanical ventilation in this group is apnea as a result of unreversed anesthetic agents (Table 17-1). The primary reasons that anesthesia is not reversed are iatrogenic hypothermia, the need to reduce cardiopulmonary stress, or the presence of altered pulmonary mechanics. Some cardiac surgeons favor cold cardioplegia to reduce the likelihood of hypoxic injury. These patients receive narcotic anesthesia throughout the procedure and may require 8 to 16 hours for warming and full reversal of anesthesia. Transplant recipients (heart or lung) are ventilated for longer periods to insure cardiopulmonary stress is mini-mized during the initial acclimation period and to minimize any adverse effects of an increased work-of-breathing in the immediate postoperative period. The most difficult group of patients are those with pre-existing lung disease whose pulmon-ary mechanics are adversely affected by surgery, who require ventilatory support because of compromised cardiopulmonary reserve and bronchial hygiene.

Table 17-1 Indications for ventilation in postoperative patients

- Apnea – unreversed anesthetic agents
- Minimize postoperative cardiopulmonary stress
- Pre-existing lung disease compromising cardiopulmonary reserve

Ventilator Settings

Minimal or no prior pulmonary disease It is usually easy to ventilate these patients. Most simply require postanesthesia recovery. Volume or pressure ventilation in the A/C (CMV) mode is acceptable (Figure 17-1). Tidal volume may be large (10 to 12 mL/kg) since lung function is normal. The rate can be set at 8 to 12/min. F_{IO_2} is titrated to maintain a normal Pa_{O_2} (> 80 mm Hg) and low levels of PEEP (5 cm H_2O) may be applied to maintain functional residual capacity (Table 17-2). In hypothermic patients, minute ventilation is decreased to avoid hypocarbia and alkalosis. As a result, the initial rate may need to be set low and increased as body temperature increases.

Prior pulmonary disease Patients with a history of chronic pulmonary disease are ventilated in the same manner as any patient with chronic pulmonary disease. Air-trapping is the foremost concern with COPD. Tidal volume and rate should be low and expiratory time is increased. PEEP is applied to counterbalance auto-PEEP when spontaneous breathing resumes. Moderate V_T (8 to 10 mL/kg) and low peak alveolar pressures (< 30 cm H_2O) should be used in patients with COPD. In patients with chronic restrictive pulmonary disease, air trapping is not a problem. Because of reduced lung volumes, however, smaller V_T (< 8 mL/kg) and rapid rates (15 to 25/min) are set to avoid high peak alveolar pressures.

Single lung transplant Of all the patients ventilated postoperatively, this group is the most troublesome if one lung has relatively normal pulmonary mechanics (transplanted lung) and the other has mechanics reflecting either obstructive or restrictive disease (native lung). In these patients, the ventilator should be set to insure the maximum function of the native lung, since this will be the lung presenting the greatest challenge. If the native lung has chronic obstruction, ventilate with moderate volume and slow rates. With pulmonary fibrosis in the native lung, a smaller V_T and more rapid rate are indicated. In the case of pulmonary fibrosis, there is less concern about air trapping. However, peak alveolar pressure may be high due to reduced compliance.

  The greatest ventilatory challenge is the patient with a single lung transplant where the native lung is obstructed and the transplanted lung has become stiff because of fluid, infection, rejection or acute lung injury. In this setting, it is difficult to dictate ideal ventilator settings because of the differing pathologies

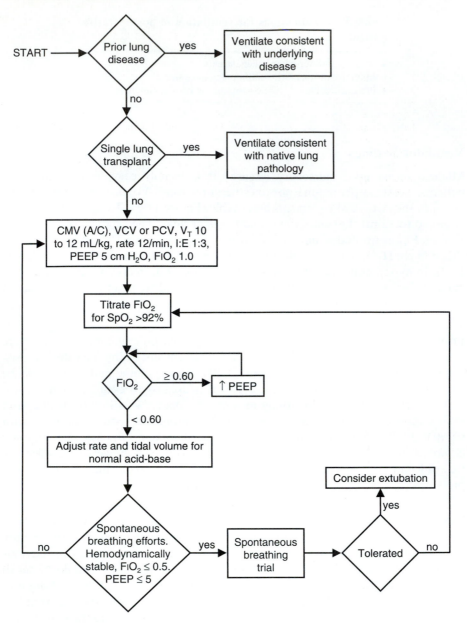

Figure 17-1 An algorithm for mechanical ventilation of the postoperative patient.

in each lung. Careful attention needs to be paid to two variables as adjustments are made. First, concern about peak alveolar pressure because of ventilator imposed lung injury and damage to the surgical site and second, air trapping in the obstructed lung resulting in grossly compromised ventilation/perfusion ratios.

Table 17-2 Initial ventilator settings for postoperative patients

A. Postoperative Patients with no prior disease.

Setting	Recommendation
Mode	A/C (CMV)
Rate	10 to 16/min
Volume/pressure control	Pressure or volume
Tidal volume	10 to 12 mL/kg and plateau pressure < 30 cm H_2O
Inspiratory time	1 s
PEEP	$\leq$ 5 cm H_2O
F_{IO_2}	Sufficient to maintain Pa_{O_2} > 80 mm Hg
Flow waveform	Descending ramp

B. Postoperative patients with prior obstructive lung disease.

Setting	Recommendation
Mode	A/C (CMV)
Rate	8–12/min
Volume/pressure control	Pressure or volume
Tidal volume	8 to 10 mL/kg and plateau pressure < 30 cm H_2O
Inspiratory time	0.6 to 1.2 s
PEEP	5 cm H_2O; counterbalance auto-PEEP
F_{IO_2}	Sufficient to maintain Pa_{O_2} > 60 mm Hg
Flow waveform	Descending ramp

C. Postoperative patients with prior restrictive lung disease

Setting	Recommendation
Mode	A/C (CMV)
Rate	15–25/min
Volume/pressure control	Pressure or volume
Tidal volume	< 8 mL/kg and plateau pressure < 30 cm H_2O
Inspiratory time	1 s
PEEP	5 cm H_2O
F_{IO_2}	Sufficient to maintain Pa_{O_2} > 60 mm Hg
Flow waveform	Descending ramp

In this setting, permissive hypercapnia is often necessary with the final ventilator settings being a compromise between conflicting needs.

Monitoring

For the majority of postoperative patients, monitoring of gas exchange (pulse oximetry and arterial blood gases), level of consciousness, pulmonary mechanics, and the ability to cough and deep breathe are sufficient to determine if there is a need for continued ventilatory support (Table 17-3). However, in patients with COPD, monitoring of auto-PEEP is also important. These patients are often fluid positive, which can affect respiratory function. Monitoring fluid balance, includ-

Table 17-3 Monitoring of the mechanically ventilated postoperative patient

- Pulse oximetry
- Level of consciousness
- Pulmonary mechanics, maximal inspiratory pressure
- Auto-PEEP and peak alveolar pressure
- Fluid balance
- Hemodynamics

ing central venous pressure, is often useful. In patients with hemodynamic instability or severe cardiac disease, careful monitoring of pulmonary and systemic hemodynamics is also indicated.

Weaning

Weaning is a simple process for most postoperative patients. When gas exchange is adequate at an F_{IO_2} of 0.40, the patient is alert and oriented, able to lift the head and take a deep breath, ventilatory support can be discontinued and the patient is extubated. Many clinicians prefer short (30 min) spontaneous breathing trials, or a gradual reduction of pressure support to 5 to 10 cm H_2O before discontinuation. However, unless the baseline status is abnormal (i.e., COPD), a specific weaning protocol may extend the time ventilation is required. In patients with underlying pulmonary disease or lung transplant patients, more prolonged weaning may be necessary.

POINTS TO REMEMBER

- General anesthesia causes pulmonary vasoconstriction and a blunting of hypoxemic and hypercapnia ventilatory drive.
- Thoracic and cardiac surgery can reduce the functional residual capacity by 20 to 30%, and upper abdominal surgery can reduce the vital capacity by 60%.
- When mechanical ventilation is indicated in postoperative patients, this is likely to be due to unreversed anesthesia.
- No special ventilatory requirements are needed in postoperative patients without pulmonary disease.
- In patients with obstructive or restrictive lung disease, ventilate according to the primary disease.
- In patients with single lung transplantation, ventilate in a manner most suited for the most diseased lung (usually the native lung).
- Monitoring of postoperative mechanically ventilated patients involves indices of gas exchange, level of consciousness, and pulmonary mechanics.
- In most postoperative patients, the ventilator can be discontinued once the F_{IO_2} is reduced and general muscular capability restored.

ADDITIONAL READING

BOYSEN PG. Postoperative Ventilatory Management. In: KACMAREK RM, STOLLER JK (eds.). *Current Respiratory Care*. Toronto, BC Decker, 1988, 327–331.
BRANSON RD. Peri-operative Respiratory Care. In PIERSON DJ, KACMAREK RM (eds.) *Foundations of Respiratory Care*. New York, Churchill Livingstone, Inc., 1992, 389–395.
DAVIS K, JOHNSON DJ. Effects of Anesthesia and Surgery on the Respiratory System. In PIERSON DJ, KACMAREK RM (eds.) *Foundations of Respiratory Care*. New York, Churchill Livingstone, Inc., 1992, 389–395.

CHAPTER EIGHTEEN

NEUROMUSCULAR DISEASE AND CHEST WALL DEFORMITIES

OBJECTIVES

1. Discuss the pathophysiology of ventilatory failure in patients with neuro-muscular disease or chest wall deformities.
2. Discuss the indications for invasive and noninvasive ventilation in this patient population.
3. Discuss initial ventilator settings for invasive and noninvasive ventilatory support in this patient population.
4. Discuss monitoring during and weaning from ventilatory support for patients with neuromuscular disease.
5. Discuss the use of the in-exsufflator in patients with neuromuscular disease.

INTRODUCTION

Patients with neuromuscular disease or chest wall deformities represent a small percentage of patients receiving ventilatory support. However, they also represent a large percentage of the patients requiring long-term ventilatory support. Since these patients usually have normal lungs and the reason for ventilatory assistance is an inability to generate sufficient muscular effort to ventilate, providing mechanical ventilation is much easier in this group than with other groups of patients.

OVERVIEW

Based on pathophysiology, this group of patients can be divided into two general categories – those with a relatively rapid (days to weeks) onset of neuromuscular weakness and those in which neuromuscular weakness is progressive and not reversible.

Rapid Onset

The two primary diseases in this category are myasthenia gravis and Guillain-Barré syndrome. This category also includes patients with prolonged paralysis following the use of neuromuscular blocking agents in the ICU and patients with high spinal cord injury. These patients do not have lung disease, but reversible neuromuscular weakness requiring ventilatory support for varying periods of time prior to return to a stable state where spontaneous breathing is feasible. The exception to this may be the spinal cord injured patient who may require long-term ventilatory support. Of concern with these patients is their perception that their lungs are being ventilated. As a result, they require large tidal volumes – sometimes exceeding 15 mL/kg. However, since they do not have intrinsic lung disease, peak alveolar pressures are easily kept below 30 cm H_2O.

Gradual Onset

Patients with muscular dystrophy, amyotrophic lateral sclerosis, thoracic deformities (severe scoliosis, kyphosis, or kyphoscoliosis), or post-polio syndrome frequently develop gradual muscular weakness over time, in some cases progressing over years. Many require periodic mechanical ventilation because of acute pulmonary infections and others require acute, then chronic, ventilatory support because of progressive deterioration in neuromuscular function. For most of these patients, mechanical ventilation is required at some point in their disease. These patients are candidates for non-invasive ventilation. The need for periodic support is a result of muscular weakness, usually without intrinsic lung disease.

MECHANICAL VENTILATION

Indications

Ventilatory support in most cases is indicated because of progressive ventilatory muscle weakness leading to acute ventilatory failure (Table 18-1). Oxygenation is not usually an issue. Exceptions are the patient with an acquired neuropathy or myopathy following prolonged mechanical ventilation (polyneuropathy or myopathy of critical illness), pneumonia, atelectasis or pulmonary edema. Oxygenation may be an issue in these patients because of the primary pathophysiology leading to ventilatory support.

Noninvasive Ventilation

Of all the groups of patients requiring ventilatory support, this is the group that is most capable of being managed with noninvasive ventilation. Noninvasive positive pressure ventilation has been successfully used in both short-term application and long-term use. Many of these patients also benefit from the use of a pneumobelt for intermittent daytime support. Noninvasive techniques are most useful in patients where the neuromuscular weakness is gradual in its development and in those requiring chronic ventilatory support.

Ventilator Settings

Invasive ventilatory support   Since these patients generally lack intrinsic lung disease, positive pressure ventilation can be accomplished with low pressures and a low F_{IO_2}. Volume ventilation with large tidal volumes and respiratory rates that the patient considers comfortable are recommended (Figure 18-1).

Unsupported spontaneous breathing (e.g., SIMV) should not be used. In most cases assist/control (CMV) is the mode of choice. If the rate and V_T are set to satisfy the patient's ventilatory demand, most patients allow the ventilator to control ventilation. Inspiratory flow waveforms may be either descending ramp or rectangular with inspiratory flows set per patient comfort. PEEP is usually not necessary, but low levels (3 to 5 cm H_2O) to maintain functional residual capacity may be beneficial in some patients. This is the only group of patients where mechanical dead space may be indicated. Since these patients desire large V_T (> 15 mL/kg) and respiratory rates are usually > 10/min, hypocarbia and alka-

Table 18-1 Indications for ventilation in patients with neuromuscular disease

- Progressive ventilatory failure
- Acute ventilatory failure

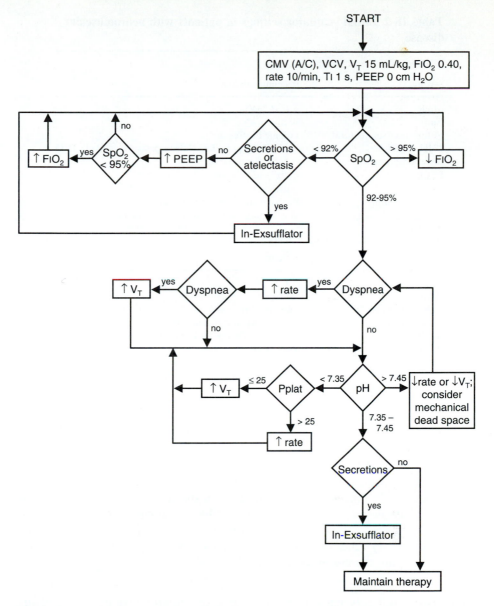

Figure 18-1 An algorithm for mechanical ventilation of the patient with neuromuscular disease who does not have underlying lung disease.

losis develop if mechanical dead space is not added. Pa_{CO_2} can be maintained at a normal level by the addition of 50 to 200 mL of dead space between the ventilator Y-piece and endotracheal tube. The addition of dead space should be considered after attempts to modify ventilatory pattern have failed (Table 18-2).

Table 18-2 Initial ventilator settings in patients with neuromuscular disease

A. Patients with normal lung volumes

Setting	Recommendation
Mode	A/C (CMV)
Rate	10 min
Volume/pressure control	Volume or pressure
Tidal volume	$\geq$ 15 mL/kg provided plateau pressure < 30 cm H_2O
Inspiratory time	$\geq$ 1 s
PEEP	Usually unnecessary
FI_{O_2}	$\geq$ 0.21
Flow waveform	Rectangular or descending ramp
Mechanical dead space	May be necessary to prevent hypocarbia

B. Patients with reduced lung volumes

Setting	Recommendation
Mode	A/C (CMV)
Rate	> 15/min
Volume/pressure control	Volume or pressure
Tidal volume	$\leq$ 10 mL/kg and plateau pressure < 30 cm H_2O
Inspiratory time	$\leq$ 1 s (peak flow $\geq$ 60 L/min with volume ventilation)
PEEP	5 cm H_2O
FI_{O_2}	usually $\leq$ 0.50
Flow waveform	Rectangular or descending ramp

The above guidelines are applicable to all patients in this group except those with reduced lung volumes (i.e., thoracic deformities or muscular dystrophies). In these patients, care must be exercised not to over-distend the lungs. Peak alveolar pressure should be maintained as low as possible (< 30 cm H_2O). This requires low tidal volumes (< 10 mL/cm H_2O) with more rapid rates (> 15/min) and shorter inspiratory times (< 1 s). These patients rarely require the use of PEEP and never require the use of mechanical dead space.

Noninvasive ventilatory support In the acute setting noninvasive positive pressure ventilation (NPPV) using either a nasal or oronasal mask is recommended. Negative pressure ventilation is not recommended. NPPV is most useful in patients where neuromuscular weakness has developed over a lengthy period of time and where lung volume has not been compromised. Ventilator settings are consistent with those designated for invasive ventilatory support. However, modification based on air leaks is necessary. The most critical factor is sizing and application of the mask. If the mask does not fit comfortably, the likelihood of intolerance is high.

Monitoring

Periodic monitoring of blood gases is necessary (Table 18-3). However, frequent blood gases are unnecessary because of the lack of intrinsic lung disease. Spontaneous V_T and respiratory rate, ventilatory pattern, vital capacity (VC), and maximum inspiratory pressure (PI_{max}) provide useful information to guide the initiation and termination of ventilatory support. Decisions to initiate ventilatory support are commonly made when VC < 10 mL/kg and PI_{max} is < −20 cm H_2O. Decisions to begin weaning occur when the above thresholds are reached, and ventilation discontinued when VC > 15 mL/kg and PI_{max} is > −30 cm H_2O with no deterioration after extended periods of spontaneous breathing (> 1 hr).

Weaning

Since these patients are committed to ventilatory support because a primary neuromuscular deficit has resulted in ventilatory muscle weakness and fatigue, weaning can only occur if these indications for ventilation have been reversed. In some patients with severe irreversible disease (e.g., high spinal cord injury, end-stage amyotrophic lateral sclerosis), weaning will not be possible and long-term ventilation strategies must be considered. In those patients where the acute process is reversible, appropriate therapy and time must be allowed for reversal of the neuromuscular deficit. In addition, retraining of ventilatory muscles is frequently needed. This is best accomplished by interposing periods of spontaneous breathing between periods of ventilatory support. Those patients with weaning difficulty receive a tracheostomy. The largest tracheostomy tube tolerated should be used to minimize resistive work-of-breathing. The first goal is ventilator independence during waking hours with support at night. Complete ventilatory independence is a secondary goal. Because of the nature of these diseases, weaning may take weeks, and care must be exercised not to fatigue patients during the spontaneous breathing trials. Patients should not be pushed to the point that ventilatory pattern changes, VC and PI_{max} decrease, or hypercarbia develops.

With many patients in this group, the decision to maintain long-term ventilatory support must be made at some point in their disease process. Specific guidelines for when this should occur are lacking. However, nocturnal NPPV should be considered whenever daytime baseline Pa_{CO_2} exceeds 45 mm Hg. When baseline hypercarbia is present and the patient's ventilatory reserve is

Table 18-3 Monitoring for the mechanically ventilated patient with neuromuscular disease or chest wall deformity

- Spontaneous tidal volume and respiratory rate
- Vital capacity and maximal inspiratory pressure
- Periodic arterial blood gases

markedly compromised, even small stressors may facilitate failure. These patients' ability to perform activities of daily living and to handle periodic stress is increased with nocturnal NPPV.

IN-EXSUFFLATOR, MAXIMUM INSUFFLATION CAPACITY, AND ASSISTED COUGH

Patients with neuromuscular diseases and chest wall deformities with ventilatory difficulties are ideal candidates for the in-exsufflator. This device simulates a cough by inflating the lungs with pressure, followed by a negative airway pressure to produce a high expiratory flow. This sequence can be repeated as necessary to clear secretions. Although no controlled trials of the use of the in-exsufflator are available, there is considerable anecdotal experience with neuromuscular disease. Many of these patients indicate no need for tracheal suctioning when the in-exsufflator is used. Initial application of the in-exsufflator requires low settings to allow acclimation. The inspiratory pressure is then adjusted to 25 to 35 cm H_2O applied for one to two seconds followed by an expiratory pressure up to -40 cm H_2O for about one to two seconds. Treatment periods consist of five to six breaths, followed by rest, and repeated until secretions are effectively cleared.

Hyperinflation therapy may be of benefit for patients with neuromuscular disease. This has been described as the maximum insufflation capacity (MIC). It is accomplished by the patient taking a deep breath, holding it, and then stacking consecutively delivered tidal volumes to the maximum volume that can be held with a closed glottis. The air is delivered from a manual or portable volume ventilator. This technique is limited by the ability of the patient to close the glottis (e.g., bulbar disease). Some clinicians train the patient in this technique when the vital capacity becomes < 2 L. MIC can be combined with manually assisted cough to improve secretion clearance. A manually assisted cough consists of an abdominal thrust and/or chest compression ("tussive squeeze") after a deep inflation. This can be quantified using a peak flow meter. A peak cough flow of > 160 L/min is needed to adequately clear airway secretions. The in-exsufflator may be necessary if the patient with neuromuscular disease cannot generate an unassisted or assisted peak flow > 160 L/min.

POINTS TO REMEMBER

- Most patients with decreased neuromuscular function do not have intrinsic lung disease.
- Two subgroups of patients are usually encountered – those with acute onset of weakness that is short-term and those with progressive weakness that is non-reversible.
- Most patients with a gradual onset of weakness are candidates for noninvasive ventilation.

- Mechanical ventilation is indicated with acute ventilatory failure caused by muscular weakness.
- In the gradual onset of weakness group, noninvasive positive pressure ventilation should be considered.
- In those patients without reduction in lung volumes, large tidal volumes (≥ 15 mL/kg), long inspiratory times (> 1 s) and moderate rates (≥ 10/min) are necessary for patient comfort.
- Mechanical dead space may be necessary in patients requiring large V_T and $\dot{V}_E$.
- Use small V_T (≤ 10 mL/kg), rapid rates (> 15/min) and short inspiratory times (≤ 1 s) in patients with reduced lung volumes.
- Monitor spontaneous ventilatory capabilities: V_T, rate, VC, PI_{max}, and ventilatory pattern.
- Weaning, when possible, is accomplished by increasing periods of spontaneous breathing trials interspersed with ventilatory support.
- The mechanical in-exsufflator is useful to mobilize secretions in patients with neuromuscular disease and a weak cough.
- Patients unable to maintain daytime Pa_{CO_2} < 45 mm Hg may be candidates for nocturnal chronic ventilatory support.

ADDITIONAL READING

ABOUSSOUAN LS, KHAN SU, MEEKER DP, ET AL. *Ann Intern Med* 1997; 127:450–453.

BONEKAT HW. Noninvasive ventilation in neuromuscular disease. *Crit Care Clin* 1998; 14:775–797.

DAU PC. Respiratory failure in myasthenia gravis. *Chest* 1985; 85:721.

DETROYER A, DEISSER P. The effects of intermittent positive pressure breathing in patients with respiratory muscle weakness. *Am Rev Respir Dis* 1981; 124–132.

KLEOPA KA, SHERMAN M, NEAL B, ET AL. BiPAP improves survival and rate of pulmonary function decline in patients with ALS. *J Neurol Sci* 1999; 15:82–88.

LYALL RA, DONALDSON N, FLEMING T, ET AL. A prospective study of quality of life in ALS patients treated with noninvasive ventilation. *Neurology* 2001; 57:153–156.

MCCOOL F, MAYEWSKI R, SHAYNE D, ET AL. Intermittent positive pressure breathing in patients with respiratory muscle weakness. *Chest* 1986; 90:546.

PINTO AC, EVANGELISTA T, CARVALHO M, ET AL. Respiratory assistance with a non-invasive ventilator (BiPAP) in MND/ALS patients: survival rates in a controlled trial. *J Neurol Sci* 1995; 129:19–26 (supplement).

PIRES M, CLARKIN SL, DABRIEO MA. The unique challenge of ventilator dependency in individuals with spinal cord injury. In: GILMARTIN ME, MAKE BJ. Mechanical ventilation in the home: issues for health care providers. *Problems in Respiratory Care* 1988; 1:257–268.

ROPPER AH. Severe acute Guillain-Barré syndrome. *Neurology* 1986; 36:429.

CARDIAC FAILURE

OBJECTIVES

1. Describe the effects of positive pressure ventilation on heart-lung interactions.
2. List indications for mechanical ventilation in patients with cardiac failure.
3. Discuss the role of continuous positive airway pressure in patients with cardiac failure.
4. Discuss the monitoring and weaning of patients with cardiac failure.
5. Describe the effects of positive pressure ventilation on heart-lung interactions.

INTRODUCTION

Cardiovascular disease is the leading cause of death in the United States. As a result, many patients present to the emergency department or general patient care units with congestive heart failure or acute myocardial infarction. Many of these patients benefit from the application of positive pressure ventilation.

OVERVIEW

Heart-Lung Interactions

The normal changes in intrathoracic pressure during spontaneous breathing facilitates venous return and maintains adequate preload to the right heart. In addition, the negative mean intrathoracic pressure assists left ventricular afterload. Left ventricular dysfunction with myocardial infarction or severe congestive heart failure results in increased left ventricular preload, pulmonary edema, decreased cardiac output, hypoxemia, and work-of-breathing. Of particular concern is the increase in blood flow required by the diaphragm and accessory muscles of breathing. The respiratory muscles receive as much as 40% of the cardiac output during stress, which can result in a reduction of blood flow to other vital organs.

Effects of Mechanical Ventilation

With positive pressure ventilation, the mean intrathoracic pressure is usually positive. During inspiration, intrathoracic pressure becomes more positive instead of more negative as occurs during spontaneous breathing. This decreases left ventricular preload and afterload. In the patient with acute left ventricular dysfunction, this may enhance the performance of a compromised myocardium. In the hypovolemic patient, however, these effects may compromise cardiac output.

 The response of the cardiovascular system to positive-pressure ventilation is dependent upon cardiovascular and pulmonary factors. From a pulmonary perspective, the compliance of the lungs and chest wall affects the transmission of alveolar pressure into the intrathoracic space. The most deleterious effect on hemodynamics occurs with a compliant lung and a stiff chest wall. Cardiovascular volume and tone, pulmonary vascular resistance, and right and left ventricular function determine the effect of intrathoracic pressure on hemodynamics (Table 19-1).

PEEP

Since PEEP elevates intrathoracic pressure, it reduces venous return and decreases preload. In the presence of left ventricular dysfunction with an elevated preload, PEEP may improve left ventricular function. PEEP may increase pulmonary vascular resistance, thus increasing right ventricular afterload and decreasing left heart filling. PEEP may decrease the compliance of the left ventricle by shifting the intra-ventricular septum. By increasing the pressure outside the heart, PEEP may improve left ventricular afterload.

Table 19-1 Determinants of cardiovascular response to positive-pressure ventilation

Cardiovascular
- Vascular volume
- Vascular tone
- Pulmonary vascular resistance
- Right and left ventricular function

Respiratory
- Resistance
- Compliance
- Homogeneity of resistance and compliance

MECHANICAL VENTILATION

Indications

Severe heart failure leads to hypoxemia, increased myocardial work, and increased work-of-breathing (Table 19-2). Mechanical ventilation in this setting is indicated to reverse the hypoxemia, reduce the work-of-breathing, and decrease myocardial work. Some patients with severe heart failure develop hypercarbia, but usually only after a considerable amount of time without treatment.

Continuous Positive Airway Pressure (CPAP)

The use of mask CPAP in the patient presenting with acute left ventricular failure and pulmonary edema reduces the work-of-breathing and the work of the myocardium. It also increases Pa_{O_2}, decreases Pa_{CO_2}, reduces the need for intubation, and may afford a survival benefit for the patient. CPAP may provide sufficient unloading while pharmacologic treatment modifies cardiovascular function to avoid invasive management. Generally, CPAP is most useful in patients who are awake, oriented and cooperative. If the CPAP mask further agitates the patient, it should be removed and invasive ventilatory support considered. Noninvasive positive pressure ventilation (NPPV) has also been used to avoid intubation of patients with acute congestive heart failure. However, NPPV should be avoided in patients with acute myocardial infarction (MI). In the patient with an acute MI and respiratory failure, invasive ventilatory support should be provided rather than NPPV.

Table 19-2 Indications for mechanical ventilation in patients with cardiovascular failure

- Increased work of the myocardium
- Increased work of breathing
- Hypoxemia

Ventilator Settings

Since spontaneous breathing potentially diverts blood flow to the respiratory muscles, CMV (A/C) should be used (Figure 19-1). Either pressure or volume ventilation is acceptable. In spite of the pulmonary edema that may be present at

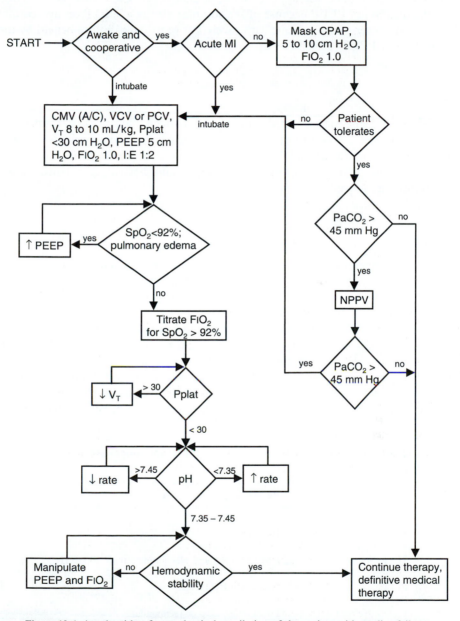

Figure 19-1 An algorithm for mechanical ventilation of the patient with cardiac failure.

the time of initiating ventilatory support, pharmacologic treatment results in rapid resolution. Tidal volumes in the 8 to 10 mL/kg range are usually adequate with respiratory rates > 10/min to achieve eucapnia. Peak alveolar pressure should be < 30 cm H_2O. Inspiratory time should be short (1 to 1.5 s). F_{IO_2} should initially be set at 1 and then titrated per Sp_{O_2} and blood gases. PEEP of 5 to 10 cm H_2O should be applied as support for the failing heart. Care must be exercised with the titration of PEEP because of the complex effects of PEEP on myocardial function. However, most patients with severe left ventricular failure benefit by the application of PEEP (Table 19-3).

Monitoring

Hemodynamics are monitored during pharmacologic therapy and mechanical ventilation (Table 19-4). Pulse oximetry is used to insure that patients are well oxygenated. Periodic arterial blood gases are needed. Peak alveolar pressure should be monitored. In addition, urine output and electrolyte balance should be carefully monitored.

Weaning

Provided no underlying chronic pulmonary disease or secondary pulmonary problems develop and the left heart failure is appropriately managed, weaning can be a relatively easy process. However, cardiovascular system function is most optimal with increased mean intrathoracic pressure in these patients. Since patients with underlying COPD generate large intrathoracic pressure swings during spontaneous breathing, the elimination of mechanical ventilatory support may result in an increase in left ventricular preload and pulmonary edema. Weaning may progress rapidly to low level pressure support and CPAP, but pulmonary edema may develop when positive pressure ventilation is discontinued. Some patients may develop ischemic changes during weaning. In this case, ventilatory support

Table 19-3 Initial ventilator settings for acute congestive heart failure

Setting	Recommendation
Mode	A/C (CMV)
Rate	10 to 15/min
Volume/pressure control	Pressure or volume
Tidal volume	8 to 10 mL/kg and plateau pressure < 30 cm H_2O
Inspiratory time	1 to 1.5 s
PEEP	5 to 10 cm H_2O
F_{IO_2}	1.0
Flow waveform	Descending ramp or rectangular

Table 19-4 Monitoring for the mechanically ventilated patient with cardiovascular failure

- Central venous pressure or pulmonary artery catheter
- Systemic hemodynamics
- Pulse oximetry and periodic arterial blood gases
- Urine output and electrolyte balance

must be continued until therapy is directed at improving cardiac function (e.g., diuresis, afterload reduction).

POINTS TO REMEMBER

- Severe left ventricular failure results in hypoxemia, increased work-of-breathing, and increased work of the myocardium.
- Positive pressure ventilation reverses the intrathoracic pressure dynamics present during spontaneous breathing, which may decrease cardiac output.
- PEEP decreases preload by increasing mean intrathoracic pressure.
- In the presence of a poorly functioning left ventricle, positive pressure ventilation and PEEP can reduce preload and afterload, improving left ventricular function.
- Mask CPAP at 5 to 10 cm H_2O with an $F_{I_{O_2}}$ of 1 may prevent mechanical ventilation.
- 100% oxygen should be administered until blood gas data indicate it can be decreased.
- PEEP of 5 to 10 cm H_2O should be used to reduce preload.
- The decreased intrathoracic pressure during weaning can result in pulmonary edema.
- Proper fluid balance, afterload reduction, and inotropic support is required for the weaning of many patients with severe left heart failure.

ADDITIONAL READING

BERSTEN AD, HOLT AW, VEDIG AE, SKOWRONSKI GA, BAGGOLEY CJ. Treatment of severe cardiogenic pulmonary edema with continuous positive airway pressure delivered by facemask. *New Eng J Med* 1991; 325: 1825–1830.

LEMAIRE F, TEBOUL J-L, CINOTTI L, ET AL. Acute left ventricular dysfunction during unsuccessful weaning from mechanical ventilation. *Anesthesiology* 1988; 69: 171–179.

POPPAS A, ROUNDS S. Congestive heart failure. *Am J Respir Crit Care Med* 2002; 165:4–48.

RAMSAY JG. Cardiac management in the ICU. *Chest* 1999; 115:138S–144S.

ASTHMA

OBJECTIVES

1. List indications for mechanical ventilation in patients with acute asthma.
2. List initial ventilator settings for the patient with acute asthma.
3. Discuss monitoring of the mechanically ventilated patient with asthma.
4. Discuss ventilator weaning of the patient with asthma.
5. Discuss the role of heliox in the management of the patient with asthma.

INTRODUCTION

Patients with a severe asthmatic attack may be markedly hypoxemic and hypercapnic. Airways resistance is so high that it appears in many patients that little gas is being delivered to the lung periphery. In fact, in some patients, peripheral breath sounds may be absent. Worldwide mortality from asthma has been rising since the 1960s. It is difficult to know if this is a result of an increase in the prevalence and the severity of the disease, or if this is a result of complacency about asthma management. The patient presenting with acute severe asthma should always be treated as a life-threatening medical emergency, potentially requiring intubation and mechanical ventilation.

OVERVIEW

Physiologic Presentation

Asthma is the presence of wheezing, chest tightness, cough and bronchial hyper-responsiveness on an intermittent basis. The patient presenting with severe asthma is distressed with labored breathing and has hyperinflation of the chest and widespread wheezing. However, in the most severe cases, obstruction may be so severe that wheezing and peripheral breath sounds are absent. The large swings in intrathoracic pressure observed in severe asthma cause large swings in the pulse amplitude (pulsus paradoxus) during inspiration and expiration. The airway may be filled with thick mucus. There is extensive broncho-spasm and mucosal edema. Spirometry indicates marked reduction in FEV_1 and peak expiratory flow.

Auto-PEEP

All patients with severe asthma develop air-trapping and auto-PEEP. The air-trapping occurs because of increased airways resistance and ball-valve obstruction by bronchospasm, inflammation, or secretions. Some lung units may have such severe obstruction and air-trapping that ventilation is impossible. This hyperin-flation and auto-PEEP can compress adjacent lung units. It is the auto-PEEP and increased resistive load that must be overcome with each breath that causes pulsus paradoxus. This, coupled with an elevated ventilatory drive by hypoxemia can result in inspiratory transpulmonary pressure gradients exceeding 25 cm H_2O. During exhalation, activation of expiratory muscles occurs in an attempt to mini-mize the functional residual capacity, auto-PEEP, and inspiratory work-of-breathing. Because of air-trapping, the functional residual capacity is increased, placing tidal breathing on a less compliant part of the pressure-volume curve of the lungs. This decreases compliance, further increasing the effort to breathe. The measured auto-PEEP in some asthmatics may not reflect the magnitude of air-trapping because of complete airway obstruction (Figure 20-1). Ideally these patients should assume a ventilatory pattern that is slow and deep to minimize air-trapping, to maximize exhaled volume, and to minimize breathing effort. However, the anxiety associated with the heightened ventilatory drive normally prevents the ideal ventilatory pattern.

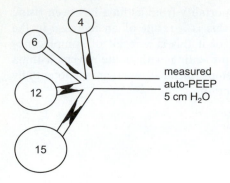

Figure 20-1 Measurement of auto-PEEP in the traditional manner (i.e., end-expiratory pause) may be an inaccurate reflection of auto-PEEP if airway closure occurs. In this example, the auto-PEEP measurement will reflect 5 cm H_2O (an average of the lung units with 4 cm H_2O and 6 cm H_2O auto-PEEP). However, some lung units have auto-PEEP levels greater than what is measured (12 cm H_2O and 15 cm H_2O).

MECHANICAL VENTILATION

Indications

Mechanical ventilation is indicated when the asthmatic patient cannot adequately maintain gas exchange. A clinical dilemma with asthma is determining when conventional therapy has failed and ventilatory support is required. Since most patients presenting with acute asthma are young and otherwise healthy, they can maintain ventilation for lengthy periods in spite of the marked increase in breathing effort. Once acute ventilatory failure develops, ventilation should be initiated (Table 20-1). However, these patients normally maintain adequate CO_2 elimination ($Pa_{CO_2} \leq 40$ mm Hg) until they are completely exhausted. As a result, once they retain CO_2, severe hypercarbia and acidosis can rapidly develop. Many clinicians believe that intubation and mechanical ventilation should occur when Pa_{CO_2} exceeds 40 mm Hg. At this point, the patient is fatiguing and waiting longer before initiating ventilation results in further hypoventilation. Although some clinicians have advocated the use of noninvasive ventilation for acute asthma, this is an area of controversy with no high level studies to support this approach.

Ventilator Settings

The major concern when ventilating the patient with severe asthma is auto-PEEP. The approach to ventilation should be focused on minimizing auto-PEEP (Table 20-2 and Figure 20-2). This usually means that permissive hypercapnia must also be accepted, particularly in the early phases of management. Appropriate bronch-

Table 20-1 Indications for ventilation in patients with asthma

- Acute ventilatory failure
- Impending acute ventilatory failure
- Severe hypoxemia

Table 20-2 Initial Ventilator settings in patients with acute asthma

Setting	Recommendation
Mode	A/C (CMV)
Rate	8 to 20/min; allow permissive hypercapnia (pH > 7.10–7.20)
Volume/pressure control	Pressure or volume; volume necessary for severe asthma
Tidal volume	4 to 8 mL/kg and plateau pressure < 30 cm H_2O
Inspiratory time	1 to 1.5 s; avoid auto-PEEP
PEEP	Use of PEEP is controversial; may attempt to counterbalance auto-PEEP
FI_{O_2}	1.0 or sufficient to maintain Pa_{O_2} > 60 mm Hg
Flow waveform	Descending ramp or rectangular

odilator therapy should be maximized. Inhaled bronchodilators and systemic steroids are an important aspect of the overall management of these patients.

Although either volume or pressure ventilation is acceptable, volume-controlled ventilation may be necessary at the onset of ventilatory support in some patients. In very severe asthma a high driving pressure may be needed to deliver the tidal volume, although a high peak alveolar pressure should be avoided. Although a peak airway pressure of 60 to 70 cm H_2O may be necessary, a plateau pressure < 30 cm H_2O may still be maintained. The difference between the peak pressure and the plateau pressure is an indication of the degree of airways resistance. Once the severity of the asthmatic attack decreases, the patient can be transitioned to pressure-control ventilation. Pressure-control ventilation is recommended since inspiratory time is not terminated by activating the high pressure limit, as frequently occurs with volume ventilation. With pressure-control ventilation, the change of delivered tidal volume at a fixed delivery pressure is a good index of changes in resistance and air trapping. As the severity of the asthmatic attack decreases, delivered V_T with pressure-controlled ventilation increases. Sufficient sedation to prevent dys-synchrony should always be used. Neuromuscular blocking agents may be necessary in some patients, although these should be avoided if possible. Prolonged paralysis may occur in some patients following neuromuscular blockade – especially those receiving high dose steroids. If adequate sedation is used, full ventilatory support can normally be achieved.

To minimize the development of auto-PEEP, a small V_T (4 to 8 mL/kg) should be used. Delivered tidal volume should always be based on peak alveolar pressure and reduced to insure plateau pressure < 30 cm H_2O. Respiratory rate should be set based on the level of air-trapping and auto-PEEP. Theoretically, a lower rate minimizes air-trapping. However, in many asthmatic patients rates can be increased to 15 to 20 breaths/min without a marked increase in auto-PEEP. Each patient responds differently. Some may require a rate of 8/min while others tolerate a rate of 20/min.

A low tidal volume with a slow rate results in CO_2 retention. Maintaining pH ≥ 7.20 is the general rule. However, in young otherwise healthy asthma

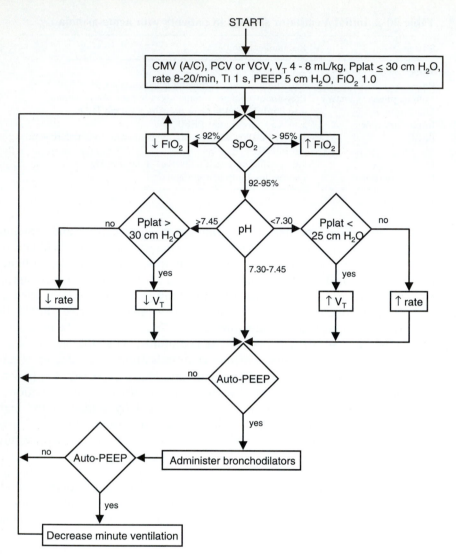

Figure 20-2 An algorithm for mechanical ventilation of the patient with asthma.

patients, a pH as low as 7.10 is often acceptable. The risk of barotrauma and hypotension usually outweighs the risks of acidosis as a result of the small V_T and minute ventilation.

Inspiratory time should be short since auto-PEEP is reduced by decreasing minute ventilation and prolonging expiratory time. However, better distribution of ventilation can be achieved by lengthening inspiratory time. Inspiratory times of 1 to 1.5 s are recommended, with evaluation of the effect of inspiratory time on auto-PEEP. In many patients, provided the rate is low, the increase in inspiratory time from 1 to 1.5 s does not significantly increase auto-PEEP. Inspiratory times greater than 1.5 s should be applied with extreme caution. A descending ramp flow pattern when volume ventilation is used should be selected to enhance distribution of ventilation. However, a shorter inspiratory time may be achieved using a rectangular flow waveform. Peak flow is selected to insure inspiratory time is maintained; frequently $\geq$ 60 L/min is necessary.

An initial F_{IO_2} of 1 should be set and then reduced when pulse oximetry and blood gas data indicate adequate oxygenation. A controversy with the management of asthma is whether PEEP should be applied. Auto-PEEP increases the pressure gradient required to trigger the ventilator. The patient must overcome the auto-PEEP level before the ventilator triggers. Applying PEEP increases ventilator circuit pressure to counterbalance auto-PEEP, eliminating the pressure differential. The applied PEEP does not increase the total PEEP if the auto-PEEP is the result of flow limitation. However, if the patient's ventilation is being controlled, does adding applied PEEP benefit the patient? Distribution of ventilation may improve with applied PEEP since those lung units without auto-PEEP may be recruited and stabilized. If applied PEEP is used, its level should not exceed the level at which total PEEP increases. If PEEP is applied in this setting, careful monitoring of gas exchange, peak alveolar pressure, auto-PEEP, and hemodynamics is necessary.

Monitoring

Barotrauma is common in asthma if peak alveolar pressures and auto-PEEP levels are excessive. Careful physical examination and chest X-rays need to be monitored (Table 20-3). With each ventilator-patient system evaluation, peak alveolar pressure, peak airway pressure, tidal volume and auto-PEEP levels should be documented and trends evaluated. Pulse oximetry monitoring is useful, since these patients' status can change quickly. Periodic blood gas monitoring is necessary. Monitoring of hemodynamics is necessary, although rarely is a pulmonary artery catheter indicated.

Weaning

Once the acute phase of asthma is adequately controlled, ventilator discontinuation should be considered. As the patient's status improves (i.e., airflow resistance

Table 20-3 Monitoring for the mechanically ventilated patient with asthma

- Presence of barotrauma
- Peak alveolar pressure and mean airway pressure
- Auto-PEEP
- Pulse oximetry and arterial blood gases
- Heart rate and blood pressure

returning to baseline, auto-PEEP eliminated and airway pressures and volumes returning to normal), sedation should be decreased, allowing the patient to resume spontaneous breathing. Once alert, oriented, and cooperative, the patient should be extubated. Assuming the only reason mechanical ventilation was necessary was acute severe asthma, once this is reversed there is no more need for ventilatory support.

HELIOX

Heliox is a mixture of helium (60% to 80%) with oxygen (20% to 40%). The use of heliox in severe asthma can improve gas exchange and decrease the work-of-breathing. Heliox can be used during spontaneous breathing or during mechanical ventilation. The low density of helium reduces the pressure required for flow through a partially obstructed airway. Ideally, a gas mixture containing 80% helium is preferred, but improved clinical status may occur with as low as 40% helium. Figure 20-3 illustrates the setup for delivery of heliox to the spontaneously breathing patient. Heliox should be considered in spontaneously breathing asthmatics not responding to initial aerosolized bronchodilator therapy. Patients with asthma requiring mechanical ventilation should be considered for heliox. Heliox can also be administered through some mechanical ventilators. Of concern is the effect of heliox on ventilator function. Ventilators are calibrated to oxygen-nitrogen mixtures (not oxygen-helium mixtures) and thus the displayed volumes are incorrect. However, pressure measurements are accurate. Before clinical use of a ventilator with heliox, its performance with heliox must be assessed to protect patient safety.

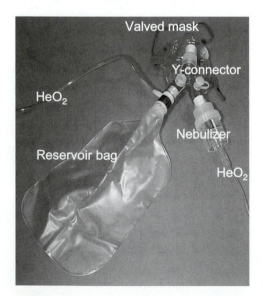

Figure 20-3 Illustration of approach to delivering heliox to a spontaneously breathing patient. The nebulizer can be operated by oxygen or heliox dependent on the required F_{IO_2}. Gas flow through the partial rebreathing mask should be sufficient to minimize entertainment of room air.

POINTS TO REMEMBER

- In the most severe cases of asthma, wheezing may be absent but pulse rate and blood pressure are elevated and pulsus paradoxus is pronounced.
- Auto-PEEP is a major problem with severe asthmatic attacks.
- Mechanical ventilation is indicated in acute or impending acute ventilatory failure; when Pa_{CO_2} rises above 40 mm Hg, mechanical ventilation should be considered.
- Either pressure-controlled or volume-controlled ventilation can be used in most patients.
- Respiratory rate should be 8 to 20/min and V_T set to keep peak alveolar pressure < 30 cm H_2O (4 to 8 mL/kg).
- Permissive hypercapnia is unavoidable until the severity of the asthma improves.
- A pH as low as 7.10 may be tolerated in many patients.
- Inspiratory time is set at 1 to 1.5 s to improve distribution of ventilation but to avoid the further development of auto-PEEP.
- Adjust $F_{I_{O_2}}$ to keep Pa_{O_2} > 60 mm Hg.
- During spontaneous breathing, use applied PEEP to offset auto-PEEP.
- During mechanical ventilation, the use of applied PEEP is controversial; when it is used, carefully monitor gas exchange, peak alveolar pressure, auto-PEEP level and hemodynamics.
- Consider the use of heliox before intubation and during ventilatory support.
- Regularly monitor auto-PEEP, peak alveolar and airway pressure, tidal volume, and the presence of barotrauma.
- Discontinue ventilatory support when volumes and pressures have returned to normal.

ADDITIONAL READING

ADNET F, DHISSI G, BORRON SW, ET AL. Complication profiles of adult asthmatics requiring paralysis during mechanical ventilation. *Intensive Care Med* 2001; 27:1729–1736.

AFESSA B, MORALES I, CURY JD. Clinical course and outcome of patients admitted to an ICU for status asthmaticus. *Chest* 2001; 120:1616–1621.

AFZAL M, THARRATT RS. Mechanical ventilation in severe asthma. *Clin Rev Allergy Immunol* 2001; 20:385–397.

KACMAREK RM, HICKLING K. Permissive hypercapnia. *Respir Care* 1993; 38:373–387.

KOH Y. Ventilatory management of patients with severe asthma. *Int Anesthesiol Clin* 2001; 39:63–73.

MANSEL JK, STOGNER SW, PETRINI MF, NORMAN JR. Mechanical ventilation in patients with acute severe asthma. *Am J Med* 1990; 89:42–48.

MARINI JJ. Should PEEP be used in airflow obstruction. *Am Rev Respir Dis* 1991; 193:9–18.

SMITH TC, MARINI JJ. Impact of PEEP on lung mechanics and work-of-breathing in severe airflow obstruction. *J Appl Physiol* 1988; 65: 1488–1499.

TUXEN D, WILLIAMS T, SCHEINKESTEL C, ET AL. Use of a measurement of pulmonary hyperinflation to control the level of mechanical ventilation in patients with severe asthma. *Am Rev Respir Dis* 1992; 146: 1136–1142.

WILLIAMS TJ, TUXEN DV, SCHEINKESTEL CD, CZARNY D, BOWES G. Risk factors for morbidity in mechanically ventilated patients with acute severe asthma. *Am Rev Respir Dis* 1992; 146: 1136–1142.

TWENTY-ONE

BURNS AND INHALATION INJURY

OBJECTIVES

1. Describe the respiratory effects of surface burns and inhalation injury.
2. Discuss issues related to airway injury in patients with inhalation injury.
3. Describe the management of carbon monoxide poisoning.
4. Discuss the indications, initial ventilator settings, monitoring, and ventilator weaning for the patient with surface burns and inhalation injury.

INTRODUCTION

Respiratory complications are common in patients with burn injuries, and respiratory failure is a common cause of mortality in these patients. Pulmonary complications can occur at a number of times along the treatment course of burned patients (Table 21-1). Pulmonary complications are often associated with inhalation injury, but may occur in patients with severe surface burns who do not have inhalation injury. Mechanical ventilation is commonly necessary in burn patients who develop respiratory failure.

OVERVIEW

Surface Burns

Respiratory failure commonly occurs in patients with major cutaneous burns. Such patients often have associated inhalation injury, and the presence of inhalation injury significantly increases the mortality related with cutaneous burns. However, respiratory failure and the need for mechanical ventilation may occur in the absence of inhalation injury. There are recognized interactions between smoke inhalation and cutaneous burns (Figure 21-1). Pain management is an important aspect of the care of patients with burn injury, and may be associated with respiratory depression. Appropriate fluid management is difficult in patients with cutaneous burns, and fluid overload with associated hypoxemia and decreased lung compliance may occur. Sepsis can also occur, resulting in respiratory failure due to ARDS. Burn patients are typically hypermetabolic, which increases the ventilation requirement and may result in respiratory failure due to fatigue.

If full thickness circumferential burns of the thorax are present, severe chest wall restriction can occur. This will typically produce respiratory failure, and can

Table 21-1 Pulmonary complications present at various times in patients with burns and smoke inhalation

Complications	Time of occurrence
Carbon monoxide poisoning	Within the first hours of exposure
Upper airway obstruction	Within the first 48 hours following injury and post extubation
Tracheobronchial obstruction	Within the first 72 hours following injury
Pulmonary edema	Hypervolemia due to fluid resuscitation – first 48 hours;
	Hypervolemia due to fluid shifts – second to fourth day;
	sepsis – after the first week
Pneumonia	After the fifth day
Pulmonary embolism	After the first week

Adapted from information in HAPONIK EF. Smoke inhalation injuries: some priorities for respiratory care professionals. *Respir Care* 1992; 37:609–629.

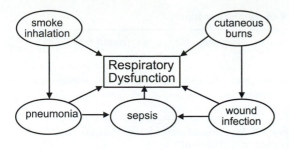

Figure 21-1 Respiratory dysfunction is central to the effects of smoke inhalation and cutaneous burns.

make mechanical ventilation difficult. High ventilating pressures may be required, but may not place the patient at risk for over-distention lung injury because the transpulmonary pressure may not be high due to the decreased chest wall compliance (Figure 21-2). Severe scarring and eschar formation can also restrict chest wall movement, and can result in difficulty weaning from mechanical ventilation. However, early surgical excision of the burn is commonly practiced, and this has reduced the need for escharotomies to improve chest wall compliance.

Inhalation Injury

Inhalation injury is associated with increased morbidity and mortality. The effects of inhalation injury can be grouped by those related to thermal injury, parenchymal injury, and system toxins. Clinical predictors of inhalation injury are listed in Table 21-2.

Thermal injury Because dry air has a low heat capacity, thermal injury to the lower respiratory tract is rare. However, inhalation of steam and explosive gases such as ether and propane can produce thermal injury to the lower respiratory tract. Thermal injury is almost always confined to the upper airway, which effec-

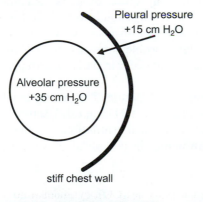

Figure 21-2 Effect of a stiff chest wall on trans-pulmonary pressure. If the chest wall is stiff, there will be a greater increase in pleural pressure. Transpulmonary pressure (the difference between the pressure inside and outside the alveolus) will be lower if the pleural pressure is increased. The amount of alveolar distention, and thus the risk of ventilator-induced lung injury, is thus decreased with a stiff chest wall. Moreover, the plateau pressure will not be a good indicator of distending pressure.

Table 21-2 Clinical predictors of inhalation injury

- Exposure characteristics: closed space or entrapment, unconscious, inhaled toxin known
- Burns to the face and neck
- Carbonaceous sputum
- Respiratory symptoms: hoarseness, sore throat, cough, dyspnea, chest pain, hemoptysis
- Respiratory signs: pharyngeal inflammation and burns, stridor, tachypnea, cyanosis, abnormal breathing sounds (wheezes, rhonchi, stridor)

Adapted from information in HAPONIK EF. Smoke inhalation injuries: some priorities for respiratory care professionals. *Respir Care* 1992; 37:609–619.

tively cools hot gas before it reaches the lower respiratory tract. Thermal injury to the upper airway results in laryngeal edema, laryngospasm, swollen vocal cords, and increased mucus production. The diagnosis is made by examination of the upper airway, often using bronchoscopy.

Problems related to thermal injury to the upper airway usually occur within the first 24 to 48 hours. Due to the risk of complete obstruction of the upper airway, the symptomatic patient should be intubated. Many of these patients also require mechanical ventilation due to other severe associated injuries. However, some patients do not require mechanical ventilation, and can breathe adequately once the endotracheal tube bypasses the upper airway obstruction. If respiratory failure does not occur, these patients can often be extubated after several days, provided the upper airway swelling has improved. Bronchoscopic examination of the upper airway may be necessary before extubation, to assess the potential for obstruction if the patient is extubated. Due to this injury of the upper airway, maintenance of a patent airway is paramount and vigilance is necessary to assure the security of the endotracheal tube. Securing the endotracheal tube can be difficult in patients with facial burns, and creative approaches for securing the airway are often necessary to prevent unplanned extubations.

Lower respiratory tract injury Although thermal injury to the lower respiratory tract is unusual, injury due to the toxic chemical composition of smoke is common. Smoke inhalation can be harmful to both the airways and lower respiratory tract. Smoke inhibits mucociliary transport and induces bronchospasm. Airway obstruction due to retained secretions is particularly problematic in patients with pre-existing lung disease, and severe bronchospasm can occur in patients with pre-existing asthma.

ARDS commonly occurs in patients with smoke inhalation. The management of ARDS in this setting is similar to the management of ARDS in other settings, and includes oxygen administration, PEEP, and mechanical ventilation. The management of ARDS resulting from smoke inhalation may be complicated by sepsis, pneumonia, and fluid overload.

Systemic toxins Systemic toxins include carbon monoxide (CO), cyanides, and a variety of nitrogen oxides. CO poisoning is the most important and the most common cause of death in fires. The toxicity of CO relates to the very high affinity of hemoglobin for CO, producing carboxyhemoglobin (COHb). COHb does not carry oxygen, and inhibits oxygen release from oxyhemoglobin (left-shifted oxyhemoglobin dissociation curve). Clinical effects of COHb are related to hypoxia (Table 21-3). The diagnosis is made based upon symptoms and measurement of blood COHb levels. Oxygen saturation and COHb levels must be measured using CO-oximetry. Arterial blood gases frequently demonstrate normal or increased Pa_{O_2}, hyperventilation, and metabolic acidosis. The lethal effects of COHb usually occur early after exposure. In patients who survive CO poisoning, symptoms may persist and occasionally get better and then worse.

The treatment for CO poisoning is oxygen administration. The half-life of COHb is four to five hrs breathing room air, 45 to 60 min breathing 100% oxygen, and 20 to 30 min breathing 100% oxygen at 3 atmospheres (hyperbaric oxygen). Use of 100% oxygen is thus mandatory in the treatment of COHb. Hyperbaric oxygen is useful if available, although its use is controversial. Hyperbaric oxygen may also be useful in patients with low COHb levels who have prolonged neurological symptoms. Airway management and mechanical ventilation may be necessary due to depressed neurological status.

MECHANICAL VENTILATION

Indications

Indications for mechanical ventilation in patients with burn injury and smoke inhalation are listed in Table 21-4. Although many of these patients require mechanical ventilation, airway management and inhalation of 100% oxygen are more important in some patients. For example, 100% oxygen is more important than mechanical ventilation in the spontaneously breathing patient with carbon

Table 21-3 Clinical effects of carbon monoxide poisoning

Carboxyhemoglobin level	Physiologic effect
< 1%	No effect
1 to 5%	Increase in blood flow to vital organs
5 to 10%	Increased visual light threshold, dyspnea on exertion, cutaneous blood vessel dilation
10 to 20%	Abnormal vision evoked response, throbbing headache
20 to 30%	Fatigue, irritability, poor judgment, diminished vision, diminished manual dexterity, nausea and vomiting
30 to 40%	Severe headache, confusion, syncope on exertion
40 to 60%	Convulsions, respiratory failure, coma and death with prolonged exposure
> 60%	Coma; rapid death

Table 21-4 Indications for mechanical ventilation in patients with burn injury and smoke inhalation

- Smoke inhalation or pulmonary burns with respiratory failure (ARDS)
- Severe burns with chest wall restriction
- Respiratory depression due to the pain control
- Respiratory depression due to inhalation of systemic toxins (carbon monoxide)
- Respiratory failure due to secondary infection – pneumonia, sepsis
- Postoperative skin grafting or escharotomy

monoxide poisoning. Moreover, mechanical ventilation without 100% oxygen in these patients may be lethal. Similarly, spontaneously breathing patients with upper airway obstruction due to smoke inhalation and thermal burns may need an artificial airway, but not necessarily mechanical ventilation.

Ventilator Settings

Recommendations for initial ventilator settings are listed in Table 21-5. An algorithm for initial ventilator management is shown in Figure 21-3. Full ventilatory support is often required initially, and can be provided by CMV (A/C). Pressure support is usually not appropriate as an initial ventilatory mode in this patient population. Many of these patients require sedation and paralysis when mechanical ventilation is initiated, and this is particularly true if chest wall compliance is decreased. High frequency percussive ventilation has been advocated in some burn centers in the management of these patients, although there is no clear evidence that this approach is superior to conventional modes of ventilation.

Oxygenation is dependant upon F_{IO_2}, mean airway pressure, and the extent of pulmonary dysfunction. If the patient has carbon monoxide poisoning, 100% oxygen is required until the measured carboxyhemoglobin level is less than

Table 21-5 Initial mechanical ventilator settings with burns and smoke inhalation

Setting	Recommendation
Mode	CMV (A/C)
Rate	15 to 20 breaths/min (lower if auto-PEEP is present)
Volume/pressure control	Either can be used, based upon bias of the clinical team
Tidal volume	8 to 12 mL/kg ideal body weight provided that plateau pressure < 30 cm H_2O; 4 to 8 mL/kg if ARDS is present
Inspiratory time	1 second
PEEP	5 cm H_2O; 10 cm H_2O if ARDS is present
F_{IO_2}	1.0 – particularly with carbon monoxide poisoning
Flow waveform	Descending ramp

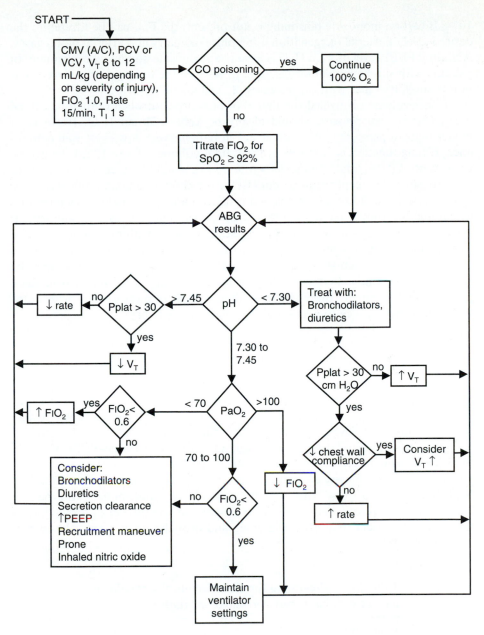

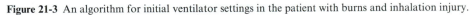

Figure 21-3 An algorithm for initial ventilator settings in the patient with burns and inhalation injury.

10%. If carbon monoxide poisoning is not present, the F_{IO_2} can be titrated to the desired level of arterial oxygenation using pulse oximetry and arterial blood gases. An initial PEEP level of 5 cm H_2O is usually appropriate and may be adequate. In patients with smoke inhalation resulting in ARDS, the management of oxygenation is similar to that with other causes of ARDS.

Either volume-controlled ventilation or pressure-controlled ventilation can be used. The plateau pressure should ideally be kept < 30 cm H_2O. However, a higher plateau pressure may be necessary in patients with low chest wall compliance. If lung function is relatively normal, tidal volumes of 8 to 12 mL/kg can be used. With ARDS, tidal volumes of 4 to 8 mL/kg should be used and the plateau pressure should be kept below 30 cm H_2O if the chest wall is not stiff. An initial respiratory rate of 15 to 20 breaths/min is usually adequate, and can be increased if required to produce the desired Pa_{CO_2}. Lower rates are necessary if auto-PEEP is present due to high airways resistance. Many patients with burn injury become hypermetabolic, and a high minute ventilation may be required to maintain a normal Pa_{CO_2}. In such patients, auto-PEEP is likely, and its presence must be monitored frequently. Permissive hypercapnia is usually well tolerated in these patients, and is usually more desirable than a high respiratory rate with auto-PEEP or a high airway pressure with associated lung injury.

Monitoring

Monitoring mechanically ventilated burn patients is similar in many aspects to that with any ventilated patient (Table 21-6). Pulse oximetry is unreliable if high carboxyhemoglobin levels are present, and should not be used in this circumstance. If minute ventilation is increased, the presence of auto-PEEP must be frequently evaluated. Chest wall compliance, and thus respiratory system compliance, can be decreased with chest wall burns and scar formation. Bronchospasm and auto-PEEP can be particularly problematic if the patient has a history of reactive airways disease. Increased production of airway secretions may also occur, requiring suctioning and bronchoscopy. Chest physiother-

Table 21-6 Monitoring for the mechanically ventilated patient with burn injury or smoke inhalation

- Auto-PEEP
- Peak pressure, plateau pressure, and mean airway pressure
- Airway resistance and respiratory system compliance
- Arterial blood gases
- Pulse oximetry if COHb < 5%
- Fluid intake and output
- Cardiac filling pressure (central venous pressure)
- Nutritional status and metabolic rate

apy should be avoided in these patients because it increases pain and metabolic rate. Fluid overload is a common problem in these patients, and can result in shunting and decreased lung compliance. Due to the high metabolic rates of these patients, nutritional support is necessary to facilitate healing and weaning from mechanical ventilation. Pulmonary embolism can occur in patients with prolonged immobility, and pulmonary infection is also common in these patients.

Weaning

If the extent of injury is not severe, discontinuation of mechanical ventilation for burn patients can occur early and quickly. For some patients, maintenance of a stable airway is a greater issue than ventilatory support. For patients with upper airway injury, a thorough evaluation of the upper airway (often including bronchoscopy) is required before extubation. If burn injury is severe and associated with ARDS, pulmonary infection, and sepsis, the mechanical ventilation course can be long and difficult. Some of these patients will be difficult to wean, particularly if they develop multi-system failure and malnutrition. These patients require prolonged weaning with periodic spontaneous breathing trials to assess the ability of the patient to breathe without assistance. For patients who are difficult to wean, the goals should be treatment of injuries and underlying pre-existing conditions, bronchodilation and bronchial hygiene, nutritional support, and strengthening and conditioning of respiratory muscles.

POINTS TO REMEMBER

- Respiratory complications are common in patients with burn injury and smoke inhalation.
- Thoracic surface burns can result in decreased chest wall compliance.
- Thermal injury can cause severe upper airway injury, but usually does not injure the lower respiratory tract.
- Smoke inhalation can cause bronchospasm and increased production of airway secretions.
- Smoke inhalation can produce ARDS.
- Carbon monoxide poisoning is a common cause of mortality in patients with smoke inhalation.
- Breathing 100% oxygen is mandatory to treat carbon monoxide poisoning, and hyperbaric oxygen may be useful.
- Ventilatory requirements of burn patients can be high due to hypermetabolism.
- Decreased chest wall compliance, decreased lung compliance, and increased airway resistance can make ventilation difficult in the patient with burn injury and smoke inhalation.

ADDITIONAL READING

BARRET JP, DESAI MH, HERNDON DN. Effects of tracheostomies on infection and airway complications in pediatric burn patients. *Burns* 2000; 26:190–193.

CORTIELLA J, MLCAK R, HERNDON D. High frequency percussive ventilation in pediatric patients with inhalation injury. *J Burn Care Rehabil* 1999; 20:232–235.

DANCEY DR, HAYES J, GOMEZ M, ET AL. ARDS in patients with thermal injury. *Intensive Care Med* 1999; 25:1231–1236.

FITZPATRICK JC, CIOFFI WG JR. Ventilatory support following burns and smoke-inhalation injury. *Respir Care Clin N Am* 1997; 3:21–49.

MLCAK R, CORTIELLA J, DESAI M, HERNDON D. Lung compliance, airway resistance, and work-of-breathing in children after inhalation injury. *J Burn Care Rehabil* 1997; 18:531–534

SELLERS BJ, DAVIS BL, LARKIN PW, ET AL. Early prediction of prolonged ventilator dependence in thermally injured patients. *J Trauma* 1997; 43:899–903.

SHERIDAN RL. Airway management and respiratory care of the burn patient. *Int Anesthesiol Clin* 2000; 38:129–145.

TWENTY-TWO

BRONCHOPLEURAL FISTULA

OBJECTIVES

1. Describe the pathophysiology of bronchopleural fistula.
2. List techniques to minimize air leak.
3. Discuss the mechanical ventilation of patients with bronchopleural fistula.

INTRODUCTION

Pneumothorax, subcutaneous emphysema, pneumomediastinum, pneumoperi-cardium and other forms of extra alveolar air are referred to as barotrauma or volutrauma. A bronchopleural fistula is a persistent leak from the lung into the pleural space, identified by either intermittent (during inspiration) or con-tinuous chest tube air leak. Most barotrauma occurs in patients with trauma,

ARDS, COPD, and asthma. Although properly treated extra-alveolar air and bronchopleural fistula are not usually life threatening problems, they do complicate ventilator management.

OVERVIEW

Pathophysiology

Extra-alveolar air can develop with trauma, surgical procedures, and vascular line placement. During mechanical ventilation, extra-alveolar air forms as a result of alveolar rupture to allow gas to enter the adjacent bronchovascular sheath and dissect into the pleural space. Pulmonary disease, high pressure and over-distention must be present for extra-alveolar gas to develop. Extra-alveolar air develops most frequently in COPD and ARDS patients, particularly if complicated by necrotizing pneumonia. Avoiding auto-PEEP and keeping peak alveolar pressure < 30 cm H_2O avoids the setting where alveolar rupture is facilitated.

Techniques to Minimize Air Leak

Pneumothorax during mechanical ventilation is treated with chest tube drainage and suction. The combination of negative pleural pressure from the chest tube (−20 cm H_2O) and positive pressure from the ventilator establishes a high pressure gradient across the lung and may facilitate the development of a bronchopleural fistula. If a fistula develops, flow through the fistula is determined by the magnitude and duration of the pressure gradient across the lung. Ideally, the approach used to provide mechanical ventilation should minimize pressure (peak inspiratory pressure, plateau pressure, PEEP, and mean alveolar pressure), inspiratory time, and chest tube suction to avoid accumulation of pleural air. Some clinicians recommend independent lung ventilation or high frequency ventilation. Others have proposed manipulation of the chest tube suction system. Two specific approaches to modify chest tube suction are intermittent inspiratory chest tube occlusion and the application of intrapleural pressure equivalent to the level of PEEP. Anecdotal experience with these maneuvers demonstrates a decrease in the air leak but collapse of lung units is common and neither technique has resulted in improved outcome.

Although leak from a bronchopleural fistula should be avoided if possible, it is important to recognize that CO_2 elimination occurs through the fistula. The CO_2 concentration leaving the fistula may be similar to that exhaled from the endotracheal tube. In most cases the fistula does not close until the underlying disease process has resolved. The presence of a bronchopleural fistula is an ominous sign. However, patients usually do not die from a bronchopleural fistula – they die with a bronchopleural fistula.

MECHANICAL VENTILATION

Indications

A bronchopleural fistula or other type of extra-alveolar air is not by itself an indication for mechanical ventilation. Its presence, however, increases the potential for problems with gas exchange. Indications for mechanical ventilation in this setting are apnea, acute ventilatory failure, impending acute ventilatory failure, or oxygenation deficit (Table 22-1).

Ventilator Settings

The goal of ventilator settings is to reduce the pressure gradient across the lung. Thus the plateau pressure, mean airway pressure, and PEEP should be minimized (Table 22-2 and Figure 22-1). A ventilatory pattern should be chosen that results in the least gas exiting the fistula, provided gas exchange targets are met. The use of pressure ventilation in this setting allows the ability to control peak alveolar pressure. However, pressure-controlled ventilation may increase the leak through the fistula because it maintains alveolar pressure constant throughout the inspiratory phase. The choice of pressure-controlled or volume-controlled ventilation should be determined by the mode that minimizes air leak through the fistula.

Some of these patients require paralysis to establish the lowest air leak across the fistula and acceptable cardiopulmonary function. Whether spontaneous breathing should be allowed depends upon the severity of the underlying disease process and the hemodynamics and gas exchange during spontaneous breathing. Pressure support ventilation should be used cautiously. With pressure support, inspiration terminates when flow decelerates to a predetermined level. If the leak across the fistula is greater than this level, the ventilator will not appropriately cycle from inspiration to exhalation during pressure support ventilation. Moreover, suction applied to the chest tube may trigger the ventilator.

Permissive hypercapnia and the acceptance of low arterial oxygenation ($Pa_{O_2} > 50$ mm Hg) are necessary for some of these patients. This is particularly

Table 22-1 Indications for mechanical ventilation

Bronchopleural fistula is not by itself an indication for mechanical ventilation but may be necessary in the following settings:
- Apnea
- Acute ventilatory failure
- Impending acute ventilatory failure
- Oxygenation deficit

Table 22-2 Mechanical ventilator settings for bronchopleural fistula

Setting	Recommendation
Mode	A/C (CMV)
Rate	6 to 20/min or greater, dependent on underlying disease and air trapping
Volume/pressure control	Pressure or volume control; avoid pressure support due to failure of expiratory cycle due to leak through fistula
Tidal volume	Plateau pressure < 30 cm H_2O; V_T 4–8 mL/kg
Inspiratory time	≤ 1 s depending on air leak
PEEP	As low as possible; dependent on oxygenation
FIO_2	High F_{IO_2} more desirable than high pressure; $Pa_{O_2} > 50$ mm Hg
Flow waveform	Descending ramp
Mean airway pressure	Lowest level to achieve $Pa_{O_2} > 50$ mm Hg; ideally < 15 cm H_2O

true if the underlying disease state is ARDS, COPD or trauma. Respiratory rate is set high enough to maximize CO_2 elimination but low enough to minimize fistula leak and air trapping. Depending on the underlying disease state, this may be a rate as low as 6/min or as high as 20/min.

Management of oxygenation is difficult with a bronchopleural fistula, since PEEP used to treat oxygenation increases the leak. As a result, a high F_{IO_2} is needed. PEEP should either not be applied or used at the minimal level necessary to recruit atelectatic areas. The goal is to minimize PEEP and mean airway pressure. However, particularly in ARDS and trauma, the oxygenation deficit may be severe and higher levels of PEEP required.

Independent Lung Ventilation

The use of a double lumen endotracheal tube with two ventilators (either synchronized or asynchronous) has been proposed for the management of severe bronchopleural fistula. This approach is only recommended when the fistula is the result of disruption of a large airway or where maintenance of an acceptable level of gas exchange is impossible and surgical intervention is planned. This should be considered a short-term solution. Of concern with independent lung ventilation is the potential damage to both the trachea and mainstem bronchi resulting from the use of a double lumen tube, the difficulty of maintaining proper position of the tube, the difficulty with suctioning and secretion clearance, and the technical issues due to the use of two ventilators. Settings on the two ventilators should be based on the pathology of the ventilated lung. Each lung may be ventilated in a similar manner but with lower pressures and volumes to the affected lung or with CPAP alone to the affected lung. The volume of the air leak, as well as hemodynamic and gas exchange stability, are the key variables used to determine the adequacy of ventilator settings.

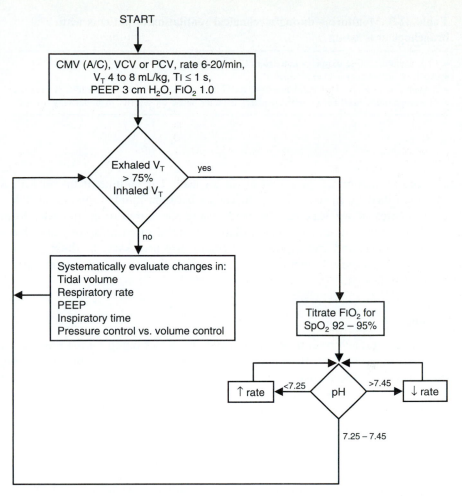

Figure 22-1 An algorithm for mechanical ventilation of the patient with bronchopleural fistula.

High Frequency Ventilation

Little data other than case studies support improved outcome with high frequency ventilation. The use of high frequency ventilation is not recommended. Lack of accepted management protocols, high cost of the equipment, a limited number of patients requiring the technology, and lack of data indicating improved outcome all support this recommendation. Many centers that frequently used high frequency ventilation for this purpose in the past have abandoned its use.

Monitoring

Key concerns during monitoring of patients with a bronchopleural fistula (Table 22-3) are assurance of adequate gas exchange (pulse oximetry and arterial blood

Table 22-3 Monitoring during mechanical ventilation of patients with bronchopleural fistula

- Gas exchange: pulse oximetry and arterial blood gases
- Air leak: inspiratory and expiratory V_T
- System pressures: peak alveolar pressure, mean airway pressure, and end-expiratory pressure
- Hemodynamics: need for pulmonary artery catheter based on severity of underlying disease

gases) and evaluation of the extent of the air leak. The volume of the air leak is easily quantified by measuring the difference between inhaled and exhaled V_T. Such estimates of air leak can be made using the monitoring and waveform capabilities of current generation ventilators. Careful monitoring of peak alveolar, mean airway, and end-expiratory pressures are necessary. In those patients with severe lung injury or hemodynamic instability, the use of a pulmonary artery catheter is indicated.

Weaning

The specific approach used to wean these patients is not based on the presence of the fistula, but rather on the underlying disease. In general, as the underlying disease improves, the fistula begins to close. The presence of a fistula is not an indication to continue mechanical ventilation. Weaning guidelines are not specific to the presence of a bronchopleural fistula.

POINTS TO REMEMBER

- Extra-alveolar air occurs most commonly in patients with trauma, ARDS, and COPD.
- Disease, high pressure and over-distention are required for extra-alveolar air to occur.
- Air leak is minimized by maintaining the lowest possible pressure (peak alveolar, mean airway and end-expiratory) and short inspiratory times.
- The CO_2 concentration in the gas from the fistula may be similar to that exhaled through the ventilator.
- The goal with ventilator settings is to maintain the lowest pressure gradient across the fistula and to achieve minimally acceptable gas exchange targets (permissive hypercapnia, $Pa_{O_2} > 50$ mm Hg).
- Independent lung ventilation is only indicated in the presence of bronchial air leaks, where gas exchange is impossible, and only for short-term use.
- Monitor system pressures, volume of the air leak, gas exchange and hemodynamics.
- Weaning guidelines are based on the underlying disease state.

ADDITIONAL READING

BISHOP MJ, BENSON MS, SATO P, PIERSON DJ. Comparison of high-frequency jet ventilation with conventional mechanical ventilation for bronchopleural fistula. *Anesth Anal* 1987; 66:833–838.

PETERSON HP, BAIER H. Incidence of pulmonary barotrauma in a medical ICU. *Crit Care Med* 1983; 11:786–791.

PIERSON DJ. Barotrauma and bronchopleural fistula. In: TOBIN MJ, ed. *Principles and Practice of Mechanical Ventilation*. New York, McGraw-Hill Inc., 1994, 813–836.

TWENTY-THREE

DRUG OVERDOSE

OBJECTIVES

1. Describe the presentation of a patient with acute drug overdose.
2. Discuss the initial ventilator settings for patients with acute drug overdose.
3. Describe the monitoring and ventilator weaning of patients from mechanical ventilation.

INTRODUCTION

When considering patients who require mechanical ventilation, those where the indication is drug overdose comprise a very small percentage. However, many of these patients require immediate intubation and mechanical ventilation – often by prehospital personnel.

OVERVIEW

The patient presenting with a drug overdose is frequently obtunded, stuporous and unable to effectively maintain spontaneous breathing. However, with some classes of drugs (e.g., tricyclic antidepressants) central nervous system hyperactivity may be the initial clinical presentation. If ingested in sufficient quantity, all drugs can result in respiratory depression and necessitate intubation and mechanical ventilation (Table 23-1). In addition, cardiovascular compromise commonly occurs with many types of drug overdoses. Narcotics and sedatives frequently result in hypotension, while tricyclic antidepressants and cocaine can cause life-threatening arrhythmias. The length of ventilatory support may be short or prolonged depending on the drug ingested, the quantity ingested, and the presence of underlying lung disease or complications. Patients may have periods of wakefulness and profound respiratory depression. Even when the quantity of ingested drug is insufficient to depress spontaneous breathing, risk of aspiration may still be a primary concern necessitating close observation or intubation for airway protection.

MECHANICAL VENTILATION

Indications

Patients with drug overdose are intubated to facilitate mechanical ventilation and for airway protection. Mechanical ventilation is usually initiated due to apnea or acute ventilatory failure. Oxygenation is often not a concern with these patients unless aspiration has occurred.

Ventilator Settings

These patients are not difficult to ventilate unless aspiration has occurred. They tend to be young and otherwise healthy without underlying lung disease. The ventilatory mode of choice is A/C (CMV) provided with either pressure or volume ventilation (Table 23-2 and Figure 23-1). Any mode with a backup rate is acceptable. Since the lungs are normal, V_T of 8 to 12 mL/kg is usually adequate with a rate of 10/min dependent on Pa_{CO_2}. If volume ventilation is selected, an inspira-

Table 23-1 Indications for mechanical ventilation in patients with drug overdose

- Apnea
- Acute respiratory failure
- Impending acute respiratory failure

Table 23-2 Initial mechanical ventilator settings with drug overdose

Setting	Recommendation
Mode	A/C (CMV)
Rate	10/min
Volume/pressure control	Volume or pressure
Tidal volume	8 to 12 mL/kg
Inspiratory time	0.8 to 1 s
PEEP	3 to 5 cm H_2O to maintain functional residual capacity
FI_{O_2}	≤ 0.40 is usually adequate
Flow waveform	Rectangular or descending ramp
Mean airway pressure	Lowest necessary to maintain $Pa_{O_2} \geq 80$ mm Hg

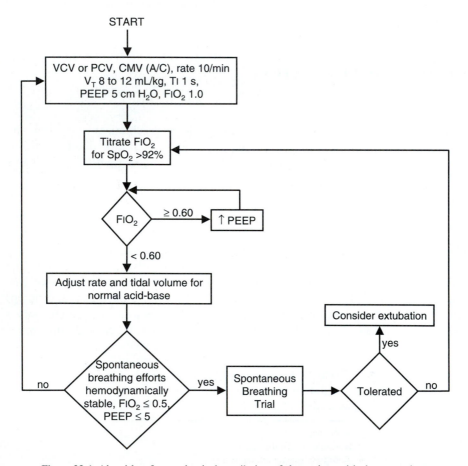

Figure 23-1 Algorithm for mechanical ventilation of the patient with drug overdose.

tory time of 0.8 to 1 s with a peak flow of ≥ 60 L/min is usually necessary. Inspiratory flow waveform may be either rectangular or ramp. With pressure ventilation, the pressure control level should be set to provide the desired V_T with inspiratory times 0.8–1 s. Since oxygenation is not a concern, $F_{IO_2} \leq 0.40$ is usually adequate to maintain normal Pa_{O_2} (> 80 mm Hg). PEEP is usually not necessary, although the use of 3–5 cm H_2O to maintain functional residual capacity is acceptable provided cardiovascular function is stable and the addition of PEEP does not adversely affect cardiac output. Since many ingested drugs produce profound peripheral vasodilation, concern regarding mean airway pressure is warranted.

Monitoring

Regurgitation and aspiration are the primary concerns with overdose patients, and precautions should be taken until the patient is ready for extubation. Nasogastric suction reduces the likelihood of aspiration. However, even with a nasogastric tube it is important that the endotracheal tube cuff is adequately inflated. Hemodynamic stability is a concern with many overdose patients and life-threatening arrhythmias may occur. Monitoring of ECG and systemic arterial blood pressure is indicated. Since underlying lung disease is not usually an issue, monitoring of arterial blood gases is needed infrequently, but frequent evaluation of acid-base balance may be necessary with some ingested drugs (e.g., salicylates). In some cases, alkalinization including respiratory alkalosis may be indicated to facilitate clearance of the ingested drug. Since mechanical ventilation is indicated for respiratory depression, careful monitoring of the level of consciousness and patient-ventilator synchrony are necessary. Many patients become agitated and combative as their level of neurologic depression decreases (Table 23-3).

Weaning

Discontinuation of ventilatory support is indicated when the drug is sufficiently cleared to allow spontaneous ventilation. Once patients are awake and concern regarding neurologic relapse is eliminated, discontinuation of mechanical ventilation is indicated. Since many overdoses are intentional, patients frequently awake agitated, angry or depressed. Of concern are sedative overdoses where the drug is

Table 23-3 Monitoring of the mechanically ventilated patients with drug overdose

- Observation for regurgitation and aspiration
- ECG and arterial pressure
- Acid-base balance
- Level of consciousness
- Patient-ventilator synchrony

highly lipid soluble and slowly released into the systemic circulation. These patients may fluctuate between periods of wakefulness and sedation. Premature ventilator discontinuance in this setting could be disastrous.

POINTS TO REMEMBER

- Many drugs have the potential of causing respiratory depression if sufficient quantity is ingested.
- In some patients, airway protection may be a greater issue than ventilation.
- Oxygenation is rarely a concern unless the patient has aspirated.
- Because of the potential for hemodynamic instability, PEEP may not be useful.
- Monitoring for aspiration, hemodynamic stability, and arrhythmias is critical.
- Inflation of the endotracheal tube cuff is necessary.
- Discontinue ventilatory support when neurologic function has returned to normal.
- Some drugs may cause fluctuation between periods of wakefulness and periods of sedation.

ADDITIONAL READING

HENDERSON A, WRIGHT M, POND SM. Experience with 732 acute overdose patients admitted to an intensive care unit over six years. *Med J Aust* 1993; 158:28–30.
TAITELMAN U, ELLENHORN MJ. General management of poisoning. In: HALL JB, SCHMIDT GA, WOOD LDH. *Principles of Critical Care*. New York, McGraw-Hill, 1992, pp. 2051–2060.

PART THREE

MONITORING DURING MECHANICAL VENTILATION

TWENTY-FOUR

ARTERIAL AND VENOUS BLOOD GASES

OBJECTIVES

1. List causes of hypoxemia and hypoxia.
2. Describe the oxyhemoglobin dissociation curve.
3. Describe the relationship between Pa_{CO_2}, alveolar ventilation, and carbon dioxide production.
4. Discuss the use of intra-arterial blood gas monitors and point-of-care analyzers.

5. List causes of respiratory and metabolic acid-base disturbances.
6. Use the anion gap to differentiate causes of metabolic acidosis.
7. Use the strong ion difference to differentiate acid-base disturbances.
8. Discuss the controversy related to temperature adjustment of blood gases and pH.

INTRODUCTION

Blood gas and pH measurements are an important part of the care of the mechanically ventilated patient and allow evaluation of oxygenation, ventilation, and acid-base balance. Both arterial and mixed venous blood gases can be assessed. It is also possible to continuously monitor arterial blood gases via optode systems and mixed venous oxygen saturation via pulmonary artery oximetry catheters. Increasingly, point-of-care systems can be used to measure pH, blood gases, electrolytes, and hematology at the bedside.

ARTERIAL BLOOD GASES AND pH

Although an integral component of the care of mechanically ventilated patients, excessive blood gas measurements are commonly obtained in critically ill patients. In fact, the presence of an arterial catheter may encourage increased phlebotomy for blood gas and other laboratory measurements. The use of institutional guidelines may be useful to improve the effective use of blood gases; in other words, limiting the drawing of unnecessary blood gases. Blood gases only provide data at a single point in time and fluctuate in stable critically ill patients without any change in therapy or the clinical status. A trend in blood gas (as well as other laboratory) values is usually more useful than a single isolated number. Response to a single value should be avoided unless gross abnormalities are identified.

Pa_{O_2}

The total oxygen content is a combination of dissolved oxygen and that combined with hemoglobin. The amount dissolved in plasma is small and directly related to the P_{O_2}. The normal range of Pa_{O_2} is 80 to 100 mm Hg in healthy young persons breathing room air at sea level, and decreases with age and altitude. Hypoxemia occurs when the lungs fail to adequately oxygenate arterial blood. Pa_{O_2} is a reflection of lung function and not hypoxia per se. Hypoxia can occur without hypoxemia and vice versa. The adequate Pa_{O_2} in critically ill mechanically ventilated patients is unknown, but many clinicians would agree that a $Pa_{O_2} > 60$ mm Hg (producing a $Sa_{O_2} > 90\%$) is usually acceptable. The adequacy of Pa_{O_2} must be balanced against the potentially toxic effects of Fi_{O_2} and airway pressure. Causes of hypoxemia and hypoxia are listed in Table 24-1.

Table 24-1 Clinical causes of hypoxemia and hypoxia

Hypoxemia
- Decreased inspired oxygen: altitude
- Shunt: atelectasis, pneumonia, pulmonary edema, ARDS
- Diffusion defect: pulmonary fibrosis, emphysema, pulmonary resection
- Hypoventilation: respiratory center depression, neuromuscular disease
- Poor distribution of ventilation: airway secretions, bronchospasm

Hypoxia
- Hypoxemic hypoxia: a lower than normal Pa_{O_2} (hypoxemia)
- Anemic hypoxia: decreased red blood cell count, carboxyhemoglobin, hemoglobinopathy
- Circulatory hypoxia: decreased cardiac output, decreased local perfusion
- Affinity hypoxia: decreased release of oxygen from hemoglobin to the tissues
- Histotoxic hypoxia: cyanide poisoning

Sa_{O_2}

The relationship between Pa_{O_2} and oxygen saturation of hemoglobin is described by the oxyhemoglobin dissociation curve (Figure 24-1). This is a sigmoid relationship, with hemoglobin having a greater affinity for oxygen at a high P_{O_2} (e.g., in the lungs, where the P_{O_2} is high) and a lower affinity for oxygen at a lower P_{O_2} (e.g., in the tissues, where P_{O_2} is low). The affinity of hemoglobin for oxygen is also affected by the environment of the hemoglobin molecule, which can shift the curve to the left or to the right. Shifts of the curve to the right decrease the affinity of hemoglobin for oxygen (promote oxygen unloading), and shifts of the curve to the left increase the affinity of hemoglobin for oxygen (promote oxygen binding). Because of the variable relationship between hemoglobin saturation and P_{O_2}, saturation cannot be precisely predicted from P_{O_2}, and vice versa. To accurately evaluate oxygen saturation, CO-oximetry should be performed. CO-oximetry also

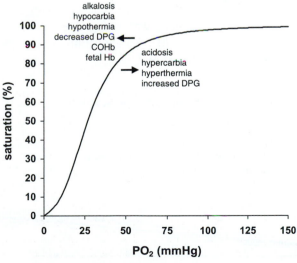

Figure 24-1 Oxyhemoglobin dissociation curve and factors that shift the curve.

allows measurement of total hemoglobin concentration, oxygen saturation, methemoglobin level, and carboxyhemoglobin level.

Pa_{CO_2}

The adequacy of alveolar ventilation is usually assessed by the Pa_{CO_2} due to the relationship between Pa_{CO_2}, $\dot{V}_A$, and $\dot{V}_{CO_2}$. Thus, Pa_{CO_2} is an indication of the body's ability to sustain alveolar ventilation adequate for $\dot{V}_{CO_2}$. $\dot{V}_{CO_2}$ is determined by the metabolic rate and is normally about 200 mL/min. An increase in $\dot{V}_{CO_2}$ requires a higher $\dot{V}_E$. Dead space affects the relationship between $\dot{V}_E$ and Pa_{CO_2}. Minute ventilation must increase to maintain the same Pa_{CO_2} in the presence of an increased dead space. Clinical causes of hypoventilation (increased Pa_{CO_2}) and hyperventilation (decreased Pa_{CO_2}) are listed in Table 24-2. Although a goal of mechanical ventilation has traditionally been to normalize Pa_{CO_2}, an elevated Pa_{CO_2} (permissive hypercapnia) may be more desirable than the high alveolar pressure required to normalize the Pa_{CO_2}.

Acid-Base Balance

Acid-base balance is explained by the Henderson-Hasselbalch Equation:

$$pH = 6.1 + \log[HCO_3^-]/(0.03 \times P_{CO_2})$$

Metabolic acid-base disturbances are those that affect the numerator of the Henderson-Hasselbalch Equation, and respiratory acid-base disturbances are those things that affect the denominator. The pH is normal (7.40) whenever the ratio $[HCO_3^-]/(0.03 \times P_{CO_2})$ is 20:1. The metabolic component of acid-base interpretation is usually given as the $[HCO_3^-]$. The metabolic component can also be expressed as base excess (BE). BE can be estimated as:

$$BE = [HCO_3^-] - 24$$

In other words, a $[HCO_3^-] < 24$ mmol/L corresponds with a negative BE, and a $[HCO_3^-] > 24$ mmol/L corresponds with a positive BE. An algorithm for classification of acid-base disturbances is shown in Figure 24-2.

Table 24-2 Clinical causes of hypoventilation and hyperventilation

Hypoventilation
- Respiratory center depression: pathologic, iatrogenic
- Disruption of neural pathways affecting respiratory muscles: neuropathy, trauma
- Neuromuscular blockade: disease, paralyzing agents
- Respiratory muscle weakness: fatigue, disease

Hyperventilation
- Respiratory center stimulation: hypoxia, anxiety, central nervous system pathology
- Metabolic acidosis
- Iatrogenic – mechanical ventilation

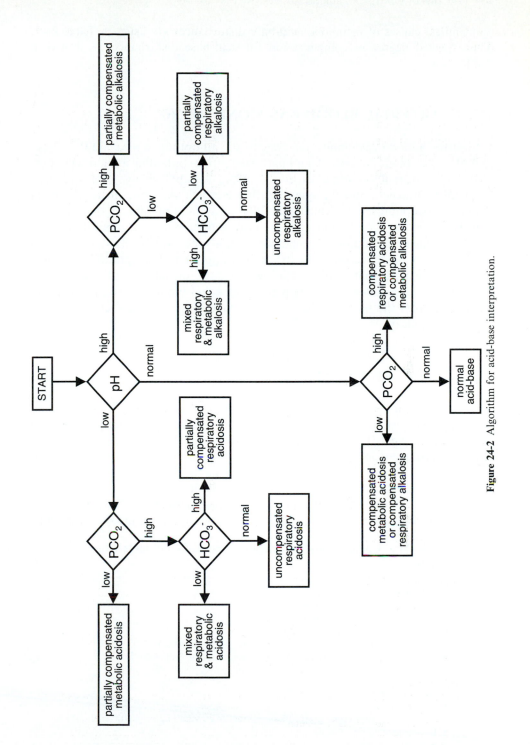

Figure 24-2 Algorithm for acid-base interpretation.

Clinical causes of metabolic acid-base disturbances are listed in Table 24-3. The expected degree of compensation for acid-base disturbances is shown in Table 24-4.

INTRA-ARTERIAL BLOOD GAS MONITORING

Intra-arterial blood gas monitoring systems use an optode to measure P_{O_2}, P_{CO_2}, and pH. The optode consists of a miniaturized probe containing a fluorescent dye. The dye changes fluorescence as the P_{O_2}, P_{CO_2} and pH change (pH and P_{CO_2} augment fluorescence and P_{O_2} quenches fluorescence). An optic fiber leads from the probe to a photosensor, which quantifies the amount of light emitted from the dye. There are two clinical approaches to intra-arterial blood gas monitoring. One approach passes the optode through an arterial line, which allows continuous monitoring of blood gases. With the second approach, the optode is attached to the proximal arterial catheter; this system does not allow continuous blood gas monitoring, but does allow frequent on-demand blood gas analysis with no blood loss from the patient. The clinical impact and cost effectiveness of these systems is unclear.

POINT-OF-CARE MONITORS

There has been increasing interest in point-of-care (POC) testing, in which blood gases are measured at or near the bedside. POC testing devices are portable and some are hand-held. They typically require only a few drops of blood for testing. Blood is introduced into a single use disposable cartridge that is introduced into the portable analyzer. The cartridge determines the specific tests (e.g., blood gases, electrolytes, hematocrit, glucose, BUN, creatinine, ionized calcium, and others). Analysis of the blood is performed by passing the sample over biosensors. The role of POC testing is evolving. Quality control and quality assurance issues must

Table 24-3 Clinical causes of metabolic acidosis and metabolic alkalosis

Metabolic acidosis
- Lactic acidosis (e.g., hypoxia)
- Ketoacidosis (e.g., uncontrolled diabetes)
- Uremic acidosis (e.g., renal failure)
- Loss of base from lower gastrointestinal tract (e.g., diarrhea)
- Loss of base from kidneys (e.g., diamox, renal tubular acidosis)
- Poisons (e.g., methanol, ethylene glycol, aspirin)

Metabolic alkalosis
- Hypokalemia
- Loss of acid from upper gastrointestinal tract (e.g., vomiting or gastric suction)
- Bicarbonate administration

Table 24-4 Expected compensation for acid-base disturbances

Respiratory acidosis	Respiratory alkalosis
$\Delta HCO_3^- = 0.10 \times \Delta Pa_{CO_2}$ (acute)	$\Delta HCO_3^- = 0.20 \times \Delta Pa_{CO_2}$ (acute)
$\Delta HCO_3^- = 0.35 \times \Delta Pa_{CO_2}$ (chronic)	$\Delta HCO_3^- = 0.5 \times \Delta Pa_{CO_2}$ (chronic)
Metabolic acidosis	**Metabolic alkalosis**
$Pa_{CO_2} = 1.5 \times HCO_3^- + 8$	$Pa_{CO_2} = 0.9 \times HCO_3^- + 15$

If the acid-base status exceeds the expected level of compensation, a mixed acid-base disturbance is present.

be appropriately addressed. The cost of the basic unit and the single use cartridges must be balanced against a more rapid turn-around time for blood gases and other tests and the smaller blood volume required for testing.

MIXED VENOUS BLOOD GASES

To assess mixed venous blood gases ($P\bar{v}_{O_2}$ and $P\bar{v}_{CO_2}$), blood is obtained from the distal port of the pulmonary artery catheter. To avoid contamination of the sample with pulmonary capillary (i.e., oxygenated) blood, the sample is withdrawn slowly with the balloon deflated. These samples are used not only to assess venous blood gases, but also to calculate shunt.

$P\bar{v}_{O_2}$

Normal $P\bar{v}_{O_2}$ is 40 mm Hg, and is a global indication of the level of tissue oxygenation. However, it has also been demonstrated that normal or supranormal values of $P\bar{v}_{O_2}$ can co-exist with severe tissue hypoxia caused primarily by arterial admixture, septicemia, hemorrhagic shock, congestive heart failure, and some febrile states. Further, $P\bar{v}_{O_2}$ reveals little about the oxygenation status of individual tissue beds. Factors affecting $P\bar{v}_{O_2}$ can be illustrated from rearrangement of the Fick Equation:

$$C\bar{v}_{O_2} = Ca_{O_2} - \dot{V}_{O_2}/\dot{Q}$$

$C\bar{v}_{O_2}$ (and its components $P\bar{v}_{O_2}$ and $S\bar{v}_{O_2}$) is decreased with decreases in Ca_{O_2} (i.e., Pa_{O_2}, O_2Hb, or Hb), decreases in $\dot{Q}$, or increases in $\dot{V}_{O_2}$. Note that an increase in $\dot{V}_{O_2}$ with a proportional increase in $\dot{Q}$ does not affect $C\bar{v}_{O_2}$ (e.g., exercise). Also note that breathing 100% oxygen by persons with normal lung function does not affect $C\bar{v}_{O_2}$ because increasing the Pa_{O_2} affects Ca_{O_2} very little (i.e., oxygen is very insoluble in blood and the hemoglobin is nearly 100% saturated when breathing room air). In patients with abnormal lung function, a decrease in $P\bar{v}_{O_2}$ may produce a decrease in Pa_{O_2}.

Venous Oximetry

Venous oximetry monitors $S\bar{v}_{O_2}$ using a system incorporated into the pulmonary artery catheter. Light is reflected off red blood cells near the pulmonary artery catheter and $S\bar{v}_{O_2}$ is determined as the ratio of transmitted and reflected light. Several commercially available systems are obtainable and differ in the number of reference wavelengths and detecting filaments. The clinical benefit of monitoring venous oximetry is unclear. This monitor is often not helpful clinically due to imprecision in the measurement system and the nonspecific nature of $S\bar{v}_{O_2}$ as discussed above.

$P\bar{v}_{CO_2}$

$P\bar{v}_{CO_2}$ is a global indication of tissue P_{CO_2}. Normal $P\bar{v}_{CO_2}$ is 45 mm Hg, which is only slightly greater than Pa_{CO_2}. Under conditions of low perfusion (e.g., cardiac arrest), there can be a great disparity between Pa_{CO_2} and $P\bar{v}_{CO_2}$. Under these conditions, a respiratory acidosis can be present at the tissue level and in the venous circulation, concurrent with a respiratory alkalosis in the arterial circulation. Pa_{CO_2} is determined by $\dot{V}_A$, whereas $P\bar{v}_{CO_2}$ is determined by perfusion (Figure 24-3).

ANION GAP AND OSMOL GAP

The anion gap (AG) is useful to differentiate causes of metabolic acidosis. Metabolic acidosis can be associated with a normal anion gap (hyperchloremic acidosis) or with an increased anion gap (normochloremic acidosis). The anion gap is calculated as:

$$AG = [Na^+] - ([Cl^-] + [HCO_3^-])$$

A normal anion gap is 8–12 mmol/L. Causes of metabolic acidosis with an increased anion gap include lactic acidosis, diabetic ketoacidosis, and azotemic (renal) acidosis. Causes of metabolic acidosis with a normal anion gap include loss

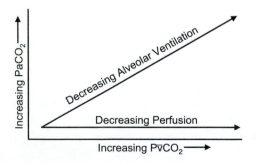

Figure 24-3 Arterial P_{CO_2} is determined by alveolar ventilation, and mixed venous P_{CO_2} is determined by perfusion.

of bicarbonate from the gastrointestinal tract (e.g., diarrhea), acetazolamide (diamox) therapy, or excessive chloride administration (e.g., HCl, NH_4Cl).

The osmol gap is the difference between the measured osmolality of the plasma and that calculated as:

$$osmol = 2[Na^+] + [glucose]/18 + [BUN]/2.8 + [ethanol]/4.6$$

where osmol is osmolality and BUN is the blood urea nitrogen. If the measured osmolality is more than 10 above that calculated, there may be unmeasured osmotically active particles present, whose metabolites may be organic acids. Metabolic acidosis with an osmol gap is consistent with the presence of the toxins methanol and ethylene glycol.

STRONG ION DIFFERENCE

The Strong Ion Difference (SID) is a method of evaluating acid-base disturbances based on Stewart's approach to acid-base chemistry. Using Stewart's approach, the only variables that affect pH are the P_{CO_2}, SID, and the concentration of unmeasured strong ions. SID is calculated as:

$$SID = [Na^+ + K^+] - [Cl^-]$$

Alternatively, SID is calculated as:

$$SID = [HCO_3^-] + 0.28 \times albumin\ (g/L) + inorganic\ phosphate\ (mmol/L)$$

The normal value for SID is 40 mmol/L. Classification of primary acid-base disturbances using SID is shown in Table 24-5. Metabolic acidosis is associated with a decreased SID and metabolic alkalosis is associated with an increased SID.

TEMPERATURE ADJUSTMENT OF BLOOD GASES AND pH

Blood gases and pH are measured at $37°C$ (normal body temperature). If the patient's temperature is abnormal, then the *in vivo* blood gas and pH values will differ from those measured and reported by the blood gas laboratory. The use of

Table 24-5 Classification of primary acid-base disturbances using Stewart's approach

	Acidosis	Alkalosis
Respiratory	$\uparrow P_{CO_2}$	$\downarrow P_{CO_2}$
Metabolic		
Water excess or deficit	$\downarrow$ SID, $\downarrow Na^+$	$\uparrow$ SID, $\uparrow Na^+$
Chloride excess or deficit	$\downarrow$ SID, $\uparrow Cl^-$	$\uparrow$ SID, $\downarrow Cl^-$
Unmeasured strong ion excess	$\downarrow$ SID, $\uparrow$ unmeasured anions	—

temperature-adjusted values for blood gases and pH is controversial. Although normal values are known for euthermia, normal values during hypothermia and hyperthermia are unknown. The acid-base changes that occur with hypothermia and hyperthermia may be homeostatic. The treatment of acid-base disturbances should be guided by the unadjusted values (i.e., those measured at $37\,^{\circ}C$). Temperature adjustment of blood gases and pH is useful to follow changes in these values with changes in body temperature. Temperature adjusted values should also be used to compare blood gases to exhaled gas values (e.g., end-tidal P_{CO_2}). Temperature adjustment allows the clinician to differentiate temperature-related changes from pathophysiologic changes.

POINTS TO REMEMBER

- Arterial blood gas and pH measurements are used to evaluate oxygenation, ventilation, and acid-base balance.
- Pa_{O_2} is a reflection of lung function.
- Hemoglobin oxygen saturation is determined by Pa_{O_2} and the position of the oxyhemoglobin dissociation curve.
- Pa_{CO_2} is determined by the relationship between alveolar ventilation and carbon dioxide production.
- Acid-base balance is explained by the Henderson-Hasselbalch equation.
- Intra-arterial blood gas monitoring systems use an optode and allow either continuous or on-demand blood gas analysis.
- Point-of-care testing uses analyzers at the bedside.
- Mixed venous oxygenation is a nonspecific indicator of the relationship between oxygen delivery and oxygen consumption.
- Mixed venous oxygen saturation can be monitored continuously using venous oximetry, but the clinical benefit of this is unclear.
- With conditions such as poor perfusion, there can be great disparity between arterial P_{CO_2} and mixed venous P_{CO_2}.
- The anion gap and osmol gap are useful to differentiate causes of metabolic acidosis.
- Blood gases and pH should not be temperature adjusted to guide treatment of acid-base disturbance.
- The Strong Ion Difference is a method of evaluating acid-base disturbances in which the only variables that affect pH are the P_{CO_2}, SID, and the concentration of unmeasured strong ions.

ADDITIONAL READING

ANDROGUE HE, ANDROGUE HJ. Acid-base physiology. *Respir Care* 2001; 46:328–341.
EPSTEIN SK, SINGH N. Respiratory acidosis. *Respir Care* 2001; 46:366–383.

FENCL V, JABOR A, KAZDA A, FIGGE J. Diagnosis of metabolic acid-base disturbances in critically ill patients. *Am J Respir Crit Care Med* 2000; 162:2246–2251.

FOSTER GT, VARZIRI ND, SASSOON CSH. Respiratory alkalosis. *Respir Care* 2001; 46:384–391.

HESS D, AGARWAL NN. Variability of blood gases, pulse oximeter saturation, and end-tidal carbon dioxide pressure in stable, mechanically ventilated patients. *J Clin Monit* 1992; 8:111–115.

HESS D, KACMAREK RM. Techniques and devices for monitoring oxygenation. *Respir Care* 1993; 38:646–671.

KHANNA A, KURTZMAN NA. Metabolic alkalosis. *Respir Care* 2001; 46:354–365.

KOST GJ, EHRMEYER SS, CHERNOW B, ET AL. The laboratory-clinical-interface. Point-of-care testing. *Chest* 1999; 115:1140–1154.

KRAUT JA, MADIAS NE. Approach to patients with acid-base disorders. *Respir Care* 2001; 46:392–403.

LARSON CP, VENDER J, SEIVER A. Multisite evaluation of a continuous intra-arterial blood gas monitoring system. *Anesthesiology* 1994; 81:543–552.

MORFEI, J. Stewart's strong ion difference approach to acid-base analysis. *Respir Care* 1999; 44:45–52.

MORGAN TJ, CLARK C, ENDRE ZH. Accuracy of base excess – an *in vitro* evaluation of the van Slyke equation. *Crit Care Med* 2000; 28:2932–2936.

PILON CS, LEATHLEY M, LONDON R, ET AL. Practice guideline for arterial blood gas measurement in the intensive care unit decreases the numbers and increases appropriateness of test. *Crit Care Med* 1997; 25:1308–1313.

SCHLICHTIG R, GROGONO AW, SEVERINGHAUS JW. Human P_{CO_2} and standard base excess compensation of acid-base imbalance. *Crit Care Med* 1998; 26:1173–1179.

SHAPIRO BA. *In vivo* monitoring of arterial blood gases and pH. *Respir Care* 1992; 37:165–169.

SIGGAARD-ANDERSON O, FOGH-ANDERSEN N, GØTHGEN IH, LARSEN VH. Oxygen status of arterial and mixed venous blood. *Crit Care Med* 1995; 23:1284–1293.

SWENSON ER. Metabolic acidosis. *Respir Care* 2001; 46:342–353.

WILKES P. Hypoproteinemia, strong ion difference, and acid-base status in critically ill patients. *J Appl Physiol* 1998; 84:1740–1748.

TWENTY-FIVE

INDICES OF OXYGENATION AND VENTILATION

OBJECTIVES

1. Calculate alveolar P_{O_2}.
2. Calculate the following indices of oxygenation: $P(A-a)_{O_2}$, Pa_{O_2}/PA_{O_2}, Pa_{O_2}/FI_{O_2}, respiratory index, oxygenation index.
3. Discuss the clinical usefulness of various indices of oxygenation.
4. Calculate pulmonary shunt.
5. Calculate dead space and alveolar ventilation.

INTRODUCTION

A number of calculated indices of oxygenation and ventilation are used for a variety of purposes. The principal reasons that these indices are used is more thoroughly to evaluate oxygenation and ventilation and to determine better the causes of abnormalities in oxygenation or ventilation. Although some of these indices are strongly endorsed by various clinicians, in general they are not necessary to evaluate oxygenation and ventilation at the bedside. An understanding of these indices, however, does lead to a better understanding of gas exchange during mechanical ventilation.

OXYGENATION

Alveolar P_{O_2}

Alveolar P_{O_2} $(P_{A_{O_2}})$ is a mathematically derived value using the alveolar gas equation:

$$P_{A_{O_2}} = \left(F_{I_{O_2}}\right) \times \left(Pb - P_{H_2O}\right) - \left(P_{a_{CO_2}} \times \left(F_{I_{O_2}} + \left(1 - F_{I_{O_2}}\right)/R\right)\right)$$

where $F_{I_{O_2}}$ is the inspired O_2 fraction, Pb is barometric pressure, P_{H_2O} is water vapor pressure (47 mm Hg at $37\,^{\circ}C$) and R is the respiratory quotient $(\dot{V}_{CO_2}/\dot{V}_{O_2})$. For calculation of $P_{A_{O_2}}$, $R = 0.8$ is commonly used. Note that the effect of R on $P_{A_{O_2}}$ depends on the $F_{I_{O_2}}$. For $F_{I_{O_2}} \geq 0.60$, the effect of R on $P_{A_{O_2}}$ becomes negligible. For a high $F_{I_{O_2}} \geq (0.60)$, the alveolar gas equation thus becomes:

$$P_{A_{O_2}} = \left(Pb - P_{H_2O}\right) \times F_{I_{O_2}} - P_{a_{CO_2}}$$

For $F_{I_{O_2}} < 0.60$, the alveolar P_{O_2} is estimated by:

$$P_{A_{O_2}} = \left(Pb - P_{H_2O}\right) - 1.25 \times P_{a_{CO_2}}$$

Tension-based Indices

There are several oxygen-tension-based indices. Each of these relates $P_{a_{O_2}}$ to either the $P_{A_{O_2}}$ or the $F_{I_{O_2}}$.

$P(A\text{-}a)_{O_2}$ The $P(A\text{-}a)_{O_2}$ is calculated by subtracting the $P_{a_{O_2}}$ from the $P_{A_{O_2}}$. An increase in $P(A\text{-}a)_{O_2}$ can result from $\dot{V}/\dot{Q}$ disturbances, shunt, or diffusion limitation. Changes in $P_{a_{CO_2}}$ will not affect the $P(A\text{-}a)_{O_2}$ because $P_{a_{CO_2}}$ is included in the calculation of $P_{A_{O_2}}$. A problem with the use of the $P(A\text{-}a)_{O_2}$ is its tendency to change as the $F_{I_{O_2}}$ changes. The normal $P(A\text{-}a)_{O_2}$ is 5 to 10 mm Hg breathing room air, but 30–60 mm Hg when breathing 100% O_2. This variability when the $F_{I_{O_2}}$ is changed limits its usefulness as an indicator of pulmonary function with $F_{I_{O_2}}$ changes and invalidates it as a predictor of the change in $P_{a_{O_2}}$ if the $F_{I_{O_2}}$ is changed. The $P(A\text{-}a)_{O_2}$ is affected not only by the $F_{I_{O_2}}$, but by the degree of

intrapulmonary shunt and $\dot{V}/\dot{Q}$ mismatch. In critically ill patients, the $P(\text{A-a})_{O_2}$ does not correlate well with the degree of pulmonary shunt. The $P(\text{A-a})_{O_2}$ is also affected by changes in mixed venous oxygen content.

Pa_{O_2}/PA_{O_2} The Pa_{O_2}/PA_{O_2} is calculated by dividing the Pa_{O_2} by PA_{O_2}. Unlike the $P(\text{A-a})_{O_2}$, the Pa_{O_2}/PA_{O_2} remains relatively stable with $F_{I_{O_2}}$ changes. A $Pa_{O_2}/PA_{O_2} < 0.75$ indicates pulmonary dysfunction due to $\dot{V}/\dot{Q}$ abnormality, shunt, or diffusion abnormality. The Pa_{O_2}/PA_{O_2} is most stable when it is less than 0.55, when the $F_{I_{O_2}}$ is greater than 0.30, and when the Pa_{O_2} is less than 100 mm Hg. The Pa_{O_2}/PA_{O_2} is more useful than the $P(\text{A-a})_{O_2}$ for comparing the pulmonary function of patients on different $F_{I_{O_2}}$ and for following a patient's pulmonary function as $F_{I_{O_2}}$ is changed. The Pa_{O_2}/PA_{O_2} can be used to predict the $F_{I_{O_2}}$ needed for a desired Pa_{O_2}:

$$F_{I_{O_2}} \text{ needed} = \left[(\text{desired } Pa_{O_2})/(Pa_{O_2}/PA_{O_2}) + Pa_{CO_2}\right]/(Pb - 47)$$

This relationship is seldom used in practice, however, because pulse oximetry can be used to quickly adjust the $F_{I_{O_2}}$ to an estimated Pa_{O_2}.

$Pa_{O_2}/F_{I_{O_2}}$ The $Pa_{O_2}/F_{I_{O_2}}$ (oxygenation index) is easier to calculate than $P(\text{A-a})_{O_2}$ and Pa_{O_2}/PA_{O_2} because it does not require calculation of PA_{O_2}. Due to its ease of calculation, this may be the most commonly used oxygenation index. A $Pa_{O_2}/F_{I_{O_2}} < 200$ is associated with significant shunt in patients with acute respiratory failure. The $Pa_{O_2}/F_{I_{O_2}}$ is affected by changes in Pa_{CO_2}. However, it has been shown to correlate with pulmonary shunt as well as Pa_{O_2}/PA_{O_2} and it has the advantage of being easier to calculate. The $Pa_{O_2}/F_{I_{O_2}}$ is commonly used in the classification of lung injury. A $Pa_{O_2}/F_{I_{O_2}} \leq 200$ indicates ARDS and a $Pa_{O_2}/F_{I_{O_2}}$ of 200 to 300 indicates acute lung injury.

Respiratory index The respiratory index (RI) is calculated by dividing the $P(\text{A-a})_{O_2}$ by the Pa_{O_2}. This may be a better indicator of oxygenation dysfunction than $P(\text{A-a})_{O_2}$, but offers no advantage over Pa_{O_2}/PA_{O_2} and $Pa_{O_2}/F_{I_{O_2}}$.

Oxygenation index The oxygenation index (OI) relates Pa_{O_2}, $F_{I_{O_2}}$, and mean airway pressure ($\bar{P}aw$):

$$OI = \left(F_{I_{O_2}} \times \bar{P}aw \times 100\right)/Pa_{O_2}$$

Although not commonly used in adults, this index is commonly used to classify respiratory failure in infants and children.

Pulmonary Shunt

Shunting is the portion of the cardiac output that moves from the right side of the heart to the left side of the heart without participating in gas exchange. Shunt is calculated from the oxygen content of pulmonary end-capillary (Cc'_{O_2}), arterial (Ca_{O_2}) and mixed venous ($C\bar{v}_{O_2}$) blood:

$$\dot{Q}_S/\dot{Q}_T = (Cc'_{O_2} - Ca_{O_2})/(Cc'_{O_2} - C\bar{v}_{O_2})$$

where $\dot{Q}_S$ is shunted cardiac output, $\dot{Q}_T$ is total cardiac output, Cc'_{O_2} is pulmonary end-capillary oxygen content, Ca_{O_2} is arterial oxygen content, and $C\bar{v}_{O_2}$ is mixed venous oxygen content. The pulmonary end-capillary, arterial, and mixed venous oxygen content can be calculated by the following equation:

$$O_2 \text{ content (mL } O_2/100 \text{ mL blood)} = Hb \times O_2Hb \times 1.34 + 0.003 \times P_{O_2}$$

where Hb is hemoglobin content, O_2Hb is hemoglobin oxygen saturation, and P_{O_2} is the partial pressure of oxygen.

The arterial oxygen content (Ca_{O_2}) is calculated from arterial blood gas values, and mixed venous oxygen content ($C\bar{v}_{O_2}$) is calculated from pulmonary artery blood gas values. Cc'_{O_2} is calculated based on the assumption that pulmonary end-capillary P_{O_2} is equal to the alveolar P_{O_2}. When $P_{A_{O_2}} > 150$ mm Hg, it is assumed that the end-capillary blood is maximally saturated with oxygen. Because small fractions of carboxyhemoglobin (COHb) and methemoglobin (metHb) are present in the blood, the end-capillary saturation becomes:

$$Sc'_{O_2} = 1 - COHb - metHb$$

Thus:

$$Cc'_{O_2} = (Hb \times Sc'_{O_2} \times 1.34) + (0.003 \times P_{A_{O_2}})$$

When a pulmonary artery catheter is not in place to sample mixed venous blood, shunt can be estimated from the equation:

$$\dot{Q}_S/\dot{Q}_t = (Cc'_{O_2} - Ca_{O_2})/(3.5 + (Cc'_{O_2} - Ca_{O_2}))$$

The 3.5 vol% can replace $Ca_{O_2} - C\bar{v}_{O_2}$ if there is cardiovascular stability and the temperature is normal. When the patient has a high Pa_{O_2} (> 150 mm Hg), the modified shunt equation can be used:

$$\dot{Q}_S/\dot{Q}_t = [(P_{A_{O_2}} - Pa_{O_2}) \times 0.003]/[3.5 + (P_{A_{O_2}} - Pa_{O_2}) \times 0.003]$$

The $Cc'_{O_2} - Ca_{O_2}$ can be replaced by $(P_{A_{O_2}} - Pa_{O_2}) \times 0.003$ in settings where it can be assumed that the Sa_{O_2} is 100%.

VENTILATION

Dead Space Ventilation

Dead space is that portion of the minute ventilation that does not participate in gas exchange. It consists of anatomic dead space and alveolar dead space. Dead space is calculated using the Bohr equation:

$$V_D/V_T = (Pa_{CO_2} - P\bar{E}_{CO_2})/Pa_{CO_2}$$

where V_D/V_T is the fraction of the total ventilation that is dead space, and $P\bar{E}_{CO_2}$ is the partial pressure of CO_2 in mixed expired gas. Normal V_D/V_T is 0.2 to 0.4.

Causes of increased V_D/V_T include pulmonary embolism, positive pressure ventilation, pulmonary hypoperfusion, and high rate-low tidal volume ventilation. To determine $P\bar{E}_{CO_2}$, mixed exhaled gas is collected for five to 15 min (Figure 25-1). During this gas collection period, the patient should be undisturbed and have a stable $\dot{V}_E$. An arterial blood sample for Pa_{CO_2} is obtained during this time. Many current-generation mechanical ventilators have a constant bias flow through the circuit, which complicates the collection of mixed exhaled gas to calculate V_D/V_T. In this case, $P\bar{E}_{CO_2}$ can be calculated from $\dot{V}_{CO_2}$ and $\dot{V}_E$:

$$P\bar{E}_{CO_2}(\dot{V}_{CO_2}/\dot{V}_E) \times P_b$$

Because dead space determinations require a leak-free system, they cannot be measured in patients with a bronchopleural fistula.

Alveolar Ventilation

From the exhaled CO_2 and $\dot{V}_E$, $\dot{V}_A$ can be calculated:

$$\dot{V}_A = \dot{V}_E \times P\bar{E}_{CO_2}/Pb.$$

$\dot{V}_A$ can also be calculated from V_D/V_T as:

$$\dot{V}_A = \dot{V}_E - (\dot{V}_E \times V_D/V_T).$$

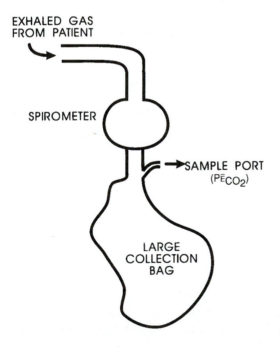

EXHALED GAS
FROM PATIENT

SPIROMETER

SAMPLE PORT
($P\bar{E}_{CO_2}$)

LARGE
COLLECTION
BAG

Figure 25-1 Schematic illustration of equipment used to collect exhaled gas for PE_{CO_2} determination.

POINTS TO REMEMBER

- $P_{A_{O_2}}$ is a function of barometric pressure, $F_{I_{O_2}}$, Pa_{CO_2}, and R.
- $P(A\text{-}a)_{O_2}$ is affected not only by pulmonary shunt, but also by $F_{I_{O_2}}$ and mixed venous oxygen content.
- $Pa_{O_2}/P_{A_{O_2}}$ is more stable than $P(A\text{-}a)_{O_2}$ when $F_{I_{O_2}}$ changes.
- $Pa_{O_2}/F_{I_{O_2}}$ is easy to calculate, and it correlates with pulmonary shunt and $Pa_{O_2}/P_{A_{O_2}}$.
- $\dot{Q}_S/\dot{Q}_T$ is calculated from Cc'_{O_2}, Ca_{O_2}, and $C\bar{v}_{O_2}$.
- V_D/V_T is calculated from Pa_{CO_2} and $P\bar{E}_{CO_2}$.
- $\dot{V}_A$ is calculated from $\dot{V}_E$ and P_{CO_2} or $\dot{V}_E$ and V_D/V_T.

ADDITIONAL READING

CANE RD, SHAPIRO BA, TEMPLIN R, WALTHER K. Unreliability of oxygen tension-based indices in reflecting intrapulmonary shunting in critically ill patients. *Crit Care Med* 1988; 16:1243–1245.

HESS D, ELSER RC, AGARWAL NN. The effects on the pulmonary shunt value of using measured versus calculated hemoglobin oxygen saturation and of correcting for the presence of carboxyhemoglobin and methemoglobin. *Respir Care* 1984; 29:1001–1005.

MAXWELL C, HESS D, SHEFET D. Use of the arterial/alveolar oxygen tension ratio to predict the $F_{I_{O_2}}$ needed for a desired Pa_{O_2}. *Respir Care* 1984; 29:1135–1139.

NELSON LD. Assessment of oxygenation: Oxygenation indices. *Respir Care* 1993; 38:631–645.

TWENTY-SIX

PULSE OXIMETRY, CAPNOGRAPHY, AND TRANSCUTANEOUS MONITORING

OBJECTIVES

1. Describe the principle of operation of pulse oximetry, capnography, and transcutaneous blood gas monitoring.
2. Discuss the appropriate use and limitations of pulse oximetry, capnography, and transcutaneous blood gas monitoring.
3. Describe the normal capnogram.
4. Discuss the relationship between noninvasive monitors of blood gases and arterial blood gases.

INTRODUCTION

Noninvasive monitoring of respiratory function is common for mechanically ventilated patients. This is particularly the case with pulse oximetry, which is now available as part of the bedside monitoring system in most critical care units. Although pulse oximetry has become a standard of care during mechanical ventilation, it is important to recognize that there are few, if any, outcome studies to demonstrate the effectiveness of this monitor. Much of the success of pulse oximetry is related to its ease of use, especially as compared to capnographs and transcutaneous monitors. Capnography is commonly used in the operating room and is popular in some critical care units, while transcutaneous monitoring has been virtually abandoned.

PULSE OXIMETRY

Principle of Operation

Pulse oximetry passes two wavelengths of light (usually 660 nm and 940 nm) through a pulsating vascular bed, and determines oxygen saturation (Sp_{O_2}) from the ratio of the amplitudes of the plethysmographic waveforms. A variety of oximeter probes are available in disposable and nondisposable designs and include finger probes, toe probes, ear probes, nasal probes, and foot probes. Most pulse oximeters provide some indication of signal strength (pulse amplitude) and some provide a display of the plethysmographic waveform. Inspection of this waveform allows the user to detect artifacts such as that which occurs with motion. Because pulse oximeters evaluate each arterial pulse, many display heart rate as well as oxygen saturation. The saturation reading should be questioned if the oximeter heart rate differs considerably from the actual heart rate. However, good agreement between the pulse oximeter heart rate and the actual heart rate does not guarantee a correct Sp_{O_2} reading.

Pulse oximeters use empirical calibration curves developed from studies of healthy volunteers. At saturations greater than 70%, the accuracy of pulse oximetry is about ±4 to 5%. To appreciate the implications of these accuracy limits, one must consider the oxyhemoglobin dissociation curve. If the pulse oximeter displays a Sp_{O_2} of 95%, the true saturation could be as low as 90% or as high as 100%. If the true saturation is 90%, the P_{O_2} will be about 60 mm Hg. However, if the true saturation is 100%, the P_{O_2} might be very high (150 mm Hg or greater). Below 70%, the accuracy of pulse oximetry is worse, but the clinical importance of this is questionable. When using Sp_{O_2}, one must understand the relationship between S_{O_2} and P_{O_2}. However, due to the variable and often unknown relationship between S_{O_2} and P_{O_2}, one should predict Pa_{O_2} from Sp_{O_2} with caution. The relationship between S_{O_2} and P_{O_2} also demonstrates the fact that pulse oximetry does not detect hyperoxemia very well.

The pulse oximeter is unique as a monitor in that it requires no user calibration. Manufacturer derived calibration curves programmed into the software of the device vary from manufacturer to manufacturer and can vary among pulse oximeters of a given manufacturer. For that reason, the same pulse oximeter and probe should be used for each Sp_{O_2} determination on a given patient. Ideally, Sp_{O_2} should be compared periodically to simultaneously obtained Sa_{O_2} measured by CO-oximetry. Spot checks of Sp_{O_2}, in which the relationship between Sp_{O_2} and Sa_{O_2} is unknown for a specific patient, should be interpreted cautiously.

Use and Limitations During Mechanical Ventilation

There are a number of performance limitations of pulse oximetry that should be understood by all clinicians who use these devices. Motion of the probe and high intensity ambient light can produce inaccurate readings. Motion artifact can be lessened by attaching the probe to an alternate site (such as the ear or toe rather than the finger) and interference by light can be minimized by wrapping the probe with a light barrier. Pulse oximeters assume that carboxyhemoglobin (COHb) and methemoglobin (metHb) concentrations are low ($< 2\%$). COHb and metHb both produce significant inaccuracy and pulse oximetry should not be used when elevated levels of these are present. Vascular dyes also affect the accuracy of pulse oximetry, with methylene blue producing the greatest effect. Because pulse oximeters require a pulsating vascular bed, they are unreliable during cardiac arrest. Nail polish can affect the accuracy of pulse oximetry and it should be removed before pulse oximetry is used. The accuracy and performance of pulse oximetry may also be affected by deeply pigmented skin. The accuracy of pulse oximetry is not affected by hyperbilirubinemia or fetal hemoglobin. Although pulse oximetry is generally considered safe, burns from defective probes and pressure necrosis may occur during monitoring by pulse oximetry.

It should be appreciated that pulse oximetry provides little indication of ventilation or acid-base status. Clinically important changes in pH and/or Pa_{CO_2} can occur with little change in Sp_{O_2}. This is particularly true when the Sp_{O_2} is $> 95\%$, as is often the case with mechanically ventilated patients. It is important to recognize that pulse oximetry is of limited value during ventilator weaning. Desaturation occurs relatively late in the course of a weaning failure and should be detectable earlier using clinical findings (e.g., tachypnea, tachycardia, accessory muscle use, diaphoresis). Because pulse oximetry also does not evaluate tissue oxygen delivery, a patient can have significant tissue hypoxia in spite of an adequate Sp_{O_2}.

Pulse oximetry is indicated in unstable patients likely to desaturate, in patients receiving a therapeutic intervention that is likely to produce hypoxemia (such as bronchoscopy), and in patients having interventions likely to produce changes in arterial oxygenation (such as changes in $F_{I_{O_2}}$ or PEEP). For the titration of $F_{I_{O_2}}$, a $Sp_{O_2} \geq 92$ to 94% in white patients (and 95% in black patients) is reliable in predicting a satisfactory level of oxygenation ($Pa_{O_2} \geq 60$ mm Hg) in most adult mechanically ventilated patients. Although pulse oximetry may decrease the number of blood gases required during the titration of F_{IO_2} or PEEP, it does not eliminate the need for periodic blood gases to measure Pa_{O_2}, Pa_{CO_2}, pH, and Sa_{O_2} by CO-oximetry.

CAPNOGRAPHY

Principle of Operation

Capnography is the measurement of CO_2 at the airway and display of a waveform called the capnogram. CO_2 can be measured using mass spectrometry, raman spectroscopy, or infrared absorption. Most bedside capnographs use infrared absorption at $4.26\,\mu m$. The measurement chamber is placed at the airway with a mainstream capnograph or gas is aspirated through fine-bore tubing to the measurement chamber inside the capnograph with the sidestream device. There are advantages and disadvantages of each design and neither is clearly superior.

There are potential technical problems related to the use of capnography. These include the need for periodic calibration and interference from gases such as N_2O. Water is particularly a problem because it occludes sample lines in the sidestream capnograph and condenses on the cell of mainstream devices. Manufacturers use a number of features to overcome these problems including water traps, purging of the sample line, construction of the sample line with water-vapor permeable nafion, heating of the mainstream cell, and automated calibration.

The Normal Capnogram

The normal capnogram is illustrated in Figure 26-1. During inspiration, P_{CO_2} is zero. At the beginning of exhalation, P_{CO_2} remains zero as gas from anatomic dead space leaves the airway (Phase I). The P_{CO_2} then sharply rises as alveolar gas

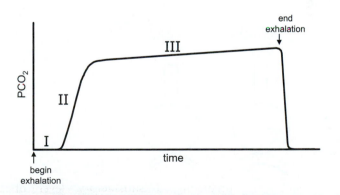

Figure 26-1 Normal capnogram. See text for details.

mixes with dead space gas (Phase II). During most of exhalation, the curve levels and forms a plateau (Phase III). This represents gas from alveoli and is called the alveolar plateau. The P_{CO_2} at the end of the alveolar plateau is called end-tidal P_{CO_2} (Pet_{CO_2}). The shape of the capnogram is abnormal in patients with abnormal lung function.

End-Tidal P_{CO_2}

The Pet_{CO_2} presumably represents alveolar P_{CO_2} (P_{ACO_2}). P_{ACO_2} is determined by the ventilation-perfusion ratio ($\dot{V}/\dot{Q}$) (Figure 26-2). With a normal $\dot{V}/\dot{Q}$, the P_{ACO_2} approximates the arterial P_{CO_2} (Pa_{CO_2}). If the $\dot{V}/\dot{Q}$ decreases, P_{ACO_2} rises towards mixed venous P_{CO_2} ($P\bar{v}_{CO_2}$). With a high $\dot{V}/\dot{Q}$ (i.e., dead space), P_{ACO_2} will approach the inspired P_{CO_2}. Pet_{CO_2} can be as low as the inspired P_{CO_2} (zero) or as high as the $P\bar{v}_{CO_2}$. An increase or decrease in Pet_{CO_2} can be the result of changes in CO_2 production (i.e., metabolism), CO_2 delivery to the lungs (i.e., circulation), or alveolar ventilation. However, because of homeostasis, compensatory changes may occur so that Pet_{CO_2} does not change. In practice, Pet_{CO_2} is a nonspecific indicator of cardiopulmonary homeostasis and usually does not indicate a specific problem or abnormality.

The gradient between Pa_{CO_2} and Pet_{CO_2} [$P(a\text{-}et)CO_2$] is often calculated. This gradient is usually small (< 5 mm Hg). However, in patients with dead space-producing disease (i.e., high $\dot{V}/\dot{Q}$), the Pet_{CO_2} may be considerably less than Pa_{CO_2}. Although not commonly appreciated, the Pet_{CO_2} may occasionally be greater than the Pa_{CO_2}.

Use and Limitations During Mechanical Ventilation

There is considerable intra- and inter-patient variability in the relationship between Pa_{CO_2} and Pet_{CO_2}. The $P(a\text{-}et)_{CO_2}$ is often too variable to allow precise prediction of Pa_{CO_2} from Pet_{CO_2}. Pet_{CO_2} as a reflection of P_{ACO_2} is useful only in mechanically ventilated patients who have relatively normal lung function, such

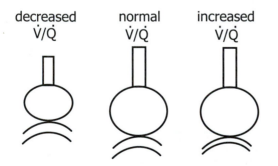

decreased $\dot{V}/\dot{Q}$ normal $\dot{V}/\dot{Q}$ increased $\dot{V}/\dot{Q}$

$PETCO_2 \approx P\bar{v}CO_2$ $PETCO_2 \approx PaCO_2$ $PETCO_2 \approx PICO_2$

Figure 26-2 Relationship between Pet_{CO_2} and $\dot{V}/\dot{Q}$.

as iatrogenic hyperventilation in head-injured patients. Pet_{CO_2} is not useful as a predictor of Pa_{CO_2} during weaning from mechanical ventilation. Use of Pet_{CO_2} as a predictor of Pa_{CO_2} is often deceiving and incorrect, and should be used with caution for this purpose in adult mechanically ventilated patients.

A useful application of capnography is the detection of esophageal intubation. Because there is normally very little CO_2 in the stomach, intubation of the esophagus and ventilation of the stomach results in a near-zero Pet_{CO_2}. A potential problem with the use of capnography to confirm endotracheal intubation occurs during cardiac arrest, with false negative results because of very low Pet_{CO_2} values related to decreased blood flow. Relatively inexpensive disposable devices that produce a color change in the presence of exhaled CO_2 are available to detect esophageal intubation. Low pulmonary blood flow results in low Pet_{CO_2} and vice versa. During resuscitation, changes in blood flow are reflected by changes in Pet_{CO_2}. However, the use of Pet_{CO_2} as a real-time objective indicator of blood flow during resuscitation is not practical.

Volumetric Capnometry

Although the traditional capnogram is time-based, it can be volume-based if expiratory flow is measured. The volume based capnogram (Figure 26-3) is displayed with P_{CO_2} on the vertical axis and volume on the horizontal axis. Airway dead space volume (i.e., anatomic dead space), alveolar dead space volume, and the volume of exhaled CO_2 (i.e., $\dot{V}_{CO_2}$) can be determined from the volume-based capnogram. Note that the determination of alveolar dead space requires knowledge of the Pa_{CO_2} in addition to the exhaled capnogram.

Technology has recently become available that uses partial rebreathing in conjunction with volumetric capnography to noninvasively measure cardiac output. A differential form of the Fick equation is used to calculate cardiac output. In brief, partial rebreathing decreases CO_2 elimination and the concentration of CO_2 in the pulmonary artery increases. By measuring the CO_2

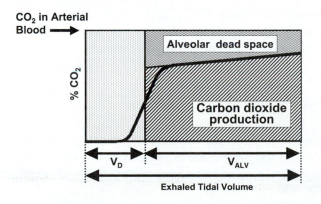

Figure 26-3 The volumetric capnogram.

elimination and end-tidal P_{CO_2} with and without rebreathing, cardiac output is calculated as:

$$\dot{Q} = \Delta \dot{V}_{CO_2}/S\Delta Pet_{CO_2}$$

where $\dot{Q}$ is cardiac output, $\Delta\dot{V}_{CO_2}$ is the difference in $\dot{V}_{CO_2}$ with and without rebreathing, S is the slope of the CO_2 dissociation curve, and ΔPet_{CO_2} is the difference in end-tidal P_{CO_2} with and without rebreathing.

TRANSCUTANEOUS P_{O_2} AND P_{CO_2}

Principle of Operation

Most commercially available transcutaneous monitors use a combination Ptc_{O_2}/Ptc_{CO_2} electrode that is fixed to the skin to measure transcutaneous P_{O_2} and P_{CO_2} (Ptc_{O_2} and Ptc_{CO_2}). The Ptc_{O_2} electrode uses a polarographic principle. To produce a Ptc_{O_2} approximating Pa_{O_2}, the electrode must be heated to approximately $44\,^{\circ}C$. The close relationship between Pa_{O_2} and Ptc_{O_2} in neonates is the result of a complex set of physiologic events. Simply stated, the increase in P_{O_2} caused by heating roughly balances the decrease in P_{O_2} caused by skin oxygen consumption and the diffusion of oxygen across the skin. It must be recognized that the close relationship between Pa_{O_2} and Ptc_{O_2} that occurs in neonates is probably more coincidental than physiological. Failure to recognize this fact creates the illusion that Ptc_{O_2} is the same a Pa_{O_2}. Particularly in adults, the Ptc_{O_2} is frequently less than Pa_{O_2}. Ptc_{O_2} is also affected by perfusion, and may reflect oxygen delivery (the product of cardiac output and arterial oxygen content) to the skin under the electrode. Ptc_{O_2} has been used in adults to monitor the results of vascular surgery, the intent being to evaluate perfusion rather than P_{O_2} per se.

Ptc_{CO_2} is measured by use of a Severinghaus electrode. Unlike the Ptc_{O_2} electrode, reasonably good correlation with Pa_{CO_2} can be obtained at a temperature of $37\,^{\circ}C$. Because Ptc_{CO_2} is consistently greater than Pa_{CO_2}, manufacturers incorporate a correction factor so that the Ptc_{CO_2} displayed approximates the Pa_{CO_2}. Like Ptc_{O_2}, the closeness with which Ptc_{CO_2} approximates Pa_{CO_2} is the result of a complex set of physiologic events and thus it is incorrect to think of Ptc_{CO_2} as Pa_{CO_2}. Decreased perfusion causes the Ptc_{CO_2} to increase.

Use and Limitations During Mechanical Ventilation

Due to the limitations listed in Table 26-1, transcutaneous monitoring has not received widespread acceptance in mechanically ventilated adults. Ptc_{O_2} monitoring is almost never used due to the widespread use of pulse oximetry. Ptc_{CO_2} may be a useful predictor of Pa_{CO_2} in neonatal, pediatric, and adult patients. However, this monitor is labor-intensive and seldom used.

Table 26-1 Limitations of transcutaneous monitoring

Frequent calibration required
Frequent position changes of electrode required
Relatively long equilibration time following electrode placement
Insufficient electrode temperature may adversely affect performance
Performance may be suboptimal over poorly perfused areas
Ptc_{O_2} tends to underestimate Pa_{O_2} and Ptc_{CO_2} tends to overestimate Pa_{CO_2}
Compromised hemodynamic status causes an underestimate of Pa_{O_2} and an overestimate of Pa_{CO_2}
Heated electrode may cause skin to blister
Ptc_{O_2} may underestimate Pa_{O_2} during hyperoxemia
Frequent membrane/electrolyte changes, and electrode maintenance required
Performance more reliable in neonates than adults (at least for Ptc_{O_2})

POINTS TO REMEMBER

- Pulse oximetry uses the principles of oximetry and plethysmography to measure Sp_{O_2}.
- Accuracy of pulse oximetry is ±4–5%, the implications of which are determined by the oxyhemoglobin dissociation curve.
- Limitations of pulse oximetry include motion artifact, high intensity ambient light, interference from COHb and metHb, interference from vascular dyes and nail polish, and inability to detect hyperoxemia.
- Pulse oximetry is indicated for patients likely to desaturate, in patients receiving therapeutic interventions likely to produce hypoxemia, and for titration of $F_{I_{O_2}}$ and PEEP.
- Capnography is the measurement of CO_2 at the airway.
- Pet_{CO_2} depends on the $\dot{V}/\dot{Q}$ ratio.
- Pet_{CO_2} is often an imprecise indicator of Pa_{CO_2}.
- Pet_{CO_2} should not be used as a noninvasive indicator of Pa_{CO_2} in critically ill, mechanically ventilated patients.
- Pet_{CO_2} may be useful to detect esophageal intubation.
- Due to technical and physiologic limitations, transcutaneous monitoring is seldom used.

ADDITIONAL READING

BHAVANI-SHANKAR K, KUMAR AY, MOSELEY HSL, AHYEE-HALLSWORTH R. Terminology and the current limitations of time capnography: A brief review. *J Clin Monit* 1995; 11:175–182.
BINDER JC, PARKIN WG. Non-invasive cardiac output determination: comparison of a new partial-rebreathing technique with thermodilution. *Anaesth Intensive Care* 2001; 29:19–23.
CARDOSO MM, BANNER MJ, MELKER RJ, BJORAKER DG. Portable devices used to detect endotracheal intubation during emergency situations: a review. *Crit Care Med* 1998; 26:957–964.

DE ABREU MG, QUINTEL M, RAGALLER M, ALBRECHT DM. Partial carbon dioxide rebreathing: a reliable technique for noninvasive measurement of nonshunted pulmonary capillary blood flow. *Crit Care Med* 1997; 25:675–683.

FRANKLIN ML. Transcutaneous measurement of partial pressure of oxygen and carbon dioxide. *Respir Care Clin N Am* 1995; 1:119–131.

GRAYBEAL JM, RUSSELL GB. Capnometry in the surgical ICU: an analysis of the arterial-to-end-tidal carbon dioxide difference. *Respir Care* 1993; 38:923–928.

HESS D. Detection and monitoring of hypoxemia and oxygen therapy. *Respir Care* 2000; 45:65–80.

HESS D, KACMAREK RM. Techniques and devices for monitoring oxygenation. *Respir Care* 1993; 38:646–671.

HESS D. Capnometry and capnography: technical aspects, physiologic aspects, and clinical applications. *Respir Care* 1990; 35:557–576.

JUBRAN A. Advances in respiratory monitoring during mechanical ventilation. *Chest* 1999; 116:1416–1425.

JUBRAN A, TOBIN MJ. Monitoring during mechanical ventilation. *Clin Chest Med* 1996; 17:453–473.

LEVINE RL. End-tidal CO_2: physiology in pursuit of clinical applications. *Intensive Care Med* 2000 Nov; 26:1595–1597.

MATHEWS PJ JR. CO-oximetry. *Respir Care Clin N Am* 1995; 1:47–68.

PALMISANO BW, SEVERINGHAUS JW. Transcutaneous P_{CO_2} and P_{O_2}: A multicenter study of accuracy. *J Clin Monit* 1990; 6:189–195.

SCHMITZ BD, SHAPIRO BA. Capnography. *Respir Care Clin N Am* 1995; 1:107–117.

SEVERINGHAUS JW, KELLEHER JF. Recent developments in pulse oximetry. *Anesthesiology* 1992; 76:1018–1038.

SINEX JE. Pulse oximetry: principles and limitations. *Am J Emerg Med* 1999; 17:59–67.

SOUBANI AO. Noninvasive monitoring of oxygen and carbon dioxide. *Am J Emerg Med* 2001; 19:141–146.

VAN DE LOUW A, CRACCO C, CERF C, ET AL. Accuracy of pulse oximetry in the intensive care unit. *Intensive Care Med* 2001; 27:1606–1613.

WAHR JA, TREMPER KK, DIAB M. Pulse oximetry. *Respir Care Clin N Am* 1995; 1:77–105.

HEMODYNAMIC MONITORING

OBJECTIVES

1. List indications for hemodynamic monitoring.
2. Describe the use of direct and derived hemodynamic measurements.
3. Describe the effect of positive pressure ventilation on hemodynamic measurements.
4. Discuss the value of measurements of oxygen delivery, oxygen consumption, and gastric tonometry.

INTRODUCTION

Invasive hemodynamic monitoring is commonly used with critically ill, mechanically ventilated patients. Due to the interactions between mechanical ventilation and hemodynamics, it is important that clinicians providing ventilatory support understand the basics of hemodynamic monitoring. Indications and complications for arterial and pulmonary artery catheters are listed in Table 27-1 and normal hemodynamic values are listed in Table 27-2. Pulmonary artery catheters have been commonly used in the care of mechanically ventilated patients – particularly those receiving high levels of PEEP. However, this practice has come under scrutiny in recent years.

HEMODYNAMIC MONITORING

Direct Measurements

Common sites for indwelling arterial catheters are the radial, brachial, axillary, and femoral arteries. The radial artery usually is the vessel of choice. Direct measurements of arterial blood pressure allow continuous display of systolic pressure, diastolic pressure, and mean arterial pressure.

Central venous pressure (CVP) is measured from a catheter located in the superior vena cava or right atrium. CVP reflects right atrial pressure, which reflects right ventricular end-diastolic pressure and the performance of the right ventricle. In patients with normal cardiac reserve and pulmonary vascular resistance, CVP reflects the ability of the myocardium to pump blood.

A pulmonary artery catheter is used to evaluate intravascular pressure and cardiac output. The pulmonary artery catheter is a special balloon tipped flow-directed catheter used for pulmonary artery pressure (PAP) and pulmonary capillary wedge pressure (PCWP) monitoring. The standard catheter consists of a proximal port (at the level of the right atrium to infuse fluids, measure CVP, and inject cold solution for cardiac output), distal port (in the pulmonary artery), a balloon (which is inflated for PCWP measurements), and a thermistor (to measure temperature and calculate cardiac output). Pulmonary artery catheters

Table 27-1 Indications and contraindications for arterial and venous cannulation

Arterial cannulation
- Indications: continuous blood pressure monitoring, frequent blood gases, continuous blood gas monitoring
- Complications: hemorrhage, infection, ischemia (embolus, thrombus, spasm)

Central venous catheter
- Indications: fluid administration, nutritional support, CVP measurements
- Complications: pneumothorax, embolus and thrombus formation, infection

Pulmonary artery cannulation
- Indications: PCWP measurements, cardiac output measurements, mixed venous blood gases
- Complications: pneumothorax, arrhythmias, embolus and thrombus formation, infection, cardiovascular injury

Table 27-2 Normal values for direct measured and derived hemodynamic values

Direct measurements

Central venous pressure	< 6 mm Hg
Pulmonary capillary wedge pressure	4–12 mm Hg
Pulmonary artery pressure	
systolic	20–30 mm Hg
diastolic	6–15 mm Hg
mean	10–20 mm Hg
Systemic arterial blood pressure	
systolic/diastolic	120/80 mm Hg
mean	80–100 mm Hg
Cardiac output	4–8 L/min
Heart rate	60–100 beats/min

Derived measurements

Cardiac index	2.5–4 L/min/m^2
Stroke volume	60–130 mL
Stroke volume index	30–50 mL/min^2
Pulmonary vascular resistance	110–250 dynes $\times$ s $\times$ cm^{-5}
Pulmonary vascular resistance index	225–314 dynes $\times$ s $\times$ cm^{-5}
Systemic vascular resistance	900–1400 dynes $\times$ s $\times$ cm^{-5}
Systemic vascular resistance index	1950–2400 dynes $\times$ s $\times$ cm^{-5}
Right ventricular stroke work index	8–10 g-m/m^2/beat
Left ventricular stroke work index	50–60 g-m/m^2/beat

can also be used to monitor mixed venous oxygen saturation, right ventricular ejection fraction, and to provide temporary cardiac pacing. The position of the catheter determines the pressure being measured. With the catheter tip in the pulmonary artery, pulmonary artery pressure is measured. An elevated PAP may indicate left-to-right shunt, left ventricular failure, mitral stenosis, or pulmonary hypertension. When the balloon is inflated, the catheter floats forward to a small branch of the pulmonary artery. Blood flow past the balloon is thus obstructed, and PCWP is measured (Figure 27-1). PCWP (also called pulmonary artery wedge pressure or pulmonary artery occlusion pressure) is a reflection of left atrial pressure. An elevated PCWP may indicate left ventricular failure, mitral stenosis, or cardiac insufficiency.

Thermodilution cardiac output is measured by injecting a cold solution into the central circulation (right atrium). The downstream temperature change in the pulmonary artery allows cardiac output to be calculated. A thermistor located near the tip of the pulmonary artery catheter measures the blood temperature in the pulmonary artery. The temperature of the patient, the temperature of the injection solution, and the change in blood temperature are the variables used to compute cardiac output. A continuous thermodilution cardiac output technique has recently become available that emits a safe amount of heat into the blood without using a fluid injectate, and cardiac output is computed by analysis of

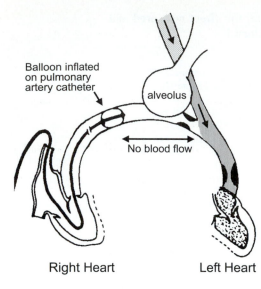

Balloon inflated on pulmonary artery catheter

alveolus

No blood flow

Right Heart

Left Heart

Figure 27-1 Illustration of the measurement of PCWP. When the balloon is inflated, the catheter floats to a distal wedge position. In this position, there is no flow past the catheter tip, and thus the pressure measured from the distal catheter tip reflects downstream (i.e., left atrial) pressure. (From O'QUIN R, MARINI JJ. Pulmonary artery occlusion pressure: Clinical physiology, measurement, and interpretation. *Am Rev Respir Dis* 1983; 128:319–326.)

temperature changes in the pulmonary artery using stochastic signal processing techniques.

Derived Measurements

Cardiac output is often normalized to patient size by dividing cardiac output ($\dot{Q}c$) by body surface area (BSA):

$$CI = \dot{Q}c/BSA$$

where CI is cardiac index. The volume of blood ejected from the ventricle with each contraction, stroke volume (SV), can be calculated by dividing cardiac output by heart rate (f_c):

$$SV = \dot{Q}c/f_c$$

Stroke volume can also be normalized to patient size:

$$SVI = CI/f_c$$

where SVI is stroke volume indexed.

Hemodynamic monitoring allows preload, afterload, and contractility to be assessed. This provides the clinician with the information necessary to assess cardiac output (Figure 27-2). Preload is determined by the amount of myocardial stretch at end-diastole (end-diastolic tension). Preload can be manipulated by controlling the volume in the ventricle. An increase in blood volume and an increase in venous tone will increase preload. A decrease in blood volume (e.g., diuretic administration) will decrease preload. The CVP is an indicator of right ventricular preload, and PCWP is an indicator of left ventricular preload.

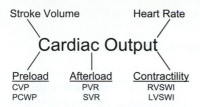

Preload   Afterload   Contractility
CVP   PVR   RVSWI
PCWP   SVR   LVSWI

Figure 27-2 The relationship between measured and derived hemodynamic parameters, and cardiac output.

Excessive preload is associated with cardiac failure and insufficient preload is associated with hypovolemia.

Afterload is the resistance that the ventricle must overcome to eject blood. The afterload of the right ventricle is pulmonary vascular resistance:

$$PVR = [(MPAP - PCWP) \times 80]/\dot{Q}c$$

where MPAP is the mean pulmonary artery pressure. PVR can be indexed to patient size:

$$PVRI = PVR \times BSA$$

where PVRI is the pulmonary vascular resistance index. The afterload of the left ventricle is systemic vascular resistance (SVR):

$$SVR = [(MAP - CVP) \times 80]/\dot{Q}c$$

where MAP is mean systemic arterial pressure. SVR can also be indexed to patient size:

$$SVRI = SVR \times BSA$$

where SVRI is the systemic vascular resistance index. Afterload is determined primarily by vascular tone; an increase in vascular tone increases afterload and a decrease in vascular tone decreases afterload. Thus, vasodilating agents (e.g., nitroprusside, nitroglycerine, hydralazine) decrease afterload, whereas vascoconstricting agents (e.g., dopamine, norepinephrine, phenylephrine) increase afterload.

Contractility is the intrinsic ability of the myocardium to contract, independent of preload and afterload. The contractility of the right ventricle is determined by the right ventricular stroke work index:

$$RVSWI = SVI \times (MPAP - CVP) \times 0.0136$$

The contractility of the left ventricle is determined by the LVSWI:

$$LVSWI = SVI \times (MAP - PCWP) \times 0.0136$$

Contractility is manipulated by use of inotropic and beta blocking agents. Inotropic agents (e.g., dopamine, dobutamine) increase contractility, and beta blocking agents (e.g., propanolol, metoprolol) decrease contractility.

AIRWAY PRESSURE AND HEMODYNAMICS

Effect of Pressure Changes During Respiratory Cycle

Although intravascular pressures are measured, it is actually transmural pressure (the difference between intraluminal pressure and pleural pressure) that is important. Thus, changes in intrapleural pressure affect transmural pressure measurements. During spontaneous breathing, pleural pressure decreases during inspiration and increases during expiration. With positive pressure breathing, pleural pressure increases during inspiration and decreases during exhalation. At end-exhalation, pleural pressure is the same for spontaneous breathing and positive pressure breathing (Figure 27-3). For that reason, intrathoracic pressure measurements should always be recorded at end-exhalation.

Because CVP is affected by pleural pressure, changes in CVP during the respiratory cycle can be used to evaluate patient effort during spontaneous or assisted ventilation. A large decrease in CVP during inhalation suggests that the patient has a high inspiratory load and may have a high work-of-breathing. A large increase in CVP during a passive positive pressure breath means that lung compliance is high relative to chest wall compliance and thus much of the airway pressure is transmitted to the pleural space.

Effect of PEEP on Hemodynamic Measurements

Positive pressure ventilation can also affect measurements of PCWP. This may occur due to catheter tip position and because of the effect of PEEP on pleural pressure. If the catheter tip is positioned in Zone I of the lungs (Figure 27-4),

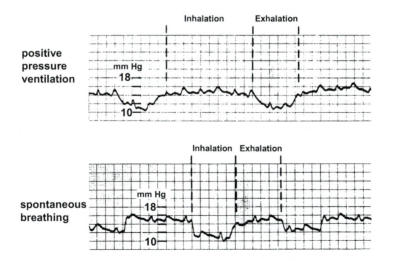

Figure 27-3 Pulmonary artery pressure waveform with spontaneous breathing (top) and positive pressure breathing (bottom). Note that end-expiratory pressure is equal for both waveforms.

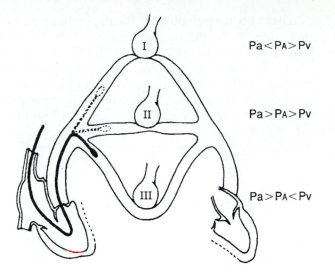

$Pa < P_A > Pv$

$Pa > P_A > Pv$

$Pa > P_A < Pv$

Figure 27-4 The effects of West Zones on PCWP measurement. In Zone I, alveolar pressure is greater than pulmonary capillary pressure. Thus, the vessel collapses and the distal catheter tip measures alveolar pressure. In Zones II and III, capillary pressure is greater than alveolar pressure, and thus the vessel remains open so that downstream (i.e., left atrium) pressure is measured. (From O'Quin R, Marini JJ. Pulmonary artery occlusion pressure: Clinical physiology, measurement, and interpretation. *Am Rev Respir Dis* 1983; 128:319–326.)

PCWP reflects alveolar pressure rather than left atrial pressure. This rarely occurs because catheter floatation will usually direct the catheter tip into Zone 3, but may occur if pulmonary artery pressure is low and PEEP is high. Techniques to determine if the catheter is wedged in Zone I are listed in Table 27-3.

The degree to which PEEP is transmitted to the pleural space is determined by the compliance of the lung and chest wall:

$$\Delta Ppl\Delta/Paw = C_L/(C_L + C_W)$$

where ΔPpl is the change in pleural pressure, ΔPaw is the change in airway pressure, C_L is lung compliance, and C_W is chest wall compliance. Because chest wall compliance and lung compliance are normally equal, only half of the PEEP pressure will be transmitted to the pleural space. When lung compliance is

Table 27-3 Indications that the pulmonary artery catheter is wedged in Zone I

- PCWP increases more than half of an increase in PEEP
- A change in airway pressure results in a change in PCWP greater than half the change in airway pressure
- PCWP is greater than pulmonary artery diastolic pressure
- Catheter tip is above level of left atrium on cross table chest X-ray

reduced, as often occurs with acute respiratory failure, less than half of the PEEP pressure will be transmitted to the pleural space and affect PCWP measurements. For example, assume that C_W is 100 mL/cm H_2O and C_L is 50 mL/cm H_2O (a typical C_L in mechanically ventilated patients). In this example, one third of the PEEP will be transmitted to the pleural space and affect PEEP. If the PEEP is 12 cm H_2O (9 mm Hg), 3 mm Hg will be transmitted to the pleural space. If the PCWP is 15 mm Hg, then the true transmural pressure is 12 mm Hg. Although this effect is usually small, it can be large when lung compliance is relatively normal, and chest wall compliance is decreased (e.g., abdominal distension).

OXYGEN DELIVERY AND OXYGEN CONSUMPTION

Oxygen delivery (D_{O_2}) is the volume of oxygen delivered to the tissues each minute and is calculated as:

$$D_{O_2} = Ca_{O_2} \times \dot{Q}c$$

Normal D_{O_2} is 1000 mL/min. Of this, the tissues normally extract 250 mL/min ($\dot{V}_{O_2}$), and 750 mL is returned to the lungs. $\dot{V}_{O_2}$ can be calculated using the Fick Equation:

$$\dot{V}_{O_2} = \dot{Q}c \times \left(Ca_{O_2} - C\bar{v}_{O_2}\right)$$

Oxygen extraction can also be calculated as the oxygen consumption divided by the oxygen delivery. Pathologic dependence of $\dot{V}_{O_2}$ on D_{O_2} has been suggested as a consequence of multiple organ system failure, and it has been recommended by some authorities to increase $\dot{Q}c$ to supranormal levels. However, such a strategy has not been shown to improve outcome in critically ill patients.

Gastric Tonometry

Under conditions of physiologic stress, the gut is one of the first regional capillary beds to suffer as blood is redirected to the brain, heart, and kidneys. Gastric tonometry measures P_{CO_2} in the gastric lumen using a balloon-tipped catheter placed into the stomach. Gastric P_{CO_2} is used to calculate gastric intraluminal pH (pHi) from the Henderson-Hasselbalch equation. In its original design, saline was placed into a gastric balloon attached to a nasogastric tube. After an equilibration period of 30 to 90 min, the saline is withdrawn and P_{CO_2} is measured. A simultaneous arterial blood sample is required to calculate plasma HCO_3^-. An automated system uses air instead of saline and measures P_{CO_2} with an infrared analyzer, pumps air in and out of the balloon, and performs the measurement every 10 to 15 min. Low pHi has been associated with failure to wean from mechanical ventilation. However, it is not widely used in the care of mechanically ventilated patients.

POINTS TO REMEMBER

- Direct hemodynamic measurements include arterial blood pressure, CVP, pulmonary artery pressure, pulmonary capillary wedge pressure, and cardiac output.
- Derived hemodynamic measurements include stroke volume, pulmonary vascular resistance, systemic vascular resistance, right ventricular stroke work, and left ventricular stroke work.
- Hemodynamic measurements are used to evaluate preload, afterload, and contractility.
- Due to vascular pressure fluctuations that occur during breathing, vascular pressures should always be recorded at end-exhalation.
- The effect of PEEP on PCWP measurements is determined by lung compliance and chest wall compliance.
- Oxygen delivery is the amount of oxygen that is delivered to the tissues each minute, and oxygen consumption is the amount of oxygen used by the tissues each minute.
- Gastric tonometry measures P_{CO_2} in the gastric lumen using a balloon-tipped catheter placed into the stomach.

ADDITIONAL READING

CONNORS AF, SPEROFF T, DAWSON NV, ET AL. The effectiveness of right heart catheterization in the initial care of critically ill patients. *JAMA* 1996; 18:889–897.

GATTINONI L, BRAZZI L, PELOSI P, ET AL. A trial of goal-oriented hemodynamic therapy in critically ill patients. *N Engl J Med* 1995; 333:1025–1032.

HALLER M, ZÖLLNER C, BRIEGEL J, FORST H. Evaluation of a new continuous thermodilution cardiac output monitor in critically ill patients: A prospective criterion study. *Crit Care Med* 1995; 23:860–866.

HAMILTON MA, MYTHEN MG. Gastric tonometry: where do we stand? *Curr Opin Crit Care* 2001; 7:122–127.

LEBUFFE G, ROBIN E, VALLET B. Gastric tonometry. *Intensive Care Med* 2001; 27:317–319.

KEENAN SP, GUYATT GH, SIBBALD WJ, ET AL. How to use articles about diagnostic technology: gastric tonometry. *Crit Care Med* 1999; 27:1726–1731.

MIHALJEVIC T, VON SEGESER LK, TÖNZ M, LESKOSEK B, ET AL. Continuous versus bolus thermodilution cardiac output measurements – a comparative study. *Crit Care Med* 1995; 23:944–949.

O'QUIN R, MARINI JJ. Pulmonary artery occlusion pressure: Clinical physiology, measurement, and interpretation. *Am Rev Respir Dis* 1983; 128:319–326.

RUSSELL JA, PHANG PT. The oxygen delivery/consumption controversy. Approaches to management of the critically ill. *Am J Respir Crit Care Med* 1994; 149:533–537.

TWENTY-EIGHT

BASIC PULMONARY MECHANICS DURING MECHANICAL VENTILATION

OBJECTIVES

1. Describe the significance of peak inspiratory pressure, plateau pressure, and auto-PEEP.
2. List factors that affect peak inspiratory pressure, plateau pressure, and auto-PEEP.
3. Calculate airways resistance, respiratory system compliance, and mean airway pressure.
4. Discuss the significance of respiratory rate, tidal volume, and maximal inspiratory pressure measurements to assess the ability to breathe spontaneously.

INTRODUCTION

Pulmonary mechanics are frequently measured on mechanically ventilated patients. Some such as peak inspiratory pressure (PIP) are recorded as part of patient-ventilator system checks. Others can be easily made at the bedside with no equipment but that available on the ventilator (e.g., airway pressure, flow, and volume). Pressure, flow, and volume should ideally be measured at the proximal airway. Commercially available mechanical ventilators monitor pressure and flow at a variety of sites, which may affect the measured values obtained.

ASSESSMENT OF MECHANICS DURING MECHANICAL VENTILATION

Airway Pressure

A typical airway pressure waveform during volume ventilation is shown in Figure 28-1. With volume ventilation, pressure increases during inspiration as volume is delivered. The slope of the pressure curve depends upon the inspiratory flow pattern. If a constant flow pattern is chosen, there will be a linear increase in pressure during inspiration. With a descending ramp flow pattern, the inspiratory pressure waveform will be convex. PIP varies directly with resistance, end-inspiratory flow, tidal volume, respiratory system compliance, and PEEP. Depending upon the inspiratory flow waveform, PIP may not occur at end-inspiration.

An end-inspiratory pause of sufficient duration (0.5–2 s) will allow equilibration between proximal airway pressure and alveolar pressure (Palv). This measurement should be made on a single breath and removed immediately to prevent the development of auto-PEEP. During the end-inspiratory pause, there is no flow and a pressure plateau develops as proximal airway pressure equilibrates with Palv. The pressure during the inspiratory pause is commonly referred to as plateau pressure (P_{plat}) and represents peak Palv. The difference between PIP and P_{plat} is due to the resistive properties of the system (e.g., pulmonary airways, artificial airway), and the difference between P_{plat} and

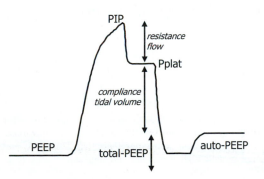

Figure 28-1 A typical airway pressure waveform during volume ventilation. Plateau pressure is determined using an end-inspiratory pause, and auto-PEEP is determined using an end-expiratory pause.

total PEEP is due to respiratory system compliance. The measurement of P_{plat} is valid only if the patient is passively ventilated – active breathing invalidates the measurement.

During pressure-controlled ventilation, PIP and peak Palv may be equal due to the flow waveform with this mode of ventilation (Figure 28-2). With pressure-controlled ventilation, flow decreases during inspiration and is often followed by a period of zero-flow at end-inspiration. During this period of no flow, proximal airway pressure should be equal to peak alveolar pressure. With all other factors held constant (e.g., tidal volume, compliance, PEEP), peak Palv is identical for volume-control and pressure-control ventilation. Because lung injury is related to peak Palv (i.e., plateau pressure), the importance of the decrease in PIP that occurs when changing from volume to pressure ventilation is questionable.

Auto-PEEP

An end-expiratory pause can be used to determine auto-PEEP (Figure 28-1). This method is only valid if the patient is not spontaneously breathing and there are no system leaks (e.g., circuit leak or bronchopleural fistula). For patients who are triggering the ventilator, an esophageal balloon is needed to measure auto-PEEP. During the end-expiratory pause, there is equilibration between end-expiratory pressure and proximal airway pressure. Auto-PEEP is the difference between set PEEP and total PEEP measured with this maneuver. All current generation ventilators have the capability of measuring auto-PEEP using an end-exhalation pause maneuver. Auto-PEEP is determined by the tidal volume, respiratory system compliance, airways resistance, and expiratory time:

$$\text{auto-PEEP} = V_T/[(C) \times (e^{K_E/T_E} - 1)]$$

where $K_E = 1/(R_E \times C)$, e is the base of the natural logarithm, T_E is expiratory time, R_E is expiratory airways resistance, and C is respiratory system compliance. Because set PEEP may counter-balance auto-PEEP, the presence of auto-PEEP is most appropriately measured with no PEEP set on the ventilator. Auto-PEEP is important because it causes hyperinflation, hemodynamic instability, and difficulty triggering the ventilator.

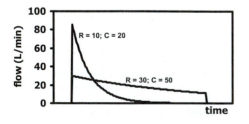

Figure 28-2 Typical airway flow waveforms for pressure controlled ventilation with low resistance and low compliance (e.g., ARDS), and with high resistance and high compliance (e.g., COPD).

Mean Airway Pressure

Many of the desired and deleterious effects of mechanical ventilation are determined by mean airway pressure ($\bar{P}aw$). Factors affecting mean airway pressure are PIP, PEEP, I:E ratio, and inspiratory pressure waveform. During pressure ventilation, the inspiratory pressure waveform is rectangular and $\bar{P}aw$ is estimated as:

$$\bar{P}aw = (PIP - PEEP)/(T_I/T_T) + PEEP$$

where T_I is inspiratory time and T_T is total cycle time. For example, with a PIP of 40 cm H_2O, PEEP of 10 cm H_2O, T_I of 1 s, rate 15/min ($T_I/T_T = 0.33$), $\bar{P}aw$ is 20 cm H_2O. During constant-flow volume ventilation, the inspiratory pressure waveform is triangular, and $\bar{P}aw$ can be estimated as

$$\bar{P}aw = 0.5 \times (PIP - PEEP)/(T_I/T_T) + PEEP$$

For example, with a PIP of 25 cm H_2O, PEEP 5 cm H_2O, Ti 1.5 s, rate 20/min ($T_I/T_T = 0.5$), $\bar{P}aw$ is 15 cm H_2O. Many current generation microprocessor ventilators display $\bar{P}aw$ from integration of the airway pressure waveform. Typical $\bar{P}aw$ for passively ventilated patients are 5–10 cm H_2O (normal), 15–25 cm H_2O (ARDS), and 10–20 cm H_2O (airflow obstruction). Because there is often an imbalance between inspiratory and expiratory resistances, mean airway pressure is not equivalent to mean alveolar pressure. The difference between mean alveolar pressure ($\bar{P}alv$) and $\bar{P}aw$ is estimated by the following relationship:

$$\bar{P}alv - \bar{P}aw = \dot{V}_E/60 \times (R_E - R_I)$$

Compliance

The difference between P_{plat} and total PEEP is determined by the compliance of the lung and chest wall. Thus, compliance can be calculated as:

$$C = V_T/(P_{plat} - PEEP)$$

The V_T used in this equation is the actual tidal volume delivered to the patient, and should be corrected for the effects of volume compressed in the ventilator circuit. PEEP should include any auto-PEEP that is present. P_{plat} should be determined from an end-inspiratory breath hold that is long enough to produce equilibration between proximal airway pressure and alveolar pressure. Causes of a decrease in compliance in mechanically ventilated patients are listed in Table 28-1.

Resistance

The difference between PIP and P_{plat} is determined by inspiratory resistance and end-inspiratory flow. During constant-flow volume ventilation, inspiratory resistance can be calculated as:

$$R_I = (PIP - P_{plat})/\dot{V}_I$$

Table 28-1 Causes of decreased compliance and increased resistance in mechanically ventilated patients

Compliance	Resistance
Pneumothorax	Bronchospasm
Mainstem intubation	Secretions
Congestive heart failure	Small endotracheal tube
ARDS	Mucosal edema
Consolidation	
Pneumonectomy	
Pleural effusion	
Abdominal distention	
Chest wall deformity	

where $\dot{V}_I$ is the inspiratory flow. Expiratory resistance can be estimated from the time constant (τ) of the lung: $R_E = \tau/C$ (Figure 28-3). Causes of increased resistance during mechanical ventilation are listed in Table 28-1. Inspiratory resistance is typically less than expiratory resistance due to the increased diameter of airways during inspiration.

Work-of-Breathing

Inspiratory work-of-breathing performed by the ventilator can be estimated during constant flow passive inflation of the lungs by the following calculation:

$$W = (PIP - 0.5 \times P_{plat})/100 \times V_T$$

For example, if PIP = 35 cm H_2O, P_{plat} = 30 cm H_2O, and tidal volume = 0.6 L, then W = 0.12 kg-m, or 0.2 kg-m/L. Note that the units for work-of-breathing are kilogram-meter (kg-m) or joules (j); 0.1 kg-m = 1.0 j. Normal work-of-breathing is 0.5 j/L. Work-of-breathing will increase with an increase in resistance, a decrease in compliance, or an increase in tidal volume. Work-of-breathing is often normalized to the tidal volume (work/L). Although work-of-breathing is not commonly calculated, it is reasonable to expect that patients with a high work-of-breathing will not wean from mechanical ventilation.

ASSESSMENT OF SPONTANEOUS BREATHING

Rate and Tidal Volume

Assessment of spontaneous respiratory rate and tidal volume is useful, particularly in patients weaning from mechanical ventilation. Tachypnea is an ominous sign and may be either a symptom or cause of respiratory muscle fatigue. Development of a pattern of rapid and shallow breathing during a spontaneous

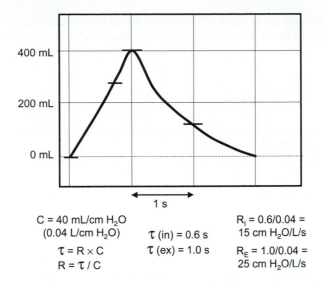

$C = 40$ mL/cm H_2O
$(0.04$ L/cm $H_2O)$

$\tau = R \times C$

$R = \tau / C$

τ (in) = 0.6 s

τ (ex) = 1.0 s

$R_I = 0.6/0.04 =$
15 cm H_2O/L/s

$R_E = 1.0/0.04 =$
25 cm H_2O/L/s

Figure 28-3 Use of the tidal volume waveform to measure time constant (τ) and calculate inspiratory and expiratory airways resistance.

breathing trial usually predicts failure. The likelihood of a patient being able to support spontaneous breathing is increased if the rate:tidal volume ratio, or rapid-shallow breathing index (RSBI), is less than 100, and decreased if the RSBI is greater than 100. For example, a patient with a spontaneous rate of 30/min with a tidal volume of 0.2 L (ratio = 150) is less likely to be ready to wean from mechanical ventilation. On the other hand, a patient with a spontaneous rate of 20/min and a tidal volume of 0.25 L (ratio = 80) is more likely to successfully wean.

The traditional technique for measuring spontaneous respiratory rate and tidal volume involved removing the patient from the ventilator, attaching a hand-held respirometer to measure minute ventilation, and counting the respiratory rate. More commonly, spontaneous respiratory rate and tidal volume are measured without removing the patient from the ventilator. This is done by setting the CPAP and pressure support to zero to remove all ventilatory assistance. Some ventilators will conveniently calculate and display the RSBI. However, it is important to appreciate that the RSBI may only be valid if the CPAP and pressure support are set to zero.

Maximal Inspiratory Pressure

The maximal inspiratory pressure (MIP or PI_{max}) is measured by attaching a manometer to the endotracheal or tracheostomy tube. The patient then forcibly inhales against an occluded airway after maximal exhalation. When PI_{max} is measured, a unidirectional valve should be used, and the airway should be completely obstructed for as long as 15 to 20 s. The patient must be closely monitored and the maneuver is terminated if signs of cardiopulmonary distress occur. A PI_{max} more negative than -30 cm H_2O usually suggests adequate inspiratory muscle strength.

POINTS TO REMEMBER

- During volume ventilation, PIP is determined by tidal volume, inspiratory flow, resistance, compliance, and PEEP.
- Peak alveolar pressure is estimated by measuring airway pressure during an end-inspiratory breath-hold.
- Auto-PEEP is estimated by measuring airway pressure during an end-expiratory breath-hold.
- Mean airway pressure is calculated from PIP, PEEP, and T_I/T_T.
- Compliance is calculated from V_T, P_{plat}, and PEEP.
- Inspiratory resistance is calculated from PIP, P_{plat} and inspiratory flow.
- Work-of-breathing is increased with increases in resistance, compliance, and V_T.
- A pattern of rapid shallow breathing may predict a failed weaning trial.
- Maximal inspiratory pressure is an indicator of inspiratory muscle strength.

ADDITIONAL READING

BRANSON RD, HURST JM, DAVIS K, CAMPBELL R. Measurement of maximal inspiratory pressure: A comparison of three methods. *Respir Care* 1989; 34:789–794.

HESS DR, MEDOFF MD, FESSLER MB. Pulmonary mechanics and graphics during positive pressure ventilation. *Int Anesthesiol Clin* 1999; 37(3):15–34.

HESS D, TABOR T. Comparison of six methods to calculate airway resistance during mechanical ventilation. *J Clin Monit* 1993; 9:275–282.

KACMAREK RM, CYCYK-CHAPMAN MC, YOUNG PJ, ROMAGNOLI DM. Determination of maximal inspiratory pressure: A clinical study literature review. *Respir Care* 1989; 34:868–878.

MARINI JJ, CROOKE PS. A general mathematical model for respiratory mechanics relevant to the clinical setting. *Am Rev Respir Dis* 1993; 147:14–24.

MARINI JJ, RAVENSCRAFT SA. Mean airway pressure: physiologic determinants and clinical importance - Part 1. Physiologic determinants and measurements. *Crit Care Med* 1992; 20:1461–1472.

MARINI JJ, RAVENSCRAFT SA. Mean airway pressure: physiologic determinants and clinical importance - Part 1. Clinical implications. *Crit Care Med* 1992; 20:1604–1616.

PRIMIANO FP, CHATBURN RL, LOUGH MD. Mean airway pressure: theoretical considerations. *Crit Care Med* 1982; 10:378–383.

TRUWITT JD, MARINI JJ. Evaluation of thoracic mechanics in the ventilated patient. Part 1: Primary measurements. *J Crit Care* 1988; 3:133–150.

TRUWITT JD, MARINI JJ. Evaluation of thoracic mechanics in the ventilated patient. Part 2: Applied mechanics. *J Crit Care* 1988; 3:199–213.

YANG KL, TOBIN MJ. A prospective study of indexes predicting the outcome of trials of weaning from mechanical ventilation. *N Engl J Med* 1991; 324:1445–1450.

TWENTY-NINE

ADVANCED PULMONARY MECHANICS DURING MECHANICAL VENTILATION

OBJECTIVES

1. Draw normal pressure, flow, and volume waveforms during mechanical ventilation.
2. Describe the effects of abnormal respiratory system mechanics on pressure, flow, and volume waveforms during mechanical ventilation.

3. Discuss the use of flow-volume and pressure-volume curves during mechanical ventilation.
4. Describe the use of esophageal pressure to measure pleural pressure changes during mechanical ventilation.
5. Discuss the usefulness of intra-abdominal pressure measurements during mechanical ventilation.

INTRODUCTION

It is useful to assess respiratory mechanics in many mechanically ventilated patients such as those using only the pressure and volume displays on the ventilator. Additional information can be gained by observing graphic waveform displays of pressure, volume, and flow. As shown in Table 29-1, the site of measurement and the mode of ventilation affect the measurements of lung mechanics during mechanical ventilation. In this chapter, mechanics based upon the waveform displays of the ventilator, pressure-volume curves, esophageal pressure, and intra-abdominal pressure are discussed.

SCALARS

Pressure

Much qualitative information can be obtained by observing the airway pressure waveform. With patient-triggered breaths, airway pressure dips below baseline to trigger the ventilator. Active patient effort often continues after the initiation of a patient-triggered breath, which produces scalloping of the airway tracing (Figure 29-1). This suggests that the inspiratory flow of the ventilator should be increased if volume-controlled ventilation is used. Alternatively, pressure-control or pressure-support ventilation may be used and the rise time can be adjusted to better meet the patient's flow demand. The depth and duration of the negative pressure deflection prior to a patient-triggered breath indicates the response of the ventilator, and the depth and duration of the negative pressure deflection during continuous positive airway pressure (CPAP) indicates the effort required to maintain flow from the ventilator.

Ideally, proximal airway pressure should be measured directly at the endotracheal tube. Some ventilator systems approximate inspiratory pressure by measuring pressure in the expiratory circuit during inspiration, and approximate expiratory pressure by measuring pressure in the inspiratory circuit during exhalation. Although this should be theoretically satisfactory, it may not allow precise reflections of proximal airway pressure throughout a dynamically changing respiratory cycle. Some ventilators measure pressure directly at the proximal airway.

Table 29.1 Influence of the site of pressure measurement and mode of ventilation on measurements of work-of-breathing and compliance

Site of pressure measurement and mode of ventilation	Area of the pressure-volume loop = work done to overcome	Slope of the pressure-volume loop
Esophageal pressure during spontaneous ventilation	Pulmonary inspiratory and expiratory resistance	Lung compliance
Esophageal pressure during mechanical ventilation	Chest-wall inspiratory and expiratory resistance	Chest-wall compliance
Pressure at tracheal (carinal) end of endotracheal tube during spontaneous ventilation	Imposed inspiratory and expiratory resistance of the total breathing apparatus (i.e., endotracheal tube, breathing circuit, and the ventilator)	Compliance of the total breathing apparatus
Pressure at the tracheal (carinal) end of endotracheal tube during mechanical ventilation	Pulmonary and chest-wall inspiratory and expiratory resistance	Compliance of the respiratory system (lungs plus chest wall)
Pressure at airway opening (between "Y" piece of breathing circuit and endotracheal tube) during spontaneous ventilation	Imposed inspiratory and expiratory resistance of the breathing circuit and ventilator	Compliance of the breathing circuitry
Pressure at airway opening during mechanical ventilation	Pulmonary and chest-wall inspiratory and expiratory resistance, plus resistance of the endotracheal tube	Compliance of the respiratory system (lungs plus chest wall)

From Banner MJ, Jaeger MJ, Kirby RR. Components of the work-of-breathing and implications for monitoring ventilator-dependent patients. *Crit Care Med* 1994; 22:515–532.

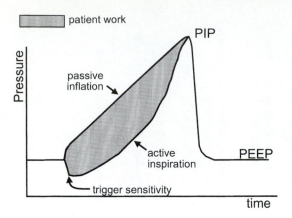

Figure 29-1 Active inspiration during positive pressure ventilation produces scalloping of the airway pressure waveform.

A typical airway pressure waveform is shown in Figure 29-2. During exhalation, the pressure should be the set PEEP level. During inhalation, the airway pressure waveform is determined by the flow delivery set on the ventilator and the patient's ventilatory demand. With constant flow volume controlled ventilation, airway pressure should increase linearly during the inspiratory phase. With pressure controlled and pressure support ventilation, airway pressure during inhalation approximates a square wave. The shape of the pressure waveform is also affected by the rise time setting on the ventilator.

Flow

Flow should ideally be measured at the proximal airway. Although some ventilators measure flow directly at the proximal endotracheal tube, most measure flow in the ventilator using inspiratory and expiratory pneumotachometers. Flow measured directly at the airway is not affected by factors such as system leaks and the compressible volume of the ventilator circuit.

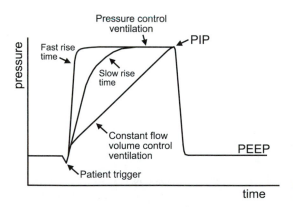

Figure 29-2 Airway pressure waveforms during mechanical ventilation.

A typical airway flow waveform is illustrated in Figure 29-3. With volume-controlled ventilation, the inspiratory flow waveform is determined by the flow setting of the ventilator. With pressure-controlled ventilation, inspiratory flow decreases according to the patient's lung mechanics. If an end-inspiratory pause is set with volume-controlled ventilation, or a long inspiratory time is used with pressure-controlled ventilation, a period of zero flow occurs at the end of the inspiratory phase.

The shape of the expiratory flow waveform is determined by lung mechanics. With a normal resistance and compliance, expiratory flow quickly reaches a peak, and then decreases throughout exhalation. Flow at end-exhalation indicates that auto-PEEP is present, but does not indicate the amount of auto-PEEP. It should also be recognized that auto-PEEP may be present even if expiratory flow is apparently zero at end-exhalation. Although useful, the end-expiratory flow is thus an insensitive and imprecise indicator of auto-PEEP.

Volume

Most monitoring systems used with mechanical ventilators do not measure volume directly. Flow is integrated to produce volume ($\int \dot{V}\,dt$). The volume waveform depends upon the flow pattern set on the ventilator. With a constant inspiratory flow, volume delivery is constant during inspiration. With pressure-controlled ventilation, most of the volume is delivered early in the inspiratory period. A leak distal to the point of volume measurement (e.g., leak around the endotracheal tube, bronchopleural fistula) produces a difference between the inspiratory and expiratory tidal volume (Figure 29-4).

LOOPS

Pressure, flow, and volume can be displayed not only as time scalars, but also as flow-volume and pressure-volume loops. This information is similar to that

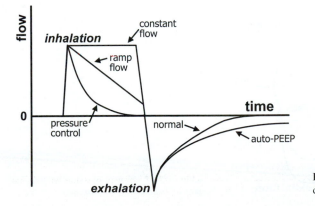

Figure 29-3 Airway flow waveforms during mechanical ventilation.

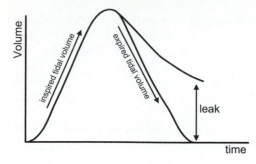

Figure 29-4 Airway volume waveforms during mechanical ventilation.

obtained in the pulmonary function laboratory with two exceptions. Loops during mechanical ventilation are obtained during tidal volume breathing, whereas loops in the pulmonary function laboratory are obtained with a vital capacity maneuver. Also, loops during mechanical ventilation are passive, whereas loops produced in the pulmonary function laboratory are with forced inhalation and exhalation.

Flow-Volume Loops

Flow-volume loops are displayed with flow as a function of volume. Some systems display expiratory flow in the positive position, whereas other systems display expiratory flow in the negative position. During inspiration, the shape of the flow-volume loop is determined by the flow setting on the ventilator. During exhalation, the shape of the flow-volume loop is determined by the characteristics of the patient's lungs. The expiratory flow-volume loop has a characteristic concavity with obstructive lung disease (Figure 29-5). With reversible airflow obstruction, the expiratory flow-volume loop may change shape following bronchodilator administration, indicating an improvement in expiratory flow.

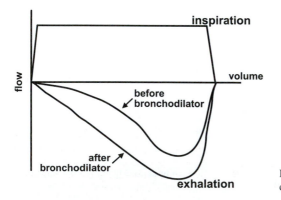

Figure 29-5 Flow-volume loops and the effect of bronchodilator therapy.

Pressure-Volume Curves

Pressure-volume curves are displayed with volume as a function of pressure. The slope of the pressure-volume loop is the lung/chest wall compliance. In recent years, there has been much enthusiasm for setting PEEP based upon inflection points determined from the inflation pressure-volume curve (Figure 29-6). The lower inflection point has been thought to represent the pressure at which a large population of alveoli are recruited. However, it has become appreciated that recruitment is likely to occur along the entire inflation pressure-volume curve. An upper inflection point on the pressure-volume loop has been thought to indicate over-distension, and there has been some enthusiasm for maintaining plateau pressure below this point. However, the upper inflection point might represent the end of recruitment rather than the point of over-distention.

The most common methods used to measure pressure-volume curves are the use of a super syringe (Figure 29-7), inflation with a constant slow flow (< 10 L/min), and the measurement of plateau pressures at various inflation volumes. Correct interpretation of the pressure-volume curve during non-constant flow ventilation (e.g., pressure-controlled ventilation), and with higher inspiratory flows, is problematic (Figure 29-8). Correct measurement of pressure-volume curves requires that the patient is relaxed and breathing in synchrony with the ventilator.

In spite of enthusiasm for the use of pressure-volume curves to set the ventilator in patients with ARDS, a number of issues preclude routine use in practice. Measurement of the pressure-volume curve requires sedation, and often paralysis, to correctly make the measurement. It is often difficult to identify the inflection points and may require mathematical curve-fitting to precisely identify the inflection points. Esophageal pressure measurement during the measurement is needed to separate lung from chest wall effects. Although the inflation limb of the pressure-volume curve is most commonly measured, the deflation limb may be more useful than inflation limb. Finally, and perhaps most important, the pres-

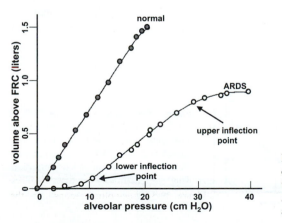

Figure 29-6 Inflation pressure-volume curves during passive mechanical ventilation. The pressure-volume curve for ARDS illustrates a lower inflection point and upper inflection point.

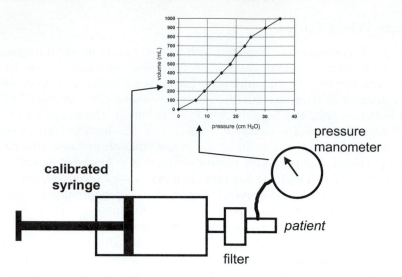

Figure 29-7 Equipment used to measure a pressure-volume curve using a super syringe.

sure-volume curve treats the lungs as a single compartment, but the lungs of patients with ARDS are heterogeneous. This likely explains why recruitment has been shown to occur along the entire inflation pressure-volume curve.

TRACHEAL PRESSURE

The effect of endotracheal tube resistance on proximal airway pressure can be overcome by measuring tracheal pressure. This can be accomplished by passing a narrow bore catheter to the distal tip of the endotracheal tube. This may allow tracheal pressures to be used to trigger the ventilator. Measurements of tracheal pressure may also be useful to titrate pressure support levels to overcome the imposed work-of-breathing through the endotracheal tube. Although measurement of tracheal pressure is attractive, the clinical feasibility of this is currently

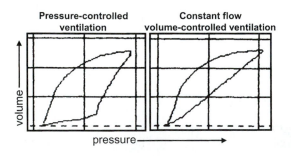

Figure 29-8 Dynamic pressure volume curves as displayed on the ventilator. The only difference between the two curves is a change from pressure controlled to volume controlled ventilation. This demonstrates that dynamic pressure-volume curves cannot be used to detect inflection points.

unclear. Due to the issues related to measurement of tracheal pressure, it has become more common to calculate tracheal pressure based on the known resistance through the endotracheal tube and flow through the tube. In fact, ventilator modes such as tube compensation calculate tracheal pressure based on this approach rather than direct measurement of tracheal pressure.

ESOPHAGEAL PRESSURE

Esophageal pressure is a reflection of intrapleural pressure, and is used to identify changes in intrapleural pressure during ventilatory maneuvers. In critically ill patients in a supine position, the absolute value for esophageal pressure often overestimates the true intrapleural pressure due to the weight of the mediastinal viscera. However, a properly placed esophageal balloon will accurately reflect changes in pleural pressure regardless of patient position. The esophageal balloon is placed in the lower third of the esophagus (about 35–40 cm from the nares in most adults). The balloon is filled and then all but 0.5–1 mL is removed.

In the spontaneously breathing subject, proper placement can be evaluated using the Baydur maneuver, in which airway and esophageal pressures are evaluated during airway occlusion. If the catheter is properly placed, equal changes will be noted for esophageal and airway pressure during airway occlusion. Proper position of the esophageal catheter can also be assessed by the observation of cardiac oscillations on the esophageal pressure waveform.

Patient versus Ventilator Work-of-Breathing

Patients often exert work during mechanical ventilation, particularly during patient-triggered modes. The work performed by the patient may be high and difficult to assess by usual means such as contraction of accessory muscles and asynchronous breathing. Measuring esophageal pressure, proximal airway pressure, and flow makes it possible to estimate the amount of inspiratory work done by the ventilator and the amount done by the patient. The sum of ventilator work and patient work is the total inspiratory work-of-breathing. Some bedside monitoring systems calculate and display these measurements on a breath-by-breath basis. Normal inspiratory work-of-breathing is 0.5 joules/L (0.05 kg-m/L). High inspiratory work (> 1.5 joule/L or > 15 joules/L/min) results in fatigue and failure to wean from mechanical ventilation. Patient effort can also be assessed by the esophageal pressure decrease during inspiration (Figure 29-9).

Auto-PEEP with Spontaneous Breathing

During passive ventilation, auto-PEEP can be assessed by use of an end-expiratory hold. During active breathing by the patient, an esophageal balloon is needed

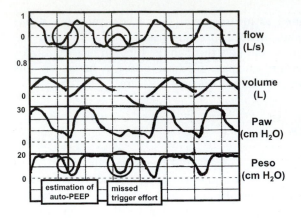

Figure 29-9 Airway pressure, flow, and volume graphics with esophageal pressure in a patient with auto-PEEP. Note the esophageal pressure decrease required to trigger the ventilator. Also note the presence of a missed trigger.

to assess auto-PEEP. With a patient-triggered breath, inspiratory flow will not occur at the proximal airway until the pleural pressure change equals the auto-PEEP level. Auto-PEEP can thus be quantified by observing the pleural pressure change required to produce flow at the proximal airway (Figure 29-10). Because auto-PEEP may be a fatiguing load for the spontaneously breathing patient, methods should be used to decrease the amount of auto-PEEP (e.g., application of external PEEP, administration of bronchodilators).

Transmission of Pressure to the Pleural Space

Esophageal pressure measurements can also be used to estimate the amount of airway pressure transmitted to the pleural space during passive positive pressure

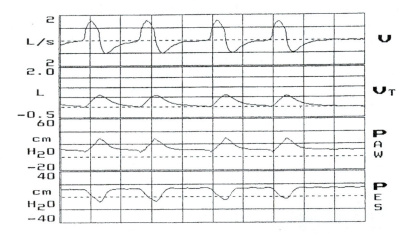

Figure 29-10 The change in esophageal pressure (bottom tracing) may be used to assess patient effort with each inspiration.

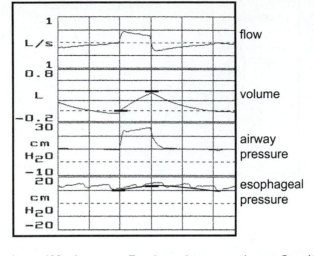

Tidal volume: 400 mL   Esophageal pressure change: 5 cm H_2O

Chest wall compliance: 400/5 = 80 mL/cm H_2O

Figure 29-11 Use of esophageal pressure to calculate chest wall compliance.

ventilation. The pleural pressure produced during passive inflation depends upon tidal volume and chest wall compliance (Figure 29-11). If the lungs are passively inflated, chest wall compliance can be calculated as the tidal volume delivered divided by the change in esophageal pressure. In the absence of an esophageal balloon, respiratory variation of the central venous pressure can be used to estimate changes in pleural pressure.

The Campbell Diagram can be used to calculate the work-of-breathing due to chest wall compliance, lung compliance, and airways resistance (Figure 29-12).

INTRA-ABDOMINAL PRESSURE

Gastric Pressure

One approach to measurement of intra-abdominal pressure is to place a balloon catheter into the stomach. The pressure in the balloon represents gastric pressure and is a reflection of intra-abdominal pressure. During spontaneous breathing, pressures can be measured simultaneously in the esophagus and the stomach. The difference between the pressure in the stomach and the esophagus is called transdiaphragmatic pressure (Pdi). Pdi is a reflection of the strength of the diaphragm. Accordingly, Pdi is used to assess diaphragm weakness.

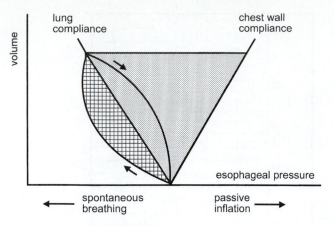

Figure 29-12 The Campbell Diagram. The slope of the pressure-volume curve during spontaneous breathing represents lung compliance. The chest wall compliance line is the slope of the esophageal pressure-volume curve generated during passive positive pressure ventilation. The area between the lung compliance line and the chest wall compliance line represents elastic work-of-breathing (shaded area). The area between the lung compliance line and the inspiratory pressure-volume curve represents the resistive work-of-breathing (cross-hatched area). The total spontaneous inspiratory work-of-breathing is the sum of the resistive work and the elastic work.

Bladder Pressure

Another method for measurement of intra-abdominal pressure is to measure bladder pressure in a patient with a Foley catheter. This is most commonly performed to assess the presence of abdominal compartment syndrome. In the mechanically ventilated patient, measurement of bladder pressure may be useful to assess the effect of abdominal pressure on chest wall compliance.

POINTS TO REMEMBER

- Much qualitative information can be obtained by observing the airway pressure waveform.
- Failure of the expiratory flow to decrease to zero indicates the presence of auto-PEEP; auto-PEEP may also be present even if expiratory flow is apparently zero at end-expiration.
- With a large leak from the lungs (around airway cuff or through a broncho-pleural fistula), expiratory volume will be less than inspiratory volume.
- Flow-volume loops can be used to assess response to bronchodilators.
- Pressure-volume loops can be used to assess trigger work, lung compliance, work performed by the ventilator during inspiration, appropriate PEEP setting, and hyperinflation.
- Esophageal pressure changes reflect pleural pressure changes.

- Esophageal pressure can be used to assess patient work-of-breathing, auto-PEEP during spontaneous breathing, and chest wall compliance.
- Measurement of intra-abdominal pressure may be useful to assess transdiaphragmatic pressure and the effect of intra-abdominal pressure on chest wall compliance.

ADDITIONAL READING

BANNER MJ, JAEGER MJ, KIRBY RR. Components of the work-of-breathing and implications for monitoring ventilator-dependent patients. *Crit Care Med* 1994; 22:515–532.

BLANCH MJ, BANNER MJ. A new respiratory monitor that enables accurate measurement of work-of-breathing: A validation study. *Respir Care* 1994; 39:897–905.

GUTTMANN J, EBERHARD L, FABRY B, ET AL. Continuous calculation of intratracheal pressure in tracheally intubated patients. *Anesthesiology* 1993; 79:503–513.

HARRIS RS, HESS DR, VENEGAS JG. An objective analysis of the pressure-volume curve in the acute respiratory distress syndrome. *Am J Respir Crit Care Med* 2000; 161:432–439.

HICKLING KG. Best compliance during a decremental, but not incremental, positive end-expiratory pressure trial is related to open-lung positive end-expiratory pressure: a mathematical model of acute respiratory distress syndrome lungs. *Am J Respir Crit Care Med* 2001; 163:69–78.

HICKLING KG. The pressure-volume curve is greatly modified by recruitment. A mathematical model of ARDS lungs. *Am J Respir Crit Care Med* 1998; 158:194–202.

JONSON B, RICHARD JC, STRAUS C, ET AL. Pressure-volume curves and compliance in acute lung injury: evidence of recruitment above the lower inflection point. *Am J Respir Crit Care Med* 1999; 159:1172–1178.

LU Q, VIEIRA SR, RICHECOEUR J, ET AL. A simple automated method for measuring pressure-volume curves during mechanical ventilation. *Am J Respir Crit Care Med* 1999; 159:275–282.

MALBRAIN ML. Abdominal pressure in the critically ill: measurement and clinical relevance. *Intensive Care Med* 1999; 25:1453–1458.

MARINI JJ. Lung mechanics determinations at the bedside: Instrumentation and clinical measurement. *Respir Care* 1990; 35:669–696.

MESSINGER G, BANNER MJ, BLANCH PB, LAYON AJ. Using tracheal pressure to trigger the ventilator and control airway pressure during continuous positive airway pressure decreases work-of-breathing. *Chest* 1995; 108:509–514.

RANIERI VM, GIULIANI R, FIORE T, DAMBROSIO M, MILIC-EMILI J. Volume-pressure curve of the respiratory system predicts effects of PEEP in ARDS: "Occlusion" versus "Constant Flow" Technique. *Am J Respir Crit Care Med* 1994; 149:19–27.

RANIERI VM, GRASSO S, FIORE T, GIULIANI R. Auto-positive end-expiratory pressure and dynamic hyperinflation. *Clin Chest Med* 1996; 17:379–394.

ROSSI A, POLESE G, BRANDI G, CONTI G. Intrinsic positive end-expiratory pressure (PEEPi). *Intensive Care Med* 1995; 21:522–536.

SERVILLO G, SVANTESSON C, BEYDON L, ET AL. Pressure-volume curves in acute respiratory failure: automated low flow inflation versus occlusion. *Am J Respir Crit Care Med* 1997; 155:1629–1636.

CHAPTER THIRTY

NUTRITIONAL ASSESSMENT

INTRODUCTION

OXYGEN CONSUMPTION, CARBON DIOXIDE PRODUCTION, AND ENERGY
EXPENDITURE

EFFECT OF STARVATION

NUTRITIONAL ASSESSMENT

INDIRECT CALORIMETRY
Open Circuit Method
Closed Circuit Method
Other Approaches
General Considerations with Indirect Calorimetry

NUTRITIONAL SUPPORT

POINTS TO REMEMBER

ADDITIONAL READING

OBJECTIVES

1. Describe the relationship between ventilation and metabolism.
2. Discuss the effects of malnutrition on respiratory function.
3. Discuss the effects of excessive caloric intake on respiratory function.
4. List markers of nutritional status in mechanically ventilated patients.
5. Compare open-circuit and closed-circuit indirect calorimetry.
6. Discuss issues related to indirect calorimetry in mechanically ventilated patients.
7. Compare enteral and parenteral approaches to nutritional support.

INTRODUCTION

Nutritional assessment and nutritional support are important considerations during mechanical ventilation (Figure 30-1). Assessment of nutritional status and determination of nutritional requirements for mechanically ventilated patients usually requires the teamwork of physicians, dietitians, respiratory therapists, and nurses. Either too few or too many calories can affect respiratory function and the ability to wean from mechanical ventilation. Too few calories causes respiratory muscle catabolism and muscle weakness. Too many calories – particularly carbohydrate calories – increases metabolic rate and can result in respiratory muscle fatigue or hypercapnia due to increased CO_2 production.

OXYGEN CONSUMPTION, CARBON DIOXIDE PRODUCTION, AND ENERGY EXPENDITURE

The relationship between metabolism, $\dot{V}_{O_2}$, and $\dot{V}_{CO_2}$ is dependent upon the substrate metabolized. $\dot{V}_{CO_2}$ divided by $\dot{V}_{O_2}$ is the respiratory quotient (RQ). The RQ is 1 for carbohydrate metabolism, 0.71 for fat metabolism, 0.81 for protein metabolism, 8.7 for lipogenesis, and 0.25 for ketogenesis. Whole body RQ is normally 0.7–1. With a balanced metabolism, RQ is 0.8, carbohydrate metabolism raises it towards 1, and fat metabolism lowers it towards 0.7. With lipogenesis, the overall RQ may be greater than one, but seldom exceeds 1.2. With ketogenesis, the overall RQ may be less than 0.7, but is seldom less than 0.65.

The principal function of the cardiopulmonary system is to provide the O_2 needed for energy production and to clear the CO_2 produced. An increase in metabolic rate increases $\dot{V}_{O_2}$ and $\dot{V}_{CO_2}$, requires an increase in ventilation, and forms the relationship between breathing ($\dot{V}_{O_2}$ and $\dot{V}_{CO_2}$) and nutrition (energy as Kcal). Excessive caloric intake, particularly with carbohydrates, can result in increased $\dot{V}_{CO_2}$.

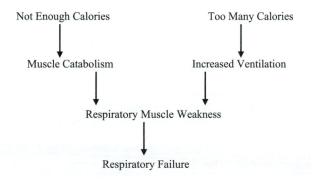

Figure **30-1** The relationship between nutrition and respiration. Either too few or too many calories can result in respiratory failure.

EFFECT OF STARVATION

Although patients are not intentionally starved, many mechanically ventilated patients receive inadequate nutritional support and thus suffer the effects of starvation. The initial response to starvation is an increase in glycogen and fat metabolism. Glycogenolysis provides glucose, which is necessary for cerebral metabolism. Glycogen stores are limited, and are depleted after four to five days of fasting. Lipolysis of adipose tissue triglycerides produces ketones, which can also be metabolized by brain cells. Gluconeogenesis also occurs, primarily due to the breakdown of muscle and visceral proteins. By the third day of fasting, ketogenesis and gluconeogenesis are at maximal rates. There is also a decrease in metabolic rate with starvation that slows the rate at which nutritional stores are depleted. There are numerous effects of starvation on respiratory function (Table 30-1), the most serious of which is loss of muscle mass due to respiratory muscle catabolism.

NUTRITIONAL ASSESSMENT

Anthropometric data are commonly used in the nutritional assessment. This includes height, weight, ideal body weight (desirable weight for height), and weight change. Upper arm anthropometric measurements such as triceps skin-folds thickness and midarm muscle circumference are also used. Skinfold thickness is an indicator of body fat, and the midarm muscle circumference is an indicator of somatic protein reserve. From height and weight, the basal energy expenditure (BEE) can be estimated using the Harris-Benedict equation:

$$BEE = 66 + 13.7 \times W + 5 \times H - 6.8 \times A \text{ (males)}$$

$$BEE = 655 + 9.66 \times W + 1.8 \times H - 4.7 \times A \text{ (females)}$$

Table 30-1 Effects of starvation on respiratory function

- Respiratory muscle function: catabolism of muscle protein results in weakening of respiratory muscles. This can result in respiratory muscle fatigue in spontaneously breathing patients, and difficulty in weaning ventilated patients.
- Surfactant production: starvation results in decreased surfactant production, which decreases lung compliance and increased work-of-breathing.
- Respiratory drive: starvation results in a decreased respiratory response to hypoxia.
- Pulmonary defense mechanisms: starvation results in an impaired immune response. The cause of death from starvation is often pneumonia.
- Colloid osmotic pressure: starvation results in a decreased circulating albumin, which decreases colloid osmotic pressure, increasing lung water and contributes to pulmonary edema.
- Airway epithelium: malnutrition may contribute to laryngeal ulceration with prolonged intubation.

where W is body mass (kg), H is height (cm), and A is age (yrs). The total daily caloric needs calculated from the Harris-Benedict equation are increased by an activity factor and an injury stress factor to determine the caloric needs of a patient. The activity factor is 20% if the patient is confined to bed and 30% if the patient is ambulatory. Typical stress factors are 10–30% for major trauma, 25–60% for sepsis, and 50–110% for burns. Although the Harris-Benedict equation is useful to estimate the caloric requirements of many patients, indirect calorimetry is superior in patients who are critically ill and have numerous nutritional stress factors. Because indirect calorimetry is labor-intensive and expensive, it should be reserved for selected patients (Table 30-2).

Biochemical data are also useful in the assessment of nutritional status (Table 30-3). Albumin levels correlate with the degree of malnutrition, and decreased levels are associated with increased risk of morbidity and mortality. Because its half-life is about 20 days, albumin levels reflect chronic rather than acute protein depletion. Albumin is not considered a specific indicator of visceral protein status in critically ill patients. Transferrin is a more sensitive indicator of acute changes in nutritional status than albumin because its half-life is about eight to 10 days. Thyroxine-binding prealbumin (transthyretin) is a sensitive indicator of visceral protein status, especially in acute stages of protein-energy malnutrition. A major advantage of prealbumin as an indicator of nutritional status is its short half-life (two to three days). Retinol binding protein is highly sensitive to changes in nutritional status, with a 12-hour half-life; however, it has limited use as an assessment parameter in renal failure because it is filtered by the glomerulus and metabolized by the kidney. The total lymphocyte count is useful as a nutrition screening parameter with non-critically ill patients, and correlates with albumin in reference to post surgery mortality and morbidity. Nitrogen balance determines the amount of nitrogen (protein) required to maintain nitrogen equilibrium, and reflects anabolism/catabolism and distribution of protein. It is determined as:

$$N \text{ balance} = \text{nitrogen intake} - \text{nitrogen output}$$

$$= \text{protein intake}/6.25 - (\text{UUN} + 4)$$

where UUN is the urine urea nitrogen. The determination of nitrogen balance requires an accurate 24-hour urine collection, an accurate assessment of protein intake, and a creatinine clearance greater than 50 mL/min. Nitrogen balance is

Table 30-2 Indications for indirect calorimetry

- Patients with several nutritional stress factors (trauma, sepsis, burns, etc.)
- Patients who are difficult to wean from mechanical ventilation
- Pediatric patients in whom caloric requirements are uncertain
- Obese patients in whom caloric requirements are uncertain
- Malnourished patients in whom caloric requirements are uncertain
- Patients who fail to respond appropriately to nutritional support

Table 30-3 Normal values for biochemical data used in nutritional assessment

Measurement	Normal	Deficient
Albumin	3.5–5 g/dL	< 2.5 g/dL
Transferrin	200–400 mg/dL	< 100 mg/dL
Prealbumin	10–20 mg/dL	≤ 10 mg/dL
Retinol binding protein	3–6 µg/dL	≤ 3 µg/dL
Total lymphocyte count	2,000–3,500 cells/mm^3	≤ 1,200 cells/mm^3
Nitrogen balance	Positive	Negative

normally positive and becomes negative with inadequate caloric and/or protein intake and metabolic stress.

INDIRECT CALORIMETRY

Indirect calorimetry is the calculation of energy expenditure by the measurement of $\dot{V}_{O_2}$ and $\dot{V}_{CO_2}$, which are converted to energy expenditure (Kcal/day) by the Weir Method:

$$\text{energy expenditure} = \dot{V}_{O_2} \times 3.941 + \dot{V}_{CO_2} \times 1.11 \times 1440$$

Indirect calorimetry also allows calculation of the RQ. Indirect calorimeters can use an open circuit method or a closed circuit method.

Open Circuit Method

The open circuit method measures the concentrations and volumes of inspired and expired gases to determine $\dot{V}_{O_2}$ and $\dot{V}_{CO_2}$. The principal components of an open circuit calorimeter (metabolic cart) are the analyzers (O_2 and CO_2), a volume-measuring device, and a mixing chamber. The analyzers must be capable of measuring small changes in gas concentrations and the volume monitor must be capable of accurately measuring volumes from 0.05 to 1 L. Exhaled gas from the patient is directed into a mixing chamber. At the outlet of the mixing chamber, a vacuum pump aspirates a small sample of gas for measurement of O_2 and CO_2. After analysis, this sample is returned to the mixing chamber. The entire volume of gas then exits through a volume monitor. Periodically, the analyzer also measures the inspired oxygen concentration. A microprocessor performs the necessary calculations. Meticulous attention to detail is required to obtain valid results using an open-circuit indirect calorimeter (Table 30-4).

Table 30-4 Important points that must be observed with the open circuit technique

---

- The $F_{I_{O_2}}$ must be stable ($\pm 0.005\%$). An air-oxygen blender is often used to prevent fluctuations caused by the instability of gas mixing systems in mechanical ventilators.
- The $F_{I_{O_2}}$ must be ≤ 0.60. Open circuit calorimeters measure $\dot{V}_{O_2}$ inaccurately at high $F_{I_{O_2}}$.
- The entire system must be leak free. This creates a problem with uncuffed airways, bronchopleural fistula, and if a sidestream capnograph is in line. Errors may also be introduced if the patient is undergoing renal dialysis.
- Inspired and expired gases must be completely separated. This can be a problem with a continuous bias flow in the system.

Closed Circuit Method

The key components of the closed circuit calorimeter are a volumetric spirometer, a mixing chamber, a CO_2 analyzer, and a CO_2 absorber. The spirometer is filled with a known volume of oxygen and is connected to the patient. As the patient rebreathes from the spirometer, oxygen is consumed and carbon dioxide is produced. The CO_2 is removed from the system by a CO_2 absorber before the gas is returned to the spirometer. The decrease in the volume of the system equals $\dot{V}_{O_2}$. Gas from the patient flows into the mixing chamber, and a sample is aspirated for $F\bar{E}_{CO_2}$ analysis. From the mixing chamber, gas flows through a CO_2 absorber and then to the spirometer. The volume of the spirometer is electronically monitored to measure tidal volume. The difference between end-expiratory volumes is calculated by a microprocessor to determine $\dot{V}_{O_2}$. If the patient is being mechanically ventilated, a bag-in-the-box system is used as a part of the inspiratory limb of the calorimeter. The bellows is pressurized by the ventilator, resulting in ventilation of the patient. Measurement time is limited by $F_{I_{O_2}}$ and the volume of the spirometer. When the volume of the spirometer decreases to a critical level, the measurement is interrupted to refill the spirometer.

Leaks from the closed circuit system will result in erroneously high $\dot{V}_{O_2}$ measurements (uncuffed airway, bronchopleural fistula, sidestream capnograph). Another problem with this technique is that compressible volume is increased and trigger sensitivity is decreased. The major advantage of the closed circuit method over the open circuit method is its ability to make measurements at a high $F_{I_{O_2}}$ (up to 1).

Other Approaches

In patients with a pulmonary artery catheter, $\dot{V}_{O_2}$ can be calculated from arterial oxygen content (Ca_{O_2}), mixed venous oxygen content ($C\bar{v}_{O_2}$), and cardiac output:

$$\dot{V}_{O_2} = \text{cardiac output} \times (Ca_{O_2} - C\bar{v}_{O_2})$$

This method can only be used if a thermodilution pulmonary artery catheter is in place. Metabolic rate can then be calculated from the $\dot{V}_{O_2}$:

$$REE = \dot{V}_{O_2} \times 4.83 \times 1440$$

Metabolic rate can also be calculated from $\dot{V}_{CO_2}$:

$$REE = \dot{V}_{CO_2} \times 5.52 \times 1440$$

General Considerations with Indirect Calorimetry

When measuring resting energy expenditure using indirect calorimetry, one must consider both the duration of each measurement and the number of measurements required to produce a reliable 24-hour estimate. Ideally, continuous 24-hour indirect calorimetry produces the best estimate of REE. For most critically ill patients, it is impossible to obtain measurements for longer than 15 to 30 min more than once every several days. It is important, however, to recognize that shorter and less frequent measurements will less reliably estimate REE. When performing indirect calorimetry, the patient should be resting, undisturbed, motionless, supine, and aware of the surroundings (unless comatose). The patient should either be on continuous nutritional support or fasting for several hours before the measurement. Before indirect calorimetry is performed, there should have been no changes in ventilation for at least 90 min, no changes that affect $\dot{V}_{O_2}$ for at least 60 min, and stable hemodynamics for at least two hours. REE is similar, but not equivalent to, basal energy expenditure (BEE). BEE is measured in a neutrothermal environment after 12 hours of fasting. Because REE is measured with the patient at rest, calories must be added due to patient activity. There may be considerable fluctuation in REE throughout the day, and from day to day.

NUTRITIONAL SUPPORT

Enteral nutrition should always be considered when a patient has a functioning gastrointestinal (GI) tract. Nutrients absorbed via the portal system with delivery to the liver may allow for better absorption and result in enhanced immune competence. The presence of nutrients in the gut prevents intestinal atrophy and maintains the absorptive capacity of the GI mucosa. Enteral nutrition also helps to preserve normal gut flora and gastric pH, which may guard against bacterial overgrowth in the small intestine and development of pneumonia. If enteral nutrition is administered appropriately, it is safer and less expensive than parenteral nutrition.

The preferred method of nutritional support is the oral route. However, it is practically impossible for most mechanically ventilated patients. In the mechanically ventilated patient, nasogastric or orogastric tubes are often used initially. These are used for short-term feeding and may be contraindicated in patients who have severe reflux, delayed gastric emptying, and are at risk of aspiration. A feeding tube placed into the small intestine should be considered for uninterrupted duodenal or jejunal feeding. It is generally assumed that feeding distal to the stomach decreases the risk of aspiration. However, because the risk of aspiration is always present with enteral feeding, patients should be placed into the semi-recumbent position (head elevated 30 degrees) to decrease the risk of aspiration. If long-term feeding is needed, tubes can be placed through the skin into the stomach or small intestine by surgical, endoscopic, radiologic, or laparoscopic techniques. These tubes are generally more comfortable than the nasogastric or enteric tubes.

Intravenous delivery of substrate may be necessary when the gastrointestinal tract is not functioning or if stimulation of the gastrointestinal or pancreatic systems would worsen the patient's condition. Placement of a central or peripheral venous catheter is required for the infusion of nutrients into the bloodstream. Central venous access is usually preferred because solutions > 600–900 mOsm/L may be infused, the volume of fluid is unrestricted, and support may continue for a long period of time. The infusion of nutrients into the central circulation, however, leaves the GI tract unstimulated which can lead to gut atrophy, mucosal compromise, weakening of the gut barrier, and increased risk of pneumonia.

POINTS TO REMEMBER

- There is a measurable relationship between metabolism (energy expenditure), $\dot{V}_{O_2}$, and $\dot{V}_{CO_2}$.
- RQ is dependent on substrate metabolized.
- Too few calories can result in respiratory muscle fatigue due to muscle catabolism, and too many calories can result in respiratory muscle fatigue due to a high ventilatory requirement.
- Methods used for nutritional assessment include anthropometric data, Harris-Benedict equation, biochemical data, and indirect calorimetry.
- Indirect calorimetry is the calculation of energy expenditure based upon measurements of $\dot{V}_{O_2}$ and $\dot{V}_{CO_2}$.
- Indirect calorimetry can be performed using open-circuit devices or closed-circuit devices.
- Caloric requirements can be determined from $\dot{V}_{O_2}$ alone, $\dot{V}_{CO_2}$ alone, or with measurements of both $\dot{V}_{O_2}$ and $\dot{V}_{CO_2}$.
- The enteral route of nutritional support is preferable to the parenteral route.

ADDITIONAL READING

BOSSCHA K, NIEUWENHUIJS VB, VOS A, ET AL. Gastrointestinal motility and gastric tube feeding in mechanically ventilated patients. *Crit Care Med* 1998; 26:1510–1517.

BRANSON RD. The measurement of energy expenditure: Instrumentation, practical considerations, and clinical application. *Respir Care* 1990; 35:640–659.

COSS-BU JA, JEFFERSON LS, WALDING D, ET AL. Resting energy expenditure and nitrogen balance in critically ill pediatric patients on mechanical ventilation. *Nutrition* 1998; 14:649–652.

EPSTEIN CD, PEERLESS JR, MARTIN JE, MALANGONI MA. Comparison of methods of measurements of oxygen consumption in mechanically ventilated patients with multiple trauma: the Fick method versus indirect calorimetry. *Crit Care Med* 2000; 28:1363–1369.

FLANCBAUM L, CHOBAN PS, SAMBUCCO S, ET AL. Comparison of indirect calorimetry, the Fick method, and prediction equations in estimating the energy requirements of critically ill patients. *Am J Clin Nutr* 1999; 69:461–466.

HUANG YC, YEN CE, CHENG CH, ET AL. Nutritional status of mechanically ventilated critically ill patients: comparison of different types of nutritional support. *Clin Nutr* 2000; 19:101–107.

JOOSTEN KF. Why indirect calorimetry in critically ill patients: what do we want to measure? *Intensive Care Med* 2001; 27:1107–1109.

KEARNS PJ, CHIN D, MUELLER L, ET AL. The incidence of ventilator-associated pneumonia and success in nutrient delivery with gastric versus small intestinal feeding: a randomized clinical trial. *Crit Care Med* 2000; 28:1742–1746.

PETROS S, ENGELMANN L. Validity of an abbreviated indirect calorimetry protocol for measurement of resting energy expenditure in mechanically ventilated and spontaneously breathing critically ill patients. *Intensive Care Med* 2001; 27:1164–1168.

SHERMAN MS. A predictive equation for determination of resting energy expenditure in mechanically ventilated patients. *Chest* 1994; 105:544–549.

FOUR

TOPICS IN MECHANICAL VENTILATION

THIRTY-ONE

AIRWAY MANAGEMENT

OBJECTIVES

1. List indications for an artificial airway.
2. List complications of artificial airways.
3. Assess patients for extubation.
4. Compare endotracheal intubation and tracheostomy.
5. Describe the use of a speaking valve.

INTRODUCTION

Although airway management and mechanical ventilation are often considered synonymous, it is possible to provide ventilatory support without an artificial airway (e.g., noninvasive positive pressure ventilation). Nonetheless, a thorough understanding of airway management is important for those providing mechanical ventilation.

INDICATIONS FOR AN ARTIFICIAL AIRWAY

There are four traditional indications for an artificial airway:

- Provide ventilatory support.
- Aid in the removal of secretions.
- Bypass upper airway obstruction.
- Prevent aspiration.

Each of these is a relative indication. For example, ventilatory support can be provided by facial mask and secretions can be removed by nasotracheal suction. It is also known that micro-aspiration commonly occurs past the cuff of the artificial airway. However, the acutely ill patient who requires ventilatory support often needs intubation to facilitate suctioning of secretions and to bypass upper airway obstruction resulting from a depressed level of consciousness.

OROTRACHEAL VERSUS NASOTRACHEAL INTUBATION

Advantages of nasotracheal intubation include improved tolerance in the patient who is awake, easier oral hygiene, ease of intubation in the patient with cervical spine injury, and decreased likelihood of self-extubation. However, the disadvantages of nasal intubation outweigh these advantages. Because nasotracheal intubation requires a narrower and longer tube, it increases airway resistance, makes suctioning and bronchoscopy more difficult, and increases the likelihood of sinusitis and otitis media. Accordingly, most patients are intubated by the oral route.

COMPLICATIONS OF AIRWAYS

A life-threatening complication of airway management is misplacement of the tube (Table 31-1). Although not all patients who experience an unplanned extubation require reintubation, there is significant morbidity and mortality associated with the need for reintubation. Efforts to avoid unplanned extubations include securing the tube (around-the-head taping procedures are preferred), restraining the patient's hands and sedation if necessary, and vigilance of the

Table 31-1 Complications of artificial airways

- Misplacement of the tube
  - unplanned extubation
  - esophageal intubation
  - mainstem intubation
- Airway trauma
  - laryngeal
  - tracheal
- Cuff leaks
- Aspiration and pneumonia
- Loss of upper airway functions
- Increased resistance of breathing
- Decreased ability to clear secretions

airway position whenever the patient or ventilator tubing is moved. The endotracheal tube can be misplaced into the esophagus or mainstem bronchus (usually the right). Although this usually occurs at the time of intubation, it can also occur anytime after intubation. The tip of the endotracheal tube can move several centimeters as the result of flexion and extension of the neck – flexion moves the endotracheal tube tip caudad and extension moves it cephalad.

As a landmark, the centimeter marking on the tube at the lip or nares should be recorded when proper tube position is determined and this landmark should be checked frequently. For the newly intubated patient, the oral endotracheal tube should generally be inserted 21 cm at the teeth for females and 23 cm for males. Tube position should be assessed frequently by auscultation and on a regular basis by chest X-ray. A thorough evaluation of endotracheal tube position should be performed immediately following intubation (Table 31-2).

The presence of the endotracheal tube is traumatic to the airway. The larynx and tracheal wall are particularly prone to injury, which will often not be recognized until after extubation. Laryngeal injuries include edema, vocal cord paralysis, glottic stenosis, and granuloma formation. Tracheal injuries include tracheal stenosis, tracheomalacia, and fistula formation to the esophagus or innominate artery. Tracheal injuries are usually related to compression of the tracheal mucosa by the endotracheal tube cuff. These injuries have decreased as the result of the common use of high-volume, low-pressure cuffs. Tracheal wall injury can be ameliorated by avoidance of cuff over-distension, which is facilitated by intra-cuff pressures of < 25 mm Hg. On the other hand, the risk of silent aspiration is increased with cuff pressures < 20 mm Hg. Accordingly, cuff pressures should be monitored at regular intervals and should be maintained in the range of 20 to 25 mm Hg.

Cuff leaks occasionally occur. This can be due to cuff rupture, accidental severing of the pilot tube, or malfunction of the pilot balloon valve mechanism (Figure 31-1). Inability to maintain cuff inflation usually results in failure to adequately ventilate the patient and necessitates re-intubation. Changing the

Table 31-2 Techniques to evaluate endotracheal tube position

- Auscultation: auscultate chest and epigastrium to differentiate tracheal versus esophageal intubation; auscultate right and left chest to differentiate tracheal versus bronchial intubation.
- Inspection: bilateral chest expansion should occur with tube in the trachea; condensation of moisture on the inside of endotracheal tube should occur with tracheal intubation.
- CO_2 detection: absent or low (< 5 mm Hg) exhaled CO_2 indicates esophageal intubation; this can be performed using a low-cost CO_2 detector and does not require the use of an expensive capnograph.
- Bronchoscopy: this allows direct visualization of tube placement and can be used to properly place the tube during difficult intubations.
- Light wand (lighted stylet): when passed to the tip of the endotracheal tube, these devices produce transillumination of the suprasternal notch when the tube is in proper position.
- Esophageal detector device: this is a squeeze bulb device which rapidly re-inflates when attached to the endotracheal tube that is in the trachea.
- Chest X-ray: the tip of the tube should be above the carina and at mid-trachea; at the level of the aortic arch.

endotracheal tube in critically ill patients is facilitated by use of a semi-rigid stylet (tube changer). Commercial tube changers are hollow and allow oxygen insufflation.

Pneumonia is common in intubated patients. Intubation bypasses the normal filtering function of the upper airway, allowing contaminated aerosols to enter the lower respiratory tract. In the past, humidifiers and ventilator circuits have been implicated in the development of pneumonia in intubated patients. It was a common practice for many years to change ventilator humidifiers and circuits at regular intervals to prevent nosocomial pneumonia. It is now recognized that contamination of the circuit is usually from the patient (rather than vice versa). The type of humidification (heated versus unheated circuits, active versus passive humidification) has little impact on the development of pneumonia in intubated patients. Moreover, the frequency of ventilator circuit changes has little impact on the development of pneumonia and changing ventilator circuits at regular intervals is unnecessary. Because sub-clinical aspiration of upper airway secretions is a common occurrence in intubated patients, pneumonia in these patients is usually the result of aspiration (rather than contamination from the ventilator circuit).

An endotracheal tube bypasses the normal glottic functions. Because this eliminates the ability of the patient to speak, special efforts must be used to communicate with the patient. Bypass of the glottis may also result in a decrease in functional residual capacity. Although a PEEP level of 3 to 5 cm H_2O may be useful to maintain functional residual capacity in intubated patients, there is no physiologic basis for the term "physiologic PEEP." Bypass of the upper airway may be problematic in the patient with COPD due to inability to control exhalation by use of pursed lips.

The flow resistance through an endotracheal tube is greater than that through the native airway. This is particularly the case with nasotracheal

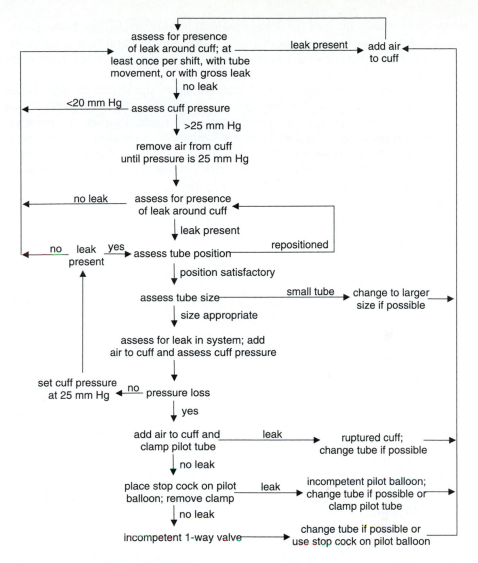

Figure 31-1 An algorithm to assess leak around the cuff of an endotracheal tube. (From HESS DR. Managing the artificial airway. *Respir Care* 1999; 44:759–772.)

tubes that are longer, have a smaller internal diameter, and may kink due to their curvature through the upper airway. A low level of pressure support (5–10 cm H_2O) may be useful to overcome the resistance through the endotracheal tube. However, with a usual adult-size endotracheal tube (e.g., 8 mm inside diameter) and a minute ventilation compatible with spontaneous breathing (e.g., < 12 L/min), the resistance of the endotracheal tube may not be clinically important. Moreover, the resistance through the endotracheal tube may be similar to the resistance through the upper airway following extubation. Nonetheless, prolonged spontaneous breathing through a small endotracheal tube is not desirable and should be supported with low-level pressure support or tube compensation.

The presence of an endotracheal tube decreases the ability to clear lower respiratory tract secretions for several reasons. Because the endotracheal tube bypasses the glottis, the patient cannot cough effectively. Further, the presence of the tube against the tracheal wall decreases mucociliary clearance. Suctioning is required to clear secretions and bronchoscopy may be needed in some patients. Because the endotracheal tube interferes with swallowing, secretions also accumulate in the upper airway and must be suctioned.

EXTUBATION

Evaluation for Extubation

Extubation should occur when there is no longer an indication for intubation. In many patients, extubation occurs when ventilatory support is no longer necessary. However, some patients need an artificial airway even though ventilatory support is no longer required. These include patients with upper airway obstruction, patients unable to adequately clear secretions, and patients unable to protect the lower respiratory tract from aspiration. One concern before extubation is whether the upper airway is free of swelling and inflammation. This is often assessed qualitatively as the amount of leak around the endotracheal tube during positive pressure ventilation with the cuff deflated (leak test). Although patients who develop upper airway obstruction after extubation usually have a failed leak test, absence of a leak with the cuff deflated may also occur in many patients who are successfully extubated (e.g., if the endotracheal tube size is large in relation to the size of the trachea). A large volume of secretions and weak cough are associated with extubation failure.

Complications of Extubation

Complications of extubation are listed in Table 31-3. Failed extubation occurs in 10 to 25% of patients. Noninvasive positive pressure ventilation is used for selected patients who cannot provide adequate ventilation to avoid re-intubation. Hoarseness is common following extubation and is usually short-term and benign. For post-extubation stridor due to upper airway swelling, cool mist therapy, aerosolized racemic epinephrine, parenteral steroids, and heliox therapy can be used. These treatments are only useful, however, for acute reversible swelling that responds relatively quickly to therapy. For irreversible post-extubation obstruction (e.g., vocal cord paralysis), the patient must be re-intubated and tracheostomy may be required.

Table 31-3 Complications of extubation

- Hoarseness
- Laryngeal edema
- Laryngospasm
- Stridor
- Vocal cord paralysis
- Glottic stenosis
- Granuloma formation

TRACHEOSTOMY

Timing of Tracheostomy

No clear consensus exists for when a tracheostomy should replace an endotracheal tube. There are both advantages and disadvantages of tracheostomy compared with translaryngeal intubation (Table 31-4). Many patients tolerate endotracheal intubation for weeks without complications. However, prolonged intubation increases the risk of glottic injury whereas tracheostomy increases the risk of tracheal stenosis. Tracheostomy is usually reserved for patients requiring long-term ventilatory support and for those needing long-term airway protection (e.g., patients with neurologic disease) or patients who cannot be weaned (multiple failed attempts to extubate). Some failure-to-wean patients may be successfully liberated from mechanical ventilation after tracheostomy. This may relate to

Table 31-4 Comparison of advantages of translaryngeal intubation and tracheostomy during prolonged ventilatory support

Advantages of translaryngeal intubation	Advantages of tracheostomy
Easy and rapid initial insertion	Ease of reinsertion if dislodged
Avoids surgical procedure	Reduced laryngeal injury
Lower cost of initial placement	Better secretion removal with suctioning
Lower risk of ventilator-associated pneumonia	Lower incidence of tube obstruction
	Less oral injury
	Improve patient comfort
	Better oral hygiene
	Improved ability to speak
	Preservation of glottic competence
	Better swallow allowing oral feeding
	Lower resistance to air flow
	Less tube dead space
	Lower work of spontaneous breathing
	More rapid weaning from mechanical ventilation

Source: JAEGER JM, LITTLEWOOD KA, DURBIN CG. The role of tracheostomy in weaning from mechanical ventilation. *Respir Care* 2002; 47:469–482.

less resistance through the tracheostomy tube, less dead space, increased ability to remove secretions, and improved patient comfort.

Percutaneous dilatational tracheostomy is a relatively new procedure that can be performed at the bedside without the risk and cost of transportation to the operating room. A small incision is performed midway between the cricoid cartilage and the sternal notch. A 14-gauge cannula is inserted into the trachea between the first and second tracheal rings. A guide wire is introduced into the trachea under direct bronchoscopic observation and the stoma is dilated with increasing sizes of specially designed plastic dilators. An appropriately sized tracheostomy tube is then inserted over a small dilator into position in the trachea. A mature tract is not formed for two weeks and attempted tracheostomy tube change during this time can lead to bleeding, tracheal injury, and death.

Weaning the Tracheostomy Tube

For patients with long-term tracheostomy, weaning with the use of a variety of airway appliances may be necessary to regain use of the upper airway. A fenestrated tracheostomy tube (Figure 31-2) can be used. These airways have one or more openings in their posterior wall. An inner cannula is removed to open the fenestrations and allow the patient to breathe through the upper airway. When the tracheostomy tube is capped, the patient is forced to breath through the upper airway. It is important that the fenestrations are properly aligned in the airway and the cuff deflated to allow breathing around the outside of the tube. The patient must be observed closely for signs of airway obstruction when the tube is capped.

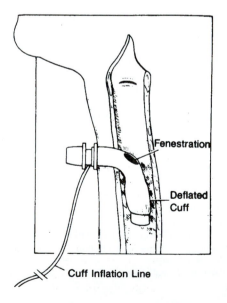

Fenestration

Deflated Cuff

Cuff Inflation Line

Figure 31-2 Schematic illustration of a fenestrated tracheostomy tube. (From WILSON DJ. Airway appliances and management. In: KACMAREK RM, STOLLER JK. *Current Respiratory Care*. Toronto, BC Decker, 1988.)

A speaking valve can be attached to the tracheostomy tube instead of a cap. These one-way valves allow the patient to inhale through the tracheostomy tube, but require exhalation through the upper airway (Figure 31-3). If the patient tolerates the fenestrated tube well, it may be replaced with a small cuffless tube. If the patient tolerates a capped cuffless tube, then the tracheostomy can usually be safely removed. For patients who require maintenance of the tracheal stoma but can breathe adequately through the upper airway, a tracheostomy button can be used. This device can be plugged to allow use of the upper airway and the plug can be removed for suctioning or to allow breathing through the tracheostomy (e.g., upper airway obstruction).

Because the upper airway is bypassed, communication is difficult for patients with artificial airways. For tracheostomized patients, a speaking tracheostomy tube can be used. With this tube, gas flow is introduced above the cuff to provide flow past the vocal cords and thus allow speech (Figure 31-4). Generally a speaking valve is preferred over a speaking tracheostomy tube. The speaking valve not only facilitates speech, but also improves swallowing and decreases the risk of aspiration.

When a speaking valve is placed, it is important that the patient can adequately exhale through the upper airway. This can be assessed by measurement of tracheal pressure when the valve is placed (Figure 31-5). If the expiratory tracheal pressure is > 10 cm H_2O, the placement of a smaller tube or upper airway pathology should be considered.

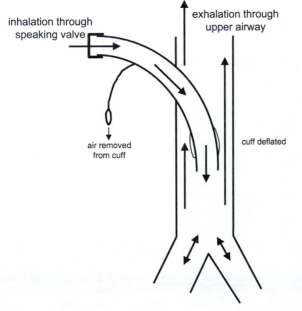

inhalation through speaking valve

exhalation through upper airway

air removed from cuff

cuff deflated

Figure 31-3 Function of a speaking valve. The patient inhales through the tracheostomy tube and exhales through the upper airway.

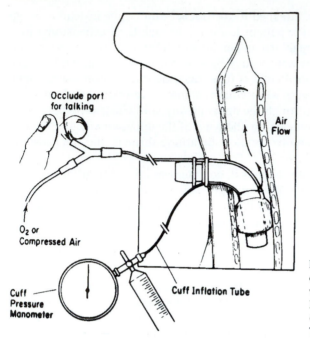

Figure 31-4 A speaking tracheostomy tube. (From WILSON DJ. Airway appliances and management. In: KACMAREK RM, STOLLER JK. *Current Respiratory Care.* Toronto, BC Decker, 1988.)

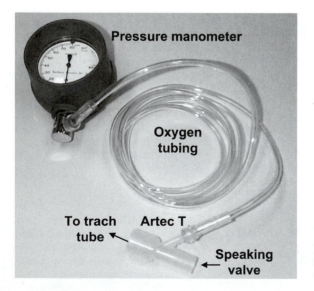

Figure 31-5 Equipment used to measure tracheal pressure when a speaking valve is used.

MISCELLANEOUS AIRWAY APPLIANCES

Alternate airway management equipment includes esophageal obturator airways, pharyngotracheal lumen airways, and esophageal-tracheal Combitubes. These devices should never be used beyond the period of initial resuscitation. An airway that has recently been popularized is the laryngeal mask airway (Figure 31-6). It is inserted without a laryngoscope and has an inflatable rim that provides a low-pressure seal over the glottic opening. This airway should be considered when the airway cannot be easily intubated. It can be used for short-term ventilation. However, it should be changed to an endotracheal tube as soon as possible. Although these devices provide a more secure airway than a facemask, they are never preferable to an endotracheal tube unless intubation is impossible.

POINTS TO REMEMBER

- The indications for an artificial airway are to provide ventilatory support, to aid in the removal of secretions, to bypass upper airway obstruction, and to prevent aspiration.
- Oral intubation is preferable to nasal intubation because a shorter tube is used, the oral endotracheal tube has a larger internal diameter, and kinking is less likely with the orotracheal tube.
- Complications of artificial airways include misplacement of the tube, trauma to the airway, cuff leaks, pneumonia, bypass of normal upper airway and glottic functions, decreased ability to clear secretions, and aspiration.
- Techniques to evaluate tracheal intubation include auscultation, inspection, CO_2 detection, bronchoscopy, lighted stylet, esophageal detector device, and chest X-ray.
- For the patient requiring intubation only for airway protection or suctioning, it is often desirable to provide a minimal level of ventilatory support until the decision is made to extubate.

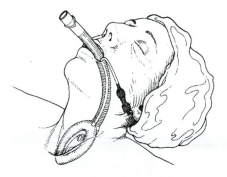

Figure 31-6 The laryngeal mask airway is inserted without a laryngoscope and has an inflatable rim that provides a low-pressure seal over the glottic opening. (From Bishop MJ. Practice guidelines for airway care during resuscitation. *Respir Care* 1995; 40:393–403.)

- Complications of extubation include hoarseness, stridor, laryngeal edema, laryngospasm, vocal cord paralysis, glottic stenosis, and granuloma formation.
- Many patients tolerate endotracheal intubation well for several weeks without complications.
- Weaning from a tracheostomy tube can be accomplished using a fenestrated tube, a small cuffless tube, or a tracheostomy button.
- A speaking valve forces exhalation through the upper airway, allows the patient to speak, and may improve swallow.
- Devices such as the laryngeal mask are never preferable to an endotracheal tube unless intubation is impossible.

ADDITIONAL READING

CAMPBELL RS. Extubation and the consequences of reintubation. *Respir Care* 1999; 44:799–806.

DUNN PF, GOULET RL. Endotracheal tubes and airway appliances. *Int Anesthesiol Clin* 2000; 38:65–94.

EPSTEIN SK. Decision to extubate. *Intensive Care Med* 2002; 28:535–546.

EPSTEIN SK. Extubation. *Respir Care* 2002; 47:483–495.

EPSTEIN SK, NEVINS ML, CHUNG J. Effect of unplanned extubation on outcome of mechanical ventilation. *Am J Respir Crit Care Med* 2000; 161:1912–1916.

FREEMAN BD, ISABELLA K, LIN N, ET AL. A meta-analysis of prospective trials comparing percutaneous and surgical tracheostomy in critically ill patients. *Chest* 2000; 118:1412–1418.

HEFFNER JE. Tracheostomy: indications and timing. *Respir Care* 1999; 44:807–815.

HESS DR. Indications for translaryngeal intubation. *Respir Care* 1999; 44:604–609.

HESS DR. Managing the artificial airway. *Respir Care* 1999; 44:759–772.

HURFORD WE. Nasotracheal intubation. *Respir Care* 1999; 44:643–647.

HURFORD WE. Techniques of endotracheal intubation. *Int Anesthesiol Clin* 2000; 38:1–28.

JAEGER JM, DURBIN CG. Special purpose endotracheal tubes. *Respir Care* 1999; 44:661–683.

JAEGER JM, LITTLEWOOD KA, DURBIN CG. The role of tracheostomy in weaning from mechanical ventilation. *Respir Care* 2002; 47:469–482.

SPIEKERMANN BF, BOGDONOFF DL, LEISURE GS, STONE DJ. Nonsurgical airway management: General considerations and specific considerations in patients with coexisting disease. *Respir Care* 1995; 40:644–654.

STAUFFER JL, SILVESTER RC. Complications of endotracheal intubation, tracheostomy, and artificial airways. *Respir Care* 1982; 27:417–434.

THIRTY-TWO

SECRETION CLEARANCE, POSITIONING, AND INHALED AEROSOL MEDICATION

OBJECTIVES

1. Describe techniques for secretion clearance in mechanically ventilated patients.
2. List complications of endotracheal suction.
3. Describe the effects of lateral and prone positioning on oxygenation.
4. Compare the use of nebulizers and metered dose inhalers in mechanically ventilated patients.

INTRODUCTION

Bronchial hygiene therapy is important in the care of mechanically ventilated patients. These therapies include suctioning, saline instillation, bronchoscopy, postural drainage therapy, positioning, and inhaled aerosol medication. Failure to adequately attend to the bronchial hygiene needs of the patient can complicate the course of mechanical ventilation.

SECRETION CLEARANCE

Secretion clearance is impaired in intubated patients due to decreased mucociliary activity and inability to cough effectively. Mucociliary activity is impaired due to the presence of the artificial airway, airway trauma due to suctioning, inadequate humidification, high $F_{I_{O_2}}$, drugs (e.g., narcotics), and underlying pulmonary disease. Cough effectiveness is impaired due to the presence of the artificial airway and depressed neurologic status. Methods commonly used to improve secretion clearance in intubated patients include suctioning, inhaled beta-agonists, postural drainage therapy with or without percussion and/or vibration, positioning, and bronchoscopy.

Hyperinflation Therapy

Hyperinflation of the lungs with a manual ventilator is a technique that has been used to facilitate secretion clearance in intubated patients. However, there is no evidence that this technique improves secretion clearance. Moreover, it may increase the likelihood of lung injury and hemodynamic sequelae.

Suctioning

Although it is not a benign procedure, suctioning is an important aspect of airway care. Complications of endotracheal suctioning are listed in Table 32-1. Suction-related complications can often be avoided by use of appropriate technique (Table 32-2). Techniques to facilitate selective endobronchial suctioning (particularly of the left) include use of curved tip catheters, turning the patient's head to the side (e.g., turning the head to the right to facilitate suctioning of the left bronchus), and lateral positioning. Of these, the use of a curved tip catheter is most successful.

The closed-suction system consists of a catheter within a protective sheath (Figure 32-1) that fits between the ventilator circuit and the airway. The catheter thus becomes part of the ventilator circuit. The sheath protects the catheter from external contamination and the patient is suctioned without removal from the ventilator. Closed suction prevents alveolar de-recruitment during suctioning and prevents contamination of clinicians during the suction procedure. Because the closed suction catheter is used repeatedly, and because it does not need to be changed at regular intervals, its use is also cost-effective.

Table 32-1 Complications of suctioning

- Hypoxemia
- Atelectasis
- Airway trauma
- Contamination
- Cardiac arrhythmias
- Selective secretion clearance from the right bronchus
- Increased intracranial pressure
- Coughing and bronchospasm

Saline Instillation

In the past, saline was often instilled during suctioning to facilitate secretion removal. However, more saline is instilled than is removed during subsequent suctioning. This may increase the volume of secretions and may worsen airway obstruction. Care must be taken to avoid contamination of the airway during saline instillation. Saline instillation can also produce airway irritation, coughing, and bronchospasm. It may be useful for selected patients with tenacious secretions, but should not be a routine procedure.

Postural Drainage Therapy

Postural drainage therapy is designed to improve the mobilization of bronchial secretions using the effects of gravity, positioning, percussion, vibration, and cough. It is as effective as bronchoscopy in the treatment of atelectasis and acute lobar collapse in intubated patients. However, there is no evidence to support the prophylactic use of postural drainage therapy in patients who do not have retained secretions. This therapy is labor intensive and expensive. Postural drainage therapy is of little benefit and potentially dangerous in acutely ill intubated patients who are producing little or no sputum. Complications of postural drainage therapy include hypoxemia, hypercapnia, increased intracranial pressure, acute hypotension, pulmonary hemorrhage, pain, vomiting and aspiration, bronchospasm, and dysrhythmias.

Table 32-2 Techniques to avoid suctioning-related complications

- Hyperoxygenation with $F_{IO_2} = 1$
- Used closed suction catheter
- Use proper catheter size (catheter size = $ID/2 \times 3$ where ID is the internal diameter of the airway)
- Use least amount of vacuum necessary to evacuate secretions (< 150 mm Hg)
- Use a gentle technique
- Limit the time of each suction attempt to ≤ 15 s
- Only suction during withdrawal of the catheter

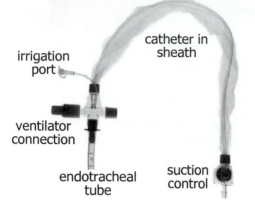

irrigation port

catheter in sheath

ventilator connection

endotracheal tube

suction control

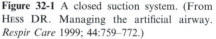

Figure 32-1 A closed suction system. (From HESS DR. Managing the artificial airway. *Respir Care* 1999; 44:759–772.)

Bronchoscopy

The most common indication for bronchoscopy in intubated patients is the diagnosis of ventilator-associated pneumonia using a protected specimen brush or bronchoalveolar lavage. Fiberoptic bronchoscopy may also be used to clear secretions in intubated patients (Table 32-3). However, it is invasive and should be reserved for cases where atelectasis persists despite conservative methods (i.e., postural drainage therapy and suctioning).

POSITIONING

Physiologic Effects

With normal lung function, ventilation is greater in the dependent lung zones due to the pleural pressure gradient (pleural pressure is more negative at the bottom of the lungs) that places dependent alveoli on a more compliant part of the pressure-volume curve. This may not be the case with diseases like ARDS, where the injury and edema are often greatest in the dorsal lung regions. When these patients are turned from a supine to a prone position, there is often an improvement in oxygenation. This is related to the gravitational effects on blood flow and the pleural pressure gradient, resulting in an improvement in $\dot{V}/\dot{Q}$. This effect does not always occur, with about 25% of patients failing to respond. For some patients, the improvement in Pa_{O_2} allows reduction of FI_{O_2} and PEEP. Unfortunately, prone positioning is technically difficult and care must be observed to avoid dislodgement of the airway and vascular lines. Chest wall compliance may decrease in the prone position, resulting in an increase in airway pressure with volume ventilation or a decrease in tidal volume with pressure ventilation. Facial edema and anterior pressure sores also may occur when the patient is placed prone. The length of time that patients should remain in the prone position is unclear. Although prone positioning improves Pa_{O_2} in many patients, its effect on survival is unclear.

Table 32-3 Indications and complications of fiberoptic bronchoscopy in intubated patients

Indications	Complications
• Obtain lower respiratory tract secretions for diagnosis of pneumonia	• Hypoxemia
	• Hypercarbia
• Clearing of secretions that are not adequately cleared by more conservative methods	• Air-trapping with bronchoscope in airway (particularly with small endotracheal tube)
• Persistent atelectasis that fails to respond to conservative treatment	• Bronchospasm
	• Contamination of lower respiratory tract
• Assess upper airway patency	• Pneumothorax
• Assess hemoptysis	• Hemoptysis
• Determine the location and extent of injury from toxic inhalation or aspiration	• Dysrhythmias
• Perform difficult intubation	
• Remove aspirated foreign body	

Lateral positioning can be useful in patients with unilateral lung disease. Positioning with the good lung down results in a higher Pa_{O_2}. Because gravity causes greater blood flow to dependent lung zones, positioning the good lung down presumably improves $\dot{V}/\dot{Q}$ by placing the more ventilated lung in the area of greatest blood flow. Positioning may be more effective than PEEP to improve Pa_{O_2} in patients with unilateral lung disease. PEEP may adversely affect arterial oxygenation with unilateral lung disease because it shunts pulmonary blood flow away from the healthy lung to the diseased lung.

Kinetic Bed Therapy

Kinetic therapy is the use of a bed that automatically and continuously turns the patient from side to side. Dependent upon the device, lateral rotation of 45–62° can be achieved. These beds have been shown to decrease the incidence of pneumonia, but have not been shown to affect outcome and cost. Indications and complications are listed in Table 32-4. Although these beds are popular in some hospitals, their impact on the management of mechanically ventilated patients remains unclear and may increase the cost of care.

INHALED AEROSOL MEDICATION

Therapeutic aerosols are often used in mechanically ventilated patients, most commonly to administer beta-agonist bronchodilators. Although these are usually considered for patients with chronic airflow obstruction, they may also be useful in patients with ARDS. Therapeutic aerosols can be delivered using a small volume nebulizer (SVN) or metered dose inhaler (MDI). A variety of factors affect aerosol delivery during mechanical ventilation (Table 32-5).

Table 32-4 Indications and complications of kinetic bed therapy in ventilated patients

Indications
- Immobilized patients (coma, spinal injury, stroke)
- Obese patients who cannot be easily turned and are at risk for complications of immobility
- Patients with unilateral lung disease who cannot be easily placed into the lateral position

Complications
- Ventilator disconnect, inadvertent extubation, accidental aspiration of circuit condensate
- Disconnection of vascular and urinary catheters
- Stretching and breakage of lines and cords
- Axial decubitus ulcer formation (occipital, sacral)
- Dysrhythmias
- Patient intolerance (awake, agitated, combative patients)
- Decreased heat loss in febrile patients
- Increased intracranial pressure
- Worsening dyspnea and hypoxemia
- Difficult examination of the posterior
- Chest X-ray artifact
- Cost

Small Volume Nebulizer

At best, about 5% of the dose placed into the SVN is deposited in the lower respiratory tract. There are a number of disadvantages associated with SVN use during mechanical ventilation. Contamination of the lower respiratory tract can occur if the SVN is the source of bacterial aerosols. The continuous flow from the SVN may increase tidal volume during volume ventilation or pressure during pressure ventilation. Continuous flow from the SVN makes triggering more difficult and increases resistance of expiratory filters and pneumotachometers. Some of these disadvantages can be offset by using the nebulizer control of the ventilator, which powers the SVN only during inspiration and may compensate for the additional flow added by the nebulizer.

Metered Dose Inhaler

Many of the complications of SVN during mechanical ventilation are avoided by use of a MDI. Pulmonary deposition from a MDI is similar to the SVN (5%). It is generally accepted that either MDI or SVN can be used effectively in mechanically ventilated patients. The MDI can be introduced into the ventilator circuit using an elbow adapter, inline adapter, or chamber adapter (Figure 32-2). However, for the same number of actuations, the greatest pulmonary deposition occurs with the chamber adapter. To maximize delivery, the MDI should be actuated at the beginning of inhalation. As with the SVN, the endotracheal tube is a formidable barrier to aerosol penetration.

Table 32-5 Factors affecting aerosol deposition during mechanical ventilation

Nebulizer or inhaler
- Endotracheal tube size: deposition is reduced by smaller endotracheal tubes
- Presence of humidification device: humidification decreases aerosol delivery by 40–50%
- Severity of disease: deposition decreases with increased airflow obstruction

Nebulizer
- Nebulizer placement: deposition is improved if the nebulizer is placed closer to the ventilator rather than at the Y-piece
- Nebulizer brand, flow, and fill volume: some nebulizer brands perform better than others; nebulizer output best at flow of 8 L/min and fill volume of 5 mL
- Treatment time: pulmonary aerosol delivery increases with longer treatment times; continuous beta agonist therapy can be used with status asthmaticus
- Duty cycle: longer inspiratory time increases aerosol delivery to the lungs
- Mechanical ventilator brand: there are differences in the ability of ventilator brands to power the inline SVN
- Bias flow: a bias flow through the ventilator circuit decreases drug delivery

Inhaler
- Type of actuator: greater dose delivered with chamber devices
- Time of actuation: MDI should be actuated at the beginning of inhalation

Dosing

The usual dose from a SVN is about ten times the dose with a MDI. Because the usual dose from the MDI is only a fraction of that with a SVN and the deposition from each is similar, more drug may be deposited in the lungs with the SVN. Thus, SVN may be more effective and convenient than MDI if high doses are required (e.g., status asthmaticus). The dose of inhaled medications (SVN or MDI) should be at least doubled in intubated patients due to the decreased pulmonary deposition secondary to the endotracheal tube.

Evaluation of Response

Response to an inhaled bronchodilator includes decreased peak airway pressure, plateau pressure, auto-PEEP, and resistive pressure (peak minus plateau pressure). More sophisticated measurements such as airway resistance and flow-volume loops may be useful in selected patients to evaluate bronchodilator response.

POINTS TO REMEMBER

- Suctioning-related complications can usually be avoided by use of appropriate technique.
- Closed suction is preferable to open suction in mechanically ventilated patients.

Inline device   Elbow device

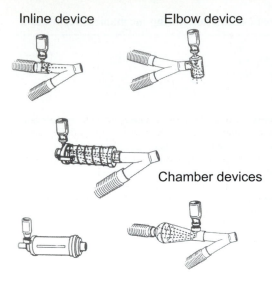

Chamber devices

Figure 32-2 MDI adapters for use in ventilator circuits. The inline adapter connects into the inspiratory limb of the ventilator circuit and uses the circuit tubing as a reservoir. The elbow adapter connects to the endotracheal tube and injects the medication directly from the MDI into the proximal endotracheal tube. The chamber adapter is a large volume device that fits into the inspiratory limb of the circuit and serves as a spacer. (Adapted from DHAND R, TOBIN MJ. Inhaled bronchodilator therapy in mechanically ventilated patients. *Am J Respir Crit Care Med* 1997; 156:3–10.)

- Saline instillation may be useful for selected patients, but should not be a routine procedure.
- Postural drainage therapy is effective in the treatment of atelectasis and acute lobar collapse in the intubated patient.
- Postural drainage therapy is of little benefit and potentially dangerous in acutely ill patients who are producing little or no sputum.
- Manual hyperinflation therapy is of little benefit and potentially dangerous as a secretion clearance technique.
- Indications for bronchoscopy in intubated patients are secretion clearance and the diagnosis of ventilator-associated pneumonia.
- When patients with ARDS are turned from a supine to a prone position, there is often an improvement in oxygenation.
- Lateral positioning with the good lung down is useful in patients with unilateral lung disease.
- Kinetic bed therapy has been shown to decrease the incidence of pneumonia, but has not been shown to affect outcome and cost.
- About 5% of the dose from SVN or MDI is deposited in the lungs of intubated patients.
- Either MDI or SVN can be used effectively in mechanically ventilated patients.
- Chamber adapters deliver a greater dose from a MDI than in-line or elbow devices.
- Response to inhaled bronchodilator therapy is assessed as a decrease in peak airway pressure, plateau pressure, and auto-PEEP.

ADDITIONAL READING

CEREDA M, VILLA F, COLONBO E, ET AL. Closed system suctioning maintains lung volume during volume-controlled mechanical ventilation. *Intensive Care Med* 2001; 27:648–654.

COMBES P, FAUVAGE B, OLEYER C. Nosocomial pneumonia in mechanically ventilated patients, a prospective randomised evaluation of the Stericath closed suctioning system. *Intensive Care Med* 2000; 26:878–882.

DHAND R. Special problems in aerosol delivery: artificial airways. *Respir Care* 2000; 45:636–645.

DHAND R, TOBIN MJ. Inhaled bronchodilator therapy in mechanically ventilated patients. *Am J Respir Crit Care Med* 1997; 156:3–10.

DUARTE AG, FINK JB, DHAND R. Inhalation therapy during mechanical ventilation. *Respir Care Clin N Am* 2001; 7:233–260.

GATTINONI L, TOGONI G, PESENTI A, ET AL. Effect of prone positioning on the survival of patients with the acute respiratory distress syndrome. *N Engl J Med* 2001; 345: 568–573.

HESS DR. Managing the artificial airway. *Respir Care* 1999; 44:759–772.

HESS DR. Nebulizers: Principles and performance. *Respir Care* 2000; 45:609–622.

HESS DR. The evidence for secretion clearance techniques. *Respir Care* 2001; 46:1276–1292.

HESS DR, AGARWAL NN, MYERS CL. Positioning, lung function, and kinetic bed therapy. *Respir Care* 1992; 37:181–197.

JOHNSON KL, KEARNERY PA, JOHNSON SB, ET AL. Closed versus open endotracheal suctioning: costs and physiologic consequences. *Crit Care Med* 1994; 22:654–666.

KOLLEF MH, PRENTICE D, SHAPIRO SD, ET AL. Mechanical ventilation with or without daily changes of in-line suction catheters. *Am J Respir Crit Care Med* 1997; 156:466–472.

CHEST TUBES

OBJECTIVES

1. Describe the clinical presentation of pneumothorax.
2. Compare pneumothorax and pleural effusion.
3. Describe the design and function of underwater seal chest drainage units.

INTRODUCTION

Accumulation of air or fluid within the pleural space can have a marked effect on ventilatory mechanics in either the spontaneously breathing or mechanically ventilated patient. In both settings, lung compliance may be markedly reduced.

Accumulation of air or fluid within the pleural space frequently requires the insertion of a chest tube with underwater seal and suction.

PNEUMOTHORAX

The accumulation of air within the pleural space is referred to as a pneumothorax. Pneumothoraces may be closed, open, or under tension. A tension pneumothorax occurs whenever a site of entry for air exists, but gas cannot exit the pleural space because of the presence of a one-way ball-valve. A closed pneumothorax is when air is trapped in the pleural space without the presence of a one-way valve. An open pneumothorax exists when a patent channel allows gas to freely move into and out of the pleural space. The development of a tension pneumothorax can be life-threatening during mechanical ventilation, since with each breath the pressure within the pneumothorax becomes greater, compromising both ventilatory and cardiovascular function. During volume ventilation, the presentation of a tension pneumothorax may be dramatic (Table 33-1). With each breath, peak airway pressure increases until the high-pressure alarm sounds, and cardiovascular compromise increases progressively to the point of collapse and cardiac arrest. During pressure ventilation, the identification of a tension pneumothorax is more difficult. With each breath, the delivered tidal volume decreases since peak airway pressure is constant. Unless the low tidal volume or minute volume alarms are set appropriately, the pneumothorax may go unnoticed during pressure ventilation, and extension of the pneumothorax is limited by the equilibration of pressure between pleura and the lung. Careful monitoring of the patient's physical condition, blood gas data, and chest X-rays are needed to identify a pneumothorax.

PLEURAL EFFUSION

Fluid accumulates within the pleural space for many reasons: cardiovascular dysfunction, tumor, post-thoracic surgery, infection, and trauma. Although a concern that requires management, pleural effusions do not present as a life-threatening medical emergency like pneumothoraces. Management requires fluid removal and frequently chest tubes are placed for fluid drainage.

CHEST TUBE INSERTION

The precise location of a chest tube is based on the reason for its insertion. Generally, chest tubes used to decompress a pneumothorax are placed anteriorly and cephalad. Emergency decompression can be performed by the insertion of a large gauge needle over the third or fourth rib. If additional decompression is needed, a small incision can be made over the third rib, followed by insertion of a

Table 33-1 Signs and symptoms of a pneumothorax during a mechanical ventilation

- Increasing difficulty ventilating:
  Volume – increasing peak airway pressure
  Pressure – decreasing tidal volume
- Deteriorating vital signs
  Initially, increasing pulse and blood pressure
  Finally, cardiovascular collapse and arrest
- Absent or diminished breath sounds on affected side
- Affected side hyperresonant to percussion
- Trachea and mediastinum shifted toward unaffected side

hemostat that is then opened to decompress the pleural space. Since blood vessels and nerves run along the lower rib border, care should be taken to make the incision over the top of the rib. In patients with multiple loculated pneumothoraces, chest tubes may be inserted at multiple locations. The anterior cephalad position is the most common, since air in the pleural space tends to migrate to the least gravity-dependent position. Chest tubes inserted for drainage of fluid also take advantage of gravity and are normally placed posteriorly and caudally.

DRAINAGE SYSTEMS

Underwater Seal

Pressure within the pleural space is normally sub-atmospheric. As a result, once the chest wall is entered, gas tends to move into the pleural space. To prevent the extension or development of a pneumothorax, a one-way valve must be attached to the chest tube to prevent air movement into the thorax. This is usually accomplished by an underwater seal (Figure 33-1). The chest tube is placed about 2 cm under a column of water. This prevents air from moving into the pleural space, but only requires a 2 cm H_2O pressure gradient for either gas or fluid to leave the chest. During spontaneous breathing, fluid moves up the chest tube from the water seal during inhalation and moves down the tube during exhalation. Gas may leak from the tube during exhalation when the pressure within the pleural space exceeds 2 cm H_2O. With positive pressure ventilation, fluid moves down the tube and gas may bubble out of the water seal during inhalation. During exhalation, gas may move up the tube or bubbling from the water seal may be continuous, dependent upon the pressure gradient and mechanics of the lungs. If fluid is draining from the chest tube, the depth that the chest tube is under water increases with drainage and tends to prevent further drainage by increasing the pressure gradient.

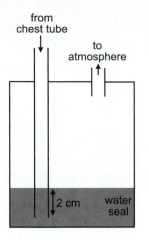

from
chest tube

to
atmosphere

2 cm   water
seal

Figure 33-1 Underwater seal chest drainage unit.

Fluid Drainage

To accommodate fluid drainage, a second container must be added to the drainage system (Figure 33-2). Fluid is allowed to drain into the collection chamber without affecting the water seal. The collection chamber must totally fill before the underwater seal would be affected. A two-bottle system allows for maintenance of the underwater seal and passive fluid drainage but is not designed to allow suction to be applied to the pleural space.

Suction

To facilitate the movement of thick, bloody pleural fluid and to prevent loculated pockets of air from accumulating, a third bottle is frequently added to the

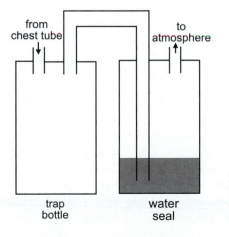

from
chest tube

to
atmosphere

trap
bottle

water
seal

Figure 33-2 Two-bottle chest drainage unit. The first bottle (attached to the chest tube) collects pleural drainage and the second chamber serves as the underwater seal.

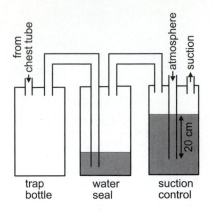

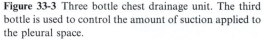

Figure 33-3 Three bottle chest drainage unit. The third bottle is used to control the amount of suction applied to the pleural space.

drainage system (Figure 33-3). This third bottle is intended to control the suction pressure applied to the thoracic space. Since central suction is high and fluctuations in central suction systems are great, and the pressure applied to the pleural space is low (≤ -20 cm H_2O), it is impossible to rely on the hospital system to regulate suction. In the third bottle, fluid to a level of ≤ 20 cm is added with a tube extending into the fluid and vented to atmospheric. The depth that this suction control tube is under water determines the amount of suction applied to the thorax. If this tube is placed 20 cm under water, no more than 20 cm H_2O of pressure can be applied to the thorax. Less suction is applied if constant bubbling is not observed from the suction control tube. When pressure within this container is < -20 cm H_2O, air from the atmosphere is drawn into the vent and bubbles under the water. This maintains a pressure of -20 cm H_2O. When suction is applied, constant bubbling from the suction control chamber should be observed.

Pop-Off

With some systems, a fourth bottle is added to act as a back-up water seal in the event that suction is disrupted or the system becomes obstructed. It is set at 2 cm H_2O to prevent excessive positive pressure from developing in the pleural space (Figure 33-4).

MAINTAINING THE SYSTEM

When evaluating a chest tube drainage system, a number of factors must be monitored. The height of the underwater seal should be 2 cm H_2O. If it is higher, gas and fluid may accumulate in the thoracic space. If the seal is not maintained, air may move into the pleural space. Bubbling should be constant in the suction control bottle. If bubbling is not present, the amount of suction

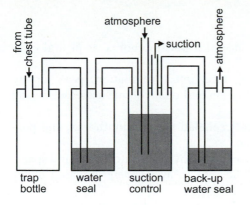

Figure 33-4 Four bottle chest drainage unit. The fourth bottle serves as a back-up water seal.

applied to the system is unknown. In addition, the suction control column should be set no higher than 20 cm H_2O. The collection bottle should be regularly drained before it fills completely. Air should not bubble from the underwater seal unless there is a persistent air leak. The extent of bubbling indicates the size of the leak. Intermittent bubbling during inhalation with positive pressure ventilation indicates a small intermittent leak, whereas vigorous continuous bubbling indicates a large leak. The site of exit of the chest tube from the wall of the thorax should be inspected regularly to insure no air leak is present that may result in the development of a pneumothorax in the spontaneously breathing patient and nullify the effects of suction. Also, any leaks in the system produce bubbling in the water seal. This may be interpreted as an air leak in the chest when none is present.

Size of Air Leak

Quantification of the air leak is impossible from observation but can be estimated by comparing the inspiratory and expiratory tidal volumes.

Clamping of Chest Tubes

Chest tube suction may need to be disrupted during transport or change of the drainage container. When positive pressure ventilation is provided, clamping of the chest tube may create a tension pneumothorax. Clamping should only occur as a monitored trial during mechanical ventilation just prior to chest tube removal. Prior to removal, tubes are frequently clamped for 30 min, followed by a chest X-ray. If no pneumothorax is noted, the chest tube is removed.

POINTS TO REMEMBER

- Chest tubes are indicated in the presence of a pneumothorax or pleural effusion.
- With a tension pneumothorax during mechanical ventilation, peak airway pressure increases during volume ventilation and tidal volume decreases during pressure ventilation.
- Chest tubes are inserted anteriorly and cephalad for pneumothorax, and posteriorly and caudal for pleural effusion.
- An underwater seal is necessary to prevent air movement into the pleural space.
- Suction is regulated by the distance the vent to atmosphere is placed under water.
- Bubbling should always be present in the suction regulating chamber.
- Chest tubes should only be clamped during a monitored trial before removal.
- Clamping of a chest tube during positive pressure ventilation may cause a tension pneumothorax.
- The size of an air leak is determined by measuring inspiratory and expiratory tidal volumes.

THIRTY-FOUR

EMERGENCY AND TRANSPORT VENTILATION

OBJECTIVES

1. Compare techniques for exhaled gas ventilation.
2. Compare self-inflating and flow-inflating manual ventilators.
3. Describe the characteristics of a transport ventilator.

INTRODUCTION

Techniques available for emergency ventilation include exhaled gas ventilation techniques, manual ventilation devices, oxygen-powered demand valves, and transport ventilators. Some of these methods (e.g., exhaled-gas techniques) may be used by non-professional laypersons. Others (e.g., manual ventilators) are used during emergency ventilation (cardiopulmonary resuscitation) and for ventilation during transport to special procedures.

EXHALED GAS VENTILATION TECHNIQUES

Mouth-to-Mouth Ventilation

Mouth-to-mouth ventilation may be the most reliable means to deliver adequate emergency ventilation by lay persons. Its advantages are ease-of-use, availability, universal application, no equipment requirement, and a large reservoir volume (the delivered volume is limited only by the rescuer's vital capacity).

Several important problems are related to mouth-to-mouth ventilation. Gastric insufflation occurs with the high pharyngeal pressures associated with high airway resistance (e.g., obstructed airway), low lung compliance, short inspiratory times (which produce high inspiratory flows), and rapid respiratory rates (which does not allow adequate time for lung deflation between breaths). Gastric insufflation during mouth-to-mouth ventilation can be decreased by the Sellick maneuver (firm pressure against the cricoid cartilage). With mouth-to-mouth ventilation, the delivered oxygen concentration is about 16% and the delivered carbon dioxide concentration is about 5%. The oxygen concentration can be increased if the rescuer breathes supplemental oxygen.

A major concern related to the use of mouth-to-mouth ventilation is the potential for disease transmission. However, health care workers are at minimal risk for Human Immunodeficiency Virus (HIV) and Hepatitis B transmission by occupational exposure and there is no evidence of HIV transmission in saliva or by casual contagion (e.g., mouth-to-mouth ventilation). Nonetheless, it is prudent to follow Centers for Disease Control and Prevention (CDC) recommendations and use a protective barrier device during emergency ventilation. Whether the risk of disease transmission during emergency ventilation is real or imagined, mouth-to-mouth ventilation is discouraged and alternative ventilation devices (mouth-to-mouth or bag-valve-mask) should be used whenever possible.

Face Shield Barrier Devices

These devices consist of a flexible plastic sheet that contains a valve and/or filter and separates the rescuer from the patient. The major advantage of these devices is that they make the task of exhaled gas ventilation more pleasant for the rescuer. Their ability to prevent disease transmission is anecdotal. The tidal volumes that can be delivered using these devices is less than those delivered during mouth-to-mouth ventilation, but greater than that with bag-valve-mask ventilation. This is probably due to the increased resistance to gas flow through the device and the decreased ability to achieve an effective seal between the rescuer and the patient. These devices may also be prone to technical error. For example, if the device is placed incorrectly (valve in wrong direction), the patient will not be ventilated.

Many of the limitations of mouth-to-mouth ventilation (e.g., gastric insufflation, low inspired oxygen) also apply to these devices.

Mouth-to-Mask Ventilation

These devices provide a barrier between the rescuer and the patient to prevent infectious disease transmission during emergency ventilation. Although this method has been used since the 1950s, it has recently become more popular due to increasing concerns related to disease transmission during CPR and increased recognition that ventilation volumes during bag-valve-mask ventilation are often inadequate. The American Heart Association recommends that mouth-to-mask ventilation be taught to health care providers as part of basic life support and many hospitals provide these near the bedsides of all patients. When combined with supplemental oxygen, mouth-to-mask ventilation is arguably the safest and most effective method of ventilatory support in the nonintubated patient when only one rescuer is present.

The mask should provide an adequate seal using an air-filled resilient cuff on the mask. The mask should have a port for administration of supplemental oxygen. It should be constructed of a transparent material to allow visual detection of regurgitation. The mask should have a standard adapter (15 mm outside diameter or a 22 mm inside diameter) to allow the attachment of a bag-valve ventilator if desired. A one-way valve or filter should be attached to the mask to protect the rescuer from contamination with the patient's exhaled gas or vomitus. An extension tube may also be used as an additional barrier between the rescuer and the patient. The exhaled gas of the patient should be vented away from the rescuer. The valve or filter should not jam in the presence of vomitus or humidity and it should have minimal airflow resistance. The dead space of the mask should be as small as possible.

Although mouth-to-mask ventilation devices typically deliver higher tidal volumes than single-operator bag-valve-mask technique, there are differences in performance between commercially available devices. Although these devices do provide a barrier between the patient and the rescuer, the one-way valves of some of these devices allow back-leak. For that reason, devices with redundant means for protection of the rescuer (e.g., one-way valve, filter, and extension tube) are desirable.

It is important that correct technique is used to hold the mask. The rescuer should be positioned at the head of the patient. The mask is placed over the patient's nose and mouth and held with the rescuer's thumbs. The first fingers of each hand are placed under the patient's mandible, and the mandible is lifted as the head is tilted back. The mask is sealed with the rescuer's thumbs. An alternative method is to hold the mask with the thumb and the first finger of each hand, using the other fingers to lift the mandible and hyper-extend the head. With either method, both of the rescuer's hands are used to hold the mask and open the patient's airway. For patients with cervical spine injury, the mandible should be lifted without tilting the head.

MANUAL VENTILATION TECHNIQUES

Self-Inflating Manual Ventilators

Manual ventilators are commonly used during resuscitation and during patient transport. Because they are self-inflating, they do not require a supplemental flow of oxygen to inflate the bag. These devices can be used with a mask or attached directly to an endotracheal or tracheostomy tube. Four critical performance criteria for manual bag-valve ventilation devices are ventilation capability (rate and tidal volume), oxygen delivery, valve performance, and durability.

The bag-valve manual ventilator consists of a self-inflating bag, an oxygen reservoir, and a non-rebreathing valve (Figure 34-1). The bag is squeezed by the operator to ventilate the patient. The bag volume varies among manufacturers and ranges from about 1 to 2 L. One-way valves are used to produce unidirectional flow from the bag, thus drawing gas into the bag when it inflates, directing gas out of the bag to the patient when it is compressed, and preventing rebreathing of exhaled gas.

The bag-valve ventilator allows the operator to feel changes in impedance such as might occur with changes in airways resistance or lung compliance. The non-rebreathing valve should have a low resistance, it should not jam with high oxygen flows, its dead space should be as low as possible, and there should be no forward or backward leak through the valve. It should be possible to attach a pressure manometer to monitor airway pressure and the exhalation port should allow attachment of a spirometer and/or PEEP valve. If the patient breathes spontaneously, the exhalation valve should close so that the patient breathes oxygen from the bag. However, allowing spontaneous breathing through the bag-valve ventilator is discouraged due to the high work imposed by the valve resistance. The patient connection should have a standard adapter (15 mm inside diameter and a 22 mm outside diameter) to attach to a mask or artificial airway.

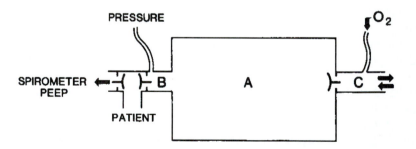

Figure 34-1 Schematic illustration of a bag-valve ventilator. A. self-inflating bag, B. Non-rebreathing valve, C. oxygen reservoir. (from HESS DR. Manual and gas-powered resuscitators. In: BRANSON RD, HESS DR, CHATBURN RL. *Respiratory Care Equipment*. Philadelphia, JB Lippincott, 1995.)

It is important to recognize that the entire volume of the bag is not delivered to the patient when the bag is compressed. A number of factors affect volume delivery from a manual bag-valve ventilator (Table 34-1).

It is difficult for a single operator to deliver large tidal volumes with a bag-valve-mask. This is probably due to inability of the operator to maintain an adequate mask seal and an open airway using one hand, while squeezing an adequate volume from the bag with the other hand. Proper bag-valve-mask ventilation requires proper technique (Figure 34-2).

Although not commonly performed, monitoring of exhaled tidal volumes during bag-valve ventilation may be desirable. Monitoring of airway pressure during manual ventilation is also important if the patient is at risk of air leak (e.g., post thoracotomy). The bag-valve ventilator should also be capable of ventilation at rapid frequencies if required during resuscitation or patient transport. There are also a variety of factors that affect the delivered oxygen concentrations from bag-valve ventilators (Table 34-2). A delivered oxygen concentration of near 100% should be available during resuscitation, suctioning, patient transport, and special procedures.

Gastric insufflation can be a significant problem during bag-valve-mask ventilation. Gastric insufflation increases with an increase in ventilation pressure, as may occur with low lung compliance. Gastric insufflation can be decreased and volume delivery to the lungs can be increased by lengthening the inspiratory time. Bedside manual ventilators can be a source of bacterial contamination. Care should be taken to avoid contamination of these devices and they should be replaced if they become grossly contaminated.

Table 34-1 Factors affecting the tidal volume delivered by bag-valve manual ventilators

Factor	Comments
Mask versus endotracheal tube	Volumes delivered during bag-valve-mask ventilation are often inadequate; gastric insufflation possible with bag-valve-mask
One hand versus two hands	Higher volumes delivered with two hands than with one hand squeezing the bag
Hand size	Higher volumes can be delivered by persons with larger hands
Lung impedance	Delivered volumes decrease with an increase in airway resistance and a decrease in lung compliance
Resuscitator brand	Differences exist for delivered volumes among commercially available devices
Fatigue	Delivered volumes may decrease during prolonged bag-valve ventilation
Gloves	Wearing medical gloves does *not* affect delivered tidal volume delivery

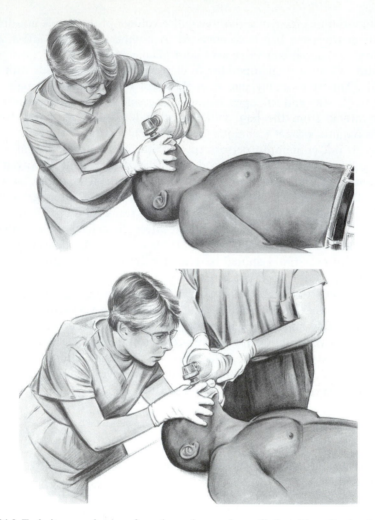

Figure 34-2 Technique used to perform bag-valve mask ventilation. Top. One-hand technique. Bottom. Two-hand technique. (From AMERICAN HEART ASSOCIATION. Adult Basic Life Support. *Circulation* 2000; 102 [Suppl I]: I-22–I-59.)

Flow-Inflating Manual Ventilators

Although they are commonly used in anesthesia, flow inflating bags are not commonly used in adult critical care. These devices are continuous flow, semi-open, breathing systems that lack a non-rebreathing valve. The circuit consists of a thin-walled anesthesia bag, an endotracheal tube or mask connector, an oxygen flow, and a bleed-off at the tail of the bag. Inflation of the bag is controlled by the oxygen flow and the bleed-off. The oxygen flow and bleed-off also control the pressure in the bag. Thus, the bag can be used to provide CPAP as well as

Table 34-2 Factors affecting oxygen concentration delivered from manual bag-valve ventilators

Factor	Comments
Oxygen flow	A low oxygen flow decreases delivered oxygen concentration; flows of 15 L/min should be used with adult bag-valve ventilators
Oxygen reservoir	A smaller reservoir volume decreases the delivered oxygen concentration; ideally, the reservoir volume should exceed the volume of the device
Oxygen supply valve	An oxygen supply valve will allow the delivery of 100% oxygen, but may impede bag reinflation
Bag recoil time	A slower bag recoil time will increase the delivered oxygen concentration
Resuscitator brand	Differences in delivered oxygen concentration exist between commercially available devices

ventilation. The bag may be fitted with a manometer and a pressure pop off. Because the patient exhales into the bag, the oxygen flow must be high enough to prevent CO_2 accumulation. The bleed-off from the bag can produce significant expiratory resistance. Disadvantages of this system are that a source of compressed gas is required, and this system is more difficult to use than a self-inflating bag-valve resuscitator.

OXYGEN-POWERED DEMAND VALVES

Although not commonly used in the hospital, oxygen-powered demand valves are used by emergency care personnel in the field. These devices are powered by a pressurized gas source and cannot be used in the absence of this gas source. These devices deliver 100% oxygen when the device is triggered by the operator (resuscitator function) or when triggered by the patient (demand-valve function). They can be used with a facemask or with an artificial airway. They do not provide the operator with a sense of lung impedance. Use of these devices is discouraged due to their likelihood to produce over-ventilation and gastric insufflation.

TRANSPORT VENTILATORS

Critically ill patients commonly require diagnostic tests and therapeutic procedures that cannot be performed at the bedside. When the critically ill patient requires transport, every effort should be made to take the ICU with the patient. For the mechanically ventilated patient, that means personnel who are familiar with the patient, monitoring equipment, airway equipment, and a means of providing ventilation (Table 34-3). Ventilation during transport can be provided either using a manual ventilator or a transport ventilator. Manual bag-valve ventilation during transport is usually adequate if provided by a clinician skilled

Table 34-3 Essential equipment for transport of the mechanically ventilated patient

Equipment	Capability
Portable monitor	ECG; pressure channels for monitoring arterial pressure, pulmonary artery pressure, or intracranial pressure; pulse oximeter
Transport ventilator and/or manual ventilator	Ideally provide ventilation similar to that provided in the ICU
Airway maintenance	Suction equipment and equipment to re-intubate if accidental extubation occurs
Drug box	All advanced cardiac life support drugs and any other drugs being administered in the ICU (e.g., sedatives, paralytics, pressors)
Infusion pumps	Must operate reliably from a battery
Stethoscope, blood pressure cuff	

Adapted from BRANSON RD. Intrahospital transport of critically ill, mechanically ventilated patients. *Respir Care* 1992; 37:775–795.

in this task (e.g., respiratory therapist or anesthesiologist) and care is exercised to maintain adequate tidal volumes, airway pressures, PEEP levels, and F_{IO_2}. Use of a transport ventilator is superior to manual ventilation because it provides a more consistent level of ventilation and frees a clinician to perform other tasks.

Characteristics of a Transport Ventilator

There are very sophisticated microprocessor-controlled transport ventilators available. Ideally, the transport ventilator should be capable of providing modes that are commonly used in the ICU. There should be separate controls for respiratory rate and tidal volume. The ventilator should provide either pressure or volume ventilation. An F_{IO_2} control may not be necessary because 100% oxygen is acceptable or desirable during transport. PEEP must be available and the trigger sensitivity must be PEEP-compensated. High pressure and disconnect alarms should be provided.

A major consideration for a transport ventilator is portability. The ventilator should be lightweight. The ventilator's dimensions should make it easy to transport with the patient (e.g., place on the bed). Transport ventilators may be either pneumatically or electronically powered. A major disadvantage of pneumatically controlled transport ventilators is that they consume gas for operation, thus depleting the gas source more quickly. Electronically controlled transport ventilators typically provide more precise control settings, are affected less by fluctuations in source-gas pressure, and do not consume as much gas for their operation.

A unique challenge occurs when mechanically ventilated patients require transport for magnetic resonance imaging. Operation of the magnetic resonance imager creates a strong magnetic field. Thus, devices (including ventilators) that have ferromagnetic components cannot be used. Patients can be ventilated using either a manual ventilator or a ventilator specifically designed for use during magnetic resonance imaging. Also, aluminum oxygen cylinders and aluminum regulators are necessary for oxygen delivery.

POINTS TO REMEMBER

- Limitations of mouth-to-mouth ventilation are its potential for disease transmission, delivery of a low oxygen concentration, and its common association with gastric insufflation.
- Mouth-to-mask devices provide a barrier between the rescuer and the patient.
- Self-inflating bag-valve ventilators are capable of delivering high oxygen concentrations.
- Due to the valve resistance, patients should not be allowed to spontaneously breathe from a bag-valve ventilator.
- Flow-inflating manual ventilators are more difficult to use than self-inflating devices.
- Use of a transport ventilator is superior to manual ventilation because it provides a more consistent level of ventilation and frees a clinician to perform other tasks.
- Transport ventilators should provide the same level of ventilation that is provided in the ICU.

ADDITIONAL READING

AMERICAN HEART ASSOCIATION in collaboration with the International Liaison Committee on Resuscitation. Adult Basic Life Support. *Circulation* 2000; 102 [Suppl I]: I-22–I-59.

AMERICAN HEART ASSOCIATION in collaboration with the International Liaison Committee on Resuscitation. Advanced Cardiovascular Life Support. Section 3: Adjuncts for Oxygenation, Ventilation, and Airway Control. *Circulation* 2000; 102 [Suppl I]: I-95–I-104.

BRANSON RD. Intrahospital transport of critically ill, mechanically ventilated patients. *Respir Care* 1992; 37:775–795.

HURST J, DAVIS K, JOHNSON D, ET AL. Cost and complications during in-hospital transport of critically ill patients: A prospective cohort study. *J Trauma* 1992; 33:582–585.

SZEM JW, HYDO LJ, FISCHER E, ET AL. High-risk intrahospital transport of critically ill patients: Safety and outcome of the necessary "road trip." *Crit Care Med* 1995; 23:1660–1666.

CHAPTER THIRTY-FIVE

NONINVASIVE POSITIVE PRESSURE VENTILATION FOR ACUTE RESPIRATORY FAILURE

OBJECTIVES

1. Discuss patient selection for noninvasive ventilation.
2. Compare interfaces for noninvasive ventilation.
3. List advantages and disadvantages of various ventilator types for noninvasive ventilation.
4. List the steps in the initiation of noninvasive ventilation.

INTRODUCTION

There has been increasing interest in providing mechanical ventilation by non-invasive means to selected patients. NPPV has been used successfully in patients with COPD, cardiogenic pulmonary edema, restrictive chest wall disease, asthma, pneumonia, post-extubation respiratory failure, post-operative respiratory failure, and solid organ transplantation. A primary outcome variable in controlled studies of NPPV is the requirement for intubation, with a lower intubation rate for patients randomized to NPPV. A lower mortality has also been reported with NPPV compared to conservative medical therapy. Because an artificial airway increases the risk of nosocomial pneumonia, it is not surprising that noninvasive ventilatory support decreases the incidence of ventilator-associated pneumonia (VAP). NPPV has also been used to achieve early extubation of selected patients and to avoid re-intubation with extubation failure. It has also been demonstrated that, from the hospital's perspective, the use of NPPV for acute severe exacerbations of COPD is less expensive than standard therapy alone.

PATIENT FACTORS

Patient Selection

Common selection criteria include acute respiratory distress (moderate to severe dyspnea, accessory muscle use, tachypnea) and acute hypercapnia (pH < 7.35 and $Pa_{CO_2} > 45$ mm Hg). Patients with a rapidly reversible process (e.g., within 48 hours) may derive the greatest benefit from NPPV. There is no benefit to the routine use of NPPV in patients with COPD and acute respiratory failure. Common exclusion criteria include apnea or need for immediate intubation, hypotension, uncontrolled arrhythmias and/or evidence of myocardial ischemia, upper airway obstruction or facial trauma, inability to clear secretions, inability to cooperate, and facial deformity or other inability to fit the mask.

The strongest evidence of effectiveness of NPPV for acute respiratory failure comes from studies of patients with acute exacerbation of COPD. Although there has been interest in the use of NPPV for the treatment of acute asthma, there is little data to support this approach. There is also some support for the use of NPPV in selected patients with acute hypoxemic respiratory failure, following solid organ transplantation, and those who are immunosuppressed.

The role of NPPV in patients with acute cardiogenic pulmonary edema is unclear. Although some have reported benefit of NPPV in this patient population, others have urged caution. Based on the available evidence, NPPV should be avoided in patients with cardiogenic pulmonary edema secondary to acute MI. There is considerable evidence for the effectiveness of mask CPAP (without NPPV) for the treatment of acute cardiogenic pulmonary edema and perhaps NPPV should be reserved for those patients who remain hypercapnic with mask CPAP therapy.

Predictors of Response

The initial response to NPPV may predict success or failure. There is a more rapid decrease in Pa_{CO_2} in patients where NPPV is successful. Unsuccessful nasal NPPV is associated with greater severity of illness, greater mouth leak, and increased difficulty acclimating to NPPV. A good level of consciousness has been associated with successful responses to NPPV for patients with COPD and acute hypercapnic respiratory failure. More severe respiratory acidosis is associated with greater likelihood of failed NPPV. In patients with acute hypoxemic respiratory failure, the likelihood of failed NPPV is greater in patients who are severely ill, are older, have a diagnosis of ARDS or pneumonia, or fail to improve after one hour of therapy.

TECHNICAL FACTORS

Patient Interface

The patient interface has a major impact on patient comfort and compliance during NPPV. A poorly fitting interface will decrease both the clinical effectiveness and the patient compliance of this therapy. The most commonly used interfaces for NPPV with acute respiratory failure are nasal masks or oronasal masks (Figure 35-1). Desirable features of a mask for noninvasive ventilation include:

A

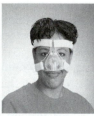

B

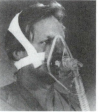

C

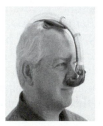

D

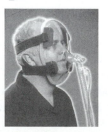

Figure 35-1 Interfaces used for noninvasive ventilation. A. Nasal mask. B. Oronasal mask (from HILL NS. Complications of noninvasive positive pressure ventilation. *Respir Care* 1997; 42:432–442). C. Nasal pillows. D. Total face mask.

- low dead space
- transparent
- lightweight
- easy to secure
- adequate seal with low facial pressure
- disposable or easy to clean
- nonirritating to the skin (non-allergenic)
- inexpensive.

   Nasal or oronasal masks designed specifically for noninvasive ventilation often use an open cushion with an inner lip. With this design, the cushion pushes against the face as pressure increases inside the mask. With a correctly sized mask, this minimizes leak and improves comfort during NPPV.

   Selecting the correct mask size is critical. The nasal mask should fit just above the junction of the nasal bone and cartilage, directly at the sides of both nares, and just below the nose above the upper lip. The oronasal mask should fit from just above the junction of the nasal bone and cartilage to just below the lower lip. A common mistake is to choose a mask that is too large. This results in leaks, decreased effectiveness, and patient discomfort. Leaks through the mouth are not uncommon when using a nasal mask. A nasal mask may be better tolerated than an oronasal mask, but ventilation is greater with an oronasal mask. When mouth leak interferes with the effectiveness of ventilation, an oronasal mask can be used. Upper airway dryness is greater with use of a nasal mask and mouth leak, which can be addressed by using heated humidification or an oronasal mask.

   Most masks designed specifically for noninvasive ventilation use cloth straps and Velcro to secure the mask. The cloth straps fit through slots at the sides and top of the mask. Use of Velcro to secure the mask allows nearly infinite adjustments of the headgear. A common mistake is to fit the headgear too tightly. It should be possible to pass one or two fingers between the headgear and the face. Fitting the headgear too tightly usually will not improve the fit and always decreases patient comfort and compliance. The design of most masks for non-invasive ventilation is such that the top of the mask is secured on the forehead rather than at the bridge of the nose. Forehead spacers are an important feature of this design. These foam cushions fill the gap between the forehead and the mask, thus reducing pressure on the bridge of the nose. This improves comfort and decreases the likelihood of pressure sores.

   Aerophagia commonly occurs with noninvasive mask ventilation, but this is usually benign because the airway pressures are less than the esophageal opening pressure. Thus, a gastric tube is not routinely necessary for mask ventilation. In fact, a gastric tube may interfere with the effectiveness of mask ventilation in several ways. It may be more difficult to achieve a mask seal if a gastric tube is present. Compression of the gastric tube against the face by the mask cushion may increase the likelihood of facial skin breakdown. A nasogastric tube will increase resistance to nasal gas flow, which may decrease the effectiveness of mask ventilation – particularly nasal ventilation.

Pressure sores on the bridge of the nose are a common complaint during noninvasive ventilation. Fortunately, ulceration and skin breakdown are avoided in many patients. Measures to reduce pressure injury should be taken as soon as signs of soreness occur at the bridge of the nose. Correct mask fit and size should be reassessed. The tension of the headgear should be reduced. A different mask style may be tried. Wound care tape such as Duoderm can be applied.

Ventilators for NPPV

Critical care ventilators are available in most hospitals to provide noninvasive ventilation. Theoretically, one should be able to attach the ventilator to a mask rather than an artificial airway to provide noninvasive ventilation. This approach has the advantages of precise control of F_{IO_2}, various modes and inspiratory flow patterns, and separation of inspiratory and expiratory gases to limit rebreathing. Critical care ventilators have extensive monitoring and alarms that are desirable during invasive ventilation, but can be a nuisance during noninvasive ventilation. The greatest disadvantage of critical care ventilators is their difficulty dealing with leaks that invariably occur during noninvasive ventilation.

Portable pressure ventilators are available from several manufacturers specifically to provide NPPV. Their major advantage is their ability to function correctly in the presence of leaks. They are blower devices that vary inspiratory and expiratory pressures in response to patient demand (Figure 35-2). These ventilators provide pressure ventilation – none provides volume ventilation. Although they can be used to provide controlled ventilation in the absence of patient effort, they are usually used to provide pressure support ventilation.

Two important issues relate to how well these ventilators trigger to the inspiratory phase and cycle to the expiratory phase. Some noninvasive ventilators automatically adjust the inspiratory trigger and expiratory cycle by tracking the patient's inspiratory and expiratory flows. Others allow the clinician to adjust the trigger and/or cycle. The ability to adjust the trigger sensitivity allows the clinician to balance the ability of the patient to initiate the inspiratory phase and the tendency of the ventilator to auto-trigger. The ability to adjust the cycle sensitivity

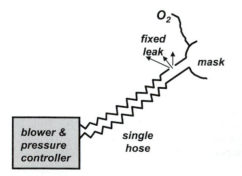

Figure 35-2 Schematic drawing illustrating the function of a portable pressure ventilator for non-invasive ventilation.

is a balance between premature termination of the inspiratory phase and expiratory muscle activity to terminate the inspiratory phase.

An issue that has generated considerable interest with the portable pressure ventilators is the potential for CO_2 rebreathing. This is of particular concern for patients with hypercapnic respiratory failure. Most of these ventilators use a single hose without a true exhalation valve. Expired gas passes through a fixed leak established in the device. Particularly with low flow from the ventilator as may occur with low PEEP levels, there may be inadequate flushing of CO_2 and subsequent rebreathing. This problem can be resolved by using higher PEEP levels (≥ 6 cm H_2O) or a valve that prevents rebreathing. Increasing the leak flow also flushes CO_2 from the system. Theoretically, a fixed leak in the mask should produce less rebreathing than a fixed leak in the hose.

Precise and constant oxygen administration is nearly impossible with portable pressure ventilators. Supplemental oxygen is typically provided by titration into the inspiratory circuit at the ventilator outlet or directly into the mask. In each case, the $F_{I_{O_2}}$ is determined by the oxygen flow and ventilatory pattern. Thus, the $F_{I_{O_2}}$ varies as the ventilatory pattern changes. Due to the high flow from the ventilator, it is generally difficult to achieve an $F_{I_{O_2}}$ greater than 0.50. Newer generation noninvasive ventilators allow the user to precisely set the $F_{I_{O_2}}$ and provide sophisticated monitoring (including graphics), alarms, and back-up ventilatory support in the event of apnea.

CAREGIVER ISSUES

If NPPV is to be successful, those caring for the patient (physicians, nurses, respiratory therapists) must be committed to this approach. This is usually achieved by familiarizing these persons with the accumulated evidence suggesting that NPPV improves outcome in selected patients. Physicians must appreciate selection criteria, respiratory therapists must understand the issues related to ventilator management and selection of an appropriate interface, and nursing personnel must appreciate issues related to mask fit and skin care. Some clinicians are reluctant to initiate NPPV due to concerns related to time requirements and difficulties encountered when NPPV is initiated. Fitting the mask, selection of appropriate ventilator settings, and patient coaching are labor intensive for the first hours of NPPV.

CLINICAL APPLICATION

The application of NPPV (Figure 35-3) requires caregiver patience and skills with both the technical aspects of mechanical ventilation and the ability to coach patients to adapt to the mask and ventilator. The primary goal when initiating NPPV is patient comfort and not an improvement in arterial blood gases *per se* (an improvement in blood gases will usually follow if patient comfort and respiratory

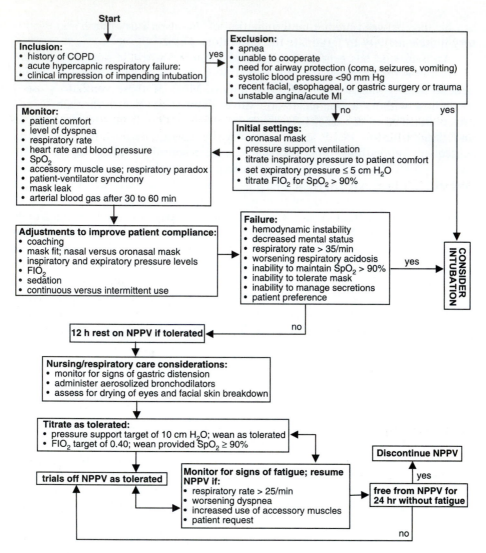

Figure 35-3 Algorithm for initiation of noninvasive ventilation for acute respiratory failure.

muscle unloading is achieved). Important steps in the clinical application of NPPV are as follows: (1) choose a ventilator capable of meeting patient needs (usually pressure ventilation), (2) choose the correct interface and avoid a mask that is too large, (3) explain therapy to the patient, (4) silence alarms and choose low settings, (5) initiate NPPV while holding mask in place, (6) secure mask, avoiding a tight fit, (7) titrate pressure to patient comfort, (8) titrate F_{IO_2} to $Sp_{O_2} > 90\%$, (9) avoid peak pressure > 20 cm H_2O, (10) titrate PEEP per trigger effort and Sp_{O_2}, (11) continue to coach and reassure patient; make adjustments to improve patient compliance.

Complications of NPPV (usually minor) include leaks, mask discomfort, facial skin breakdown, oropharyngeal drying, eye irritation, sinus congestion, patient-ventilator dys-synchrony, gastric insufflation, and hemodynamic compromise. Aerosolized bronchodilators and heliox can be administered by NPPV. The best approach to weaning from NPPV is unclear. In many cases, the patient requests removal of the mask after several hours of therapy. If the patient's condition deteriorates after removal of the mask, NPPV is resumed – otherwise it is discontinued.

POINTS TO REMEMBER

- In acute respiratory failure, the use of NPPV in appropriately selected patients decreases the need for endotracheal intubation and affords a survival benefit.
- Patients in whom the success of NPPV is the greatest are those with acute exacerbation of COPD.
- Oronasal masks provide more effective ventilation, but nasal masks are more comfortable for the patient.
- Any ventilator can be used for NPPV.
- Portable pressure ventilators compensate for leaks, but increase the risk for rebreathing of CO_2.
- The initiation of NPPV is time consuming but cost-effective.
- Aerosolized bronchodilators and heliox can be administered with NPPV.

ADDITIONAL READING

ANTONELLI M, CONTI G, MORO ML, ET AL. Predictors of failure of noninvasive positive pressure ventilation in patients with acute hypoxemic respiratory failure: a multi-center study. *Intensive Care Med* 2001; 27:1718–1728.

BACH JR, BROUGHER P, HESS DR, ET AL. Consensus statement: Noninvasive positive pressure ventilation. *Respir Care* 1997; 42:365–369.

CHATMONGKOLCHART S, KACMAREK RM, HESS DR. Heliox delivery with noninvasive positive pressure ventilation: a laboratory study. *Respir Care* 2001; 46:248–254.

CUVELIER A, MUIR J-F. Noninvasive ventilation and obstructive lung diseases. *Eur Respir J* 2001; 17:1271–1281.

DE ARAUJO MTM, VIEIRA SB, VASQUEZ EC, FLEURY B. Heated humidification or face mask to prevent upper airway dryness during continuous positive airway pressure therapy. *Chest* 2000; 117:142–147.

HESS D, CHATMONGKOLCHART S. Techniques to avoid intubation: noninvasive positive pressure ventilation and heliox therapy. *Int Anesthesiol Clin* 2000; 38:161–187.

HILL NS. Complications of noninvasive positive pressure ventilation. *Respir Care* 1997; 42:432–442.

HILL NS. *Noninvasive Positive Pressure Ventilation: Principles and Applications.* New York, Futura, 2001.

HOTCHKISS JR, ADAMS AB, DRIES DJ, ET AL. Dynamic behavior during noninvasive ventilation. Chaotic support? *Am J Respir Crit Care Med* 2001; 163:374–378.

International Consensus Conference in Intensive Care Medicine: noninvasive positive pressure ventilation in acute respiratory failure. *Am J Respir Crit Care Med* 2001; 163:283–291.

JABER S, FODIL R, CARLUCCI A, ET AL. Noninvasive ventilation with helium-oxygen in acute exacerbations of chronic obstructive pulmonary disease. *Am J Respir Crit Care Med* 2000; 161:1191–1200.

KEENAN SP, KERNERMAN PD, COOK DJ, ET AL. Effect of noninvasive positive pressure ventilation on mortality in patients admitted with acute respiratory failure: a meta-analysis. *Crit Care Med* 1997; 25:1685–1692.

MEHTA S, HILL NS. Noninvasive ventilation. *Am J Respir Crit Care Med* 2001; 163:540–577.

NAVA S, KARAKURT S, RAMPULLA C, ET AL. Salbutamol delivery during non-invasive mechanical ventilation in patients with chronic obstructive lung disease: a randomized, controlled study. *Intensive Care Med* 2001; 27:1627–1635.

PANG D, KEENAN SP, COOK DJ, SIBBALD WJ. The effect of positive pressure airway support on mortality and the need for intubation in cardiogenic pulmonary edema: a systematic review. *Chest* 1998; 114:1185–1192.

PETER JV, MORAN JL, PHILLIPS-HUGHES J, WARN D. Noninvasive ventilation in acute respiratory failure: a meta-analysis update. *Crit Care Med* 2002; 30:555–562.

WYSOCKI M, ANTONELLI M. Noninvasive mechanical ventilation in acute hypoxemic respiratory failure. *Eur Respir J* 2001; 18:209–220.

LONG-TERM MECHANICAL VENTILATION

OBJECTIVES

1. Compare the application of mechanical ventilation in the long-term care setting to that in the acute care setting.
2. List criteria to be met for the application of long-term mechanical ventilation outside the acute care setting.
3. Discuss technical considerations in the application of mechanical ventilation in alternative sites.

4. Compare the use of noninvasive and invasive ventilation for long-term ventilation.
5. Compare noninvasive positive pressure ventilation, negative pressure ventilation, pneumobelts, and rocking beds.
6. Describe the approach to invasive mechanical ventilation in the long-term setting.

INTRODUCTION

Increasing numbers of patients survive acute care and require long-term ventilatory support. This trend has resulted in the need for alternative site management of these patients. Specific approaches to ventilator management and equipment used differ outside the ICU from those commonly used in the ICU.

ALTERNATIVE SITES

There are alternatives to the ICU for the mechanically ventilated patient such as long-term ventilator facilities, congregate living centers, foster homes, and the patient's home (Table 36-1). These can be viewed from two perspectives – patient independence, or quality of life, and available medical resources or costs. Patient quality of life and independence increases as the patient moves along the spectrum from ICU to home. Paralleling this is a decrease in the cost of maintaining patients on ventilatory assistance. The cost of home ventilatory support is less than the cost of ICU care. For some patients, the ideal location for long-term ventilatory support is the home.

Table 36-1 Sites for ventilator-dependent patients, listed in order of increased patient independence and decreased cost of care

Critical care unit
Specialized respiratory care unit
General medical/surgical unit
Subacute care hospital
Long-term care hospital
Rehabilitation hospital
Skilled nursing facility
Congregate living center
Foster home
Single family home

HOME MECHANICAL VENTILATION

Home ventilatory support is not the ideal option for all patients. Not only must the patient's medical status be optimized, but they must also have appropriate coping and support structures to insure successful maintenance in the home.

Candidates

Theoretically, any patient who requires long-term ventilatory support is a candidate for home mechanical ventilation. However, patients with neuromuscular disease are the most ideal candidates for long-term ventilation or support in the home, since their overall medical status is easily stabilized and they do not have intrinsic lung disease. However, an increasing number of patients with chronic lung disease are also being maintained at home. These patients are more difficult to manage than neuromuscular/neurologically diseased patients because of their lung disease and other organ system problems.

Medical Stability

Only patients whose overall medical status is stabilized are candidates for home ventilatory support (Table 36-2). Specifically, cardiovascular, renal, metabolic, and nutritional status must be optimized. Ideally, adequate gas exchange should be maintained while the patient is ventilated with room air. At most, an $F_{I_{O_2}}$ of 0.40 should be required. In addition, PEEP should not be necessary. Patients who are able to breathe without ventilatory support for at least part of the day have an increased likelihood that home ventilatory support will be successful. This is not to say that patients who do not meet this criterion cannot be moved home, but the likelihood of success is less. However, it can be expected that as financial pressure on medical care increases, sicker and sicker patients will be moved into the home.

Table 36-2 Medical status ideal for discharge to the home

- Acceptable arterial blood gases with $F_{I_{O_2}} \leq 0.40$
- Stable ventilator settings
    $F_{I_{O_2}} \leq 0.40$
    assist/control mode
    limited use of PEEP
    stable pulmonary mechanics
- Stable cardiovascular, renal, metabolic, and nutritional status
- Absence of acute pulmonary infection
- Periods of time independent of the ventilator

Patient/Family Characteristics

In addition to medical stability, appropriate coping styles of the patient as well as adequate resources are essential for successful home ventilation (Table 36-3). Ideally, the patient should be well educated and highly motivated, optimistic, and self-directive. A strong support structure is necessary. Family and social supports need to be intact. Financial resources are also essential. Adequate personal assets and optimal health insurance coverage make it easier to move a patient to the home.

Home Care Team

Preparation, transfer, and maintenance of patients in the home must be a coordinated team effort. Ideally, a discharge coordinator (either a nurse, respiratory therapist, or social worker), case manager, primary physician, staff nurse, respiratory therapist, durable medical equipment supplier, and a home health agency should be involved in the process. These individuals are responsible for ensuring that the patient's medical status is optimized, that the home is prepared for the patient, both the patient and family are properly educated, insurance coverage is adequate, proper equipment selection is made, and appropriate support personnel are available.

TECHNICAL ISSUES

The choice of ventilatory support equipment for use in the home is important (Table 36-4). Only ventilators designed for home care should be used in the home. The complexity and technical issues associated with ICU ventilators make them unacceptable for use in the home. The ventilator chosen should be small and lightweight, simple to operate, have an internal battery capable of operating for at least one hour, and be capable of being attached to a 12-volt battery. Whether a backup ventilator is needed in the home is dependent upon the patient's ability to sustain periods of ventilator independence. Any patient who cannot breathe spontaneously for at least four hours requires a backup ventilator. In addition, all patients require a 12-volt battery with cable for travel and appropriate ventilator circuits and humidifying systems. Passover humidifiers are usually used in the home, but heat-and-moisture exchangers are more convenient during travel.

Although many patients do not require supplemental oxygen, appropriate oxygen delivery systems during mechanical ventilation and spontaneous breathing are necessary for some patients. Appropriate aerosol medication equipment may also be required. Since some home care ventilators do not produce a gas source for powering aerosol generators, a portable air compressor may be required. Finally, appropriate airway care equipment and suctioning apparatus must be available. Patients and families should be trained in the use of this equipment before discharge.

Table 36-3 Patient characteristics that may determine success in home ventilator care

Characteristic	Ideal	Acceptable	Unacceptable
Individual coping styles	Optimistic Motivated Resourceful Flexible Adaptable Sense of humor Directive	Optimistic Motivated Sense of humor	None
Support systems	Close family and social supports	Social supports	Lack of family and social supports
Education	College degree Ability to learn	Able to learn Mechanically astute	Altered mental status Unable to learn
Financial resources	Adequate personal assets Optimal health insurance coverage	Adequate health insurance coverage	Lack of personal assets Lack of health insurance
Medical condition	Stable neuromuscular disease Significant "free time" off the ventilator No other medical illnesses	Stable neuromuscular or obstructive airway disease Limited or no "free time" off the ventilator	Medically unstable
Self-care ability	Ability to provide self-care and/or direct others	Able to provide self care	Unable to care for self or direct others

From: GILMARTIN ME. Long-term mechanical ventilation: patient selection and discharge planning. *Respir Care* 1991; 36:205–216.

Table 36-4 Equipment potentially needed for home ventilatory support

- Primary and backup ventilators
- 12-volt battery and connecting cable
- Ventilator circuit and humidifier
- Manual ventilator
- Oxygen delivery system
- Suction machine and catheters
- Tracheostomy supplies
- Aerosol therapy equipment
- Monitors and alarms

NONINVASIVE VENTILATION

Noninvasive Positive Pressure Ventilation

Since the early 1980s, NPPV has been used increasingly as a method of supporting patients with chronic lung disease as well as those with neuromuscular disease. Generally, all patients requiring long-term ventilatory support are candidates for noninvasive ventilation if they do not have marked oxygenation problems, are able to manage their secretions effectively, and do not have upper airway obstruction. Although it is possible to maintain patients noninvasively for 24 hr/day, patients only requiring nocturnal ventilatory support or those capable of sustaining spontaneous ventilation for several hours daily are the most successful candidates for noninvasive techniques. The use of nocturnal NPPV is controversial, with few outcome studies to guide appropriate patient selection. Guidelines for patient selection are shown in Table 36-5.

Negative Pressure Ventilation

The iron lung has been used to provide ventilatory support since the 1940s. However, the use of negative pressure ventilation has decreased because of improvements in NPPV. Negative pressure ventilation is most effective in patients with neuromuscular causes of ventilation failure. Generally, patients with intrinsic lung disease are not adequately ventilated with negative pressure. Negative pressure ventilation has also been used in conjunction with other approaches to both noninvasive and invasive ventilatory support. The chest cuirass can be used during waking hours to allow patients who use nocturnal ventilation to communicate more effectively with caregivers. A number of factors have limited the use of negative pressure techniques. Of primary concern is the development of upper airway obstruction, body temperature regulation because of cold air being drawn over the body with each inspiratory phase, the need for assistance to get into and

Table 36-5 Clinical indications for NPPV in chronic respiratory failure

Restrictive thoracic disorders (sequelae of polio, spinal cord injury, neuropathies, myopathies and dystrophies, amyotrophic lateral sclerosis (ALS), chest wall deformities,
kyphoscoliosis)
- Symptoms: fatigue, dyspnea, morning headache
- Physiologic criteria: $Pa_{CO_2} \geq 45$ mm Hg, nocturnal oximetry demonstrating oxygen
  saturation $\leq 88\%$ for five consecutive minutes, maximal inspiratory pressures < 60
  cm H_2O or forced vital capacity $< 50\%$ predicted

Chronic obstructive pulmonary disease (chronic bronchitis, emphysema, bronchiectasis, cystic fibrosis)
- Symptoms: fatigue, dyspnea, morning headache
- Physiologic criteria: $Pa_{CO_2} \geq 55$ mm Hg, Pa_{CO_2} of 50 to 54 mm Hg and nocturnal
  oximetry demonstrating oxygen saturation $\leq 88\%$ for five consecutive minutes while
  receiving oxygen therapy ≥ 2 L/min, Pa_{CO_2} of 50 to 54 mm Hg and hospitalization
  related to recurrent episodes of hypercapnic respiratory failure

Adapted from: Clinical indications for noninvasive positive pressure ventilation in chronic
respiratory failure due to restrictive lung disease, COPD, and nocturnal hypoventilation –
a consensus conference report. *Chest* 1999; 116:521–534.

out of the negative pressure unit, and immobility during the time negative pressure is maintained.

Three approaches are available to provide negative pressure ventilation: iron
lung, chest cuirass, and pneumosuit. Of these, the chest cuirass is easiest to use
and the best tolerated. Successful use of a cuirass is increased if a unit is custom-
designed for the specific patient, which minimizes leaks. The iron lung is more
effective, since it is relatively easy to minimize leaks and the physical force available to create negative pressure is greater than with portable negative pressure
generators. The pneumosuit is a whole body suit that is difficult to fit and to seal
so as to prevent leakage.

Pneumobelts

The pneumobelt (Figure 36-1) has been available since the 1960s. It is a bladder
that fits over the abdomen between the umbilicus and pubic arch. This requires
the patient to be in the sitting position ($\geq 45°$). Inflation of the bladder pushes the
abdominal contents up, moving the diaphragm cephalad and facilitating exhalation. Decompression of the bladder allows inspiration. The increased elastic recoil
is a result of diaphragmatic displacement during expiration. Tidal volumes > 300
mL can be achieved in most adults, but rarely exceed 800 mL. The pneumobelt
can be inflated with any positive pressure ventilator that can deliver a V_T of 1.5 to
2 L. A large volume is required to pressurize the bladder. A peak bladder pressure
of about 50 cm H_2O is needed. The pneumobelt is most effective in neuromuscular diseased patients for partial ventilatory assistance.

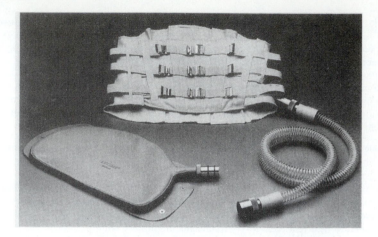

Figure 36-1 Pneumobelt with positive pressure generation. (From GILMARTIN ME: Body ventilators: equipment and techniques. *Respir Care Clin* NA 1996; 2:195–222.)

Rocking Beds

The rocking bed (Figure 36-2) has the same limited scope of use as the pneumobelt. It is generally only effective in patients without intrinsic lung disease. It supports ventilation by rhythmically moving the diaphragm and abdominal contents cephad and caudal as it moves through an arch of up to 60 degrees. Of major concern with some patients is motion sickness. If this can be medically managed during the first few days, many patients can successfully be assisted with the rocking bed. The primary group where this device has been used is patients with phrenic nerve dysfunction post cardiac surgery who require support for a limited time each day. Respiratory rates as high as 30/min can be set. Tidal volume assistance of up to about 500 mL may be achieved.

APPROACH TO INVASIVE VENTILATION

The goal of mechanical ventilation in the ICU is ventilator independence, whereas the goal in the home is to maximize the time a patient can be independent of the ventilator. Complete independence is usually not an option. Continuous mandatory ventilation (assist/control) is usually the most appropriate mode. The imposed work-of-breathing with synchronized intermittent mandatory ventilation with home care ventilators is high. In addition, the goal is to maximize ventilatory muscle rest during periods of ventilatory support in order to maximize muscle function during periods of ventilator independence. The rate is set high enough that the patient receives full ventilatory support – particularly during sleep. The rate and tidal volume settings vary dependent upon disease and individual patient

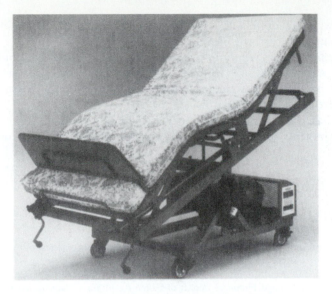

Figure 36-2 Rocking bed. (From GILMARTIN ME: Body ventilators: equipment and techniques. *Respir Care Clin* NA 1996; 2:195–222.)

status. Patients with neuromuscular disease often are most comfortable with a large tidal volume and long inspiratory time.

Monitoring

Patients at home are stable and without acute cardiopulmonary problems. As a result, the level of monitoring required is considerably less than that required of ICU patients. All invasive home care ventilators have high and low pressure alarms, disconnect alarms, and equipment failure alarms. For patients requiring supplemental oxygen, verification of $F_{I_{O_2}}$ can be performed during visits by health care providers. Pulse oximetry and capnography are not routinely indicated. Family members must, however, be able to identify the signs and symptoms associated with the development of acute cardiopulmonary dysfunction as well as dysfunction of ventilatory equipment.

POINTS TO REMEMBER

- The home affords ventilator-assisted patients the most independence and the lowest cost.
- Ideal candidates for ventilatory support in the home are those with neuromuscular disease.
- Prior to discharge, the patient must be medically stable.

- Patients who are optimistic, self-directed, and have adequate financial and personal support are most likely to succeed in the home.
- Discharge to the home requires the coordinated effort of a team of health care providers, the patient, and the family.
- Patients who cannot sustain spontaneous breathing for at least four hours should have a backup ventilator.
- Patients should receive full ventilatory support to ensure rest.
- For most patients the only monitoring required is that available on the ventilator.

ADDITIONAL READING

Clinical indications for noninvasive positive pressure ventilation in chronic respiratory failure due to restrictive lung disease, COPD, and nocturnal hypoventilation – a consensus conference. *Chest* 1999; 116:521–534.

DUNNE PJ. Demographics and Financial Impact of Home Respiratory Care. *Respir Care* 1994; 39:309–320.

GILMARTIN ME. Long-term Mechanical Ventilation: Patient selection and discharge planning. *Respir Care* 1991; 36:205–216.

LEGER P. Noninvasive Positive Pressure Ventilation at Home. *Respir Care* 1994; 39:501–514.

MAKE BJ, GILMARTIN ME. Mechanical ventilation in the home. *Crit Care Clin* 1990; 6:785–796.

MAKE BJ, HILL NS, GOLDBERG AL, ET AL. Mechanical ventilation beyond the intensive care unit. Report of a consensus conference of the American College of Chest Physicians. *Chest* 1998; 113:289S–344S.

THIRTY-SEVEN

PHARMACOLOGIC THERAPY: SEDATIVES, ANALGESICS, AND PARALYTIC AGENTS

OBJECTIVES

1. Discuss causes of sudden respiratory distress in ventilated patients.
2. Describe the approach to identify causes of sudden respiratory distress.
3. Discuss the pharmacologic effects of drugs used to control ventilation.
4. Describe the evaluation of sedation and paralysis in critically ill patients.
5. Discuss the practical approach used to provide pharmacologic control of ventilation.

INTRODUCTION

Patients requiring ventilatory support may develop sudden respiratory distress that is characterized as "out of phase with the ventilator" or "fighting the ventilator." This is due to the anxiety and stress associated with the underlying disease and the ventilatory support itself. Once oxygenation and ventilation improve, many patients require only minor sedation to acclimate to ventilatory support. Of concern is the previously calm patient who suddenly develops acute respiratory distress. Before pharmacologic therapy, the reason for the sudden change in status should be corrected if possible.

PATIENT EVALUATION: SUDDEN RESPIRATORY DISTRESS

Patient-ventilator dys-synchrony is identified by physiologic changes such as tachypnea, tachycardia, hypotension or hypertension, arrhythmia, diaphoresis, retractions, nasal flaring, use of accessory muscles, and abdominal paradox. Peak inspiratory pressure with volume-controlled ventilation or tidal volume with pressure controlled ventilation show large breath-to-breath variations. Airway pressure, flow, and volume graphics exhibit changes from baseline. Identifying the cause of sudden respiratory distress requires a systematic evaluation of the ventilator, airway, patient-ventilator interaction, and patient.

Ventilator

Table 37-1 lists the potential ventilator-related issues to be evaluated when a patient is experiencing respiratory distress. A common problem is inappropriate setting of the ventilator. Others include system leaks, circuit disconnect, malfunction of the exhalation valve, and humidifier malfunction.

Airway

With endotracheal tubes, a common cause of sudden respiratory distress is tube movement or obstruction (Table 37-2). Oral endotracheal tubes may migrate into a mainstem bronchus or the pharynx. Cephalad movement may position the cuff at the vocal cords. The tube can kink in the nasopharynx. Secretions can obstruct any airway – particularly if humidification is inadequate. The cuff may be the cause of problems due to excessive or inadequate inflation volume. The cuff may rupture or herniate over the tip of the airway. Particularly with tracheostomy tubes, the distal tip of the tube may obstruct against the tracheal wall and the tube may erode or irritate the trachea.

Table 37-1 Ventilatory causes of sudden respiratory distress

Improper setting of the ventilator
  Trigger sensitivity
  Pressure control or pressure support level
  Inspiratory time
  Peak flow
  Rise time
  Expiratory sensitivity
  Alarm settings
  F_{IO_2}
  PEEP
  Tidal volume
Circuit disconnect or leak
Malfunction of humidification system
Malfunction of exhalation valve
Overall malfunction of the ventilator
Improper function of a heat-and-moisture exchanger
Improperly set alarms

Patient-Ventilator Synchrony

Ventilator settings may be inappropriate and cause dys-synchrony between the patient and the ventilator (Table 37-3). The trigger sensitivity should be set sensitive enough to detect patient effort without causing auto-triggering. Even with a sensitive trigger, the patient may experience trigger dys-synchrony if auto-PEEP is present. With volume ventilation, flow dys-synchrony may occur if the peak flow is set too low. In the patient with a high flow demand, a peak flow of 60 to 100 L/min may be necessary. With pressure controlled ventilation, an appropriate pressure control level and inspiratory time are important. A pressure control setting that is too low and an inspiratory rise time that is too long (or too

Table 37-2 Airway causes of sudden respiratory distress

Malposition of the endotracheal tube
  Migration into mainstem bronchus
  Migration cephalad – cuff at the vocal cords
Cuff problems
  Rupture
  Herniation
Endotracheal tube kinking
Endotracheal obstruction
Airway trauma from tracheostomy tubes
  Tracheoesophageal fistula
  Tracheal stenosis at tip of tube
  Innominate artery fistula

Table 37-3 Patient ventilator dys-synchrony: causes of sudden respiratory distress

Inappropriate ventilator selection
    With volume ventilation, inappropriate V_T or T_I
    With pressure ventilation, inappropriate pressure or T_I
Inappropriate trigger sensitivity setting
Inappropriate trigger type (pressure vs. flow)
Inadequate rise time
Inappropriate expiratory cycle level with pressure support
Inadequate F_{IO_2}
Inadequate PEEP level
Inappropriate SIMV rate

short) can produce dys-synchrony. With pressure support ventilation, the pressure support setting, inspiratory rise time, and inspiratory termination criteria should be assessed. A pressure support setting that is too high and a low inspiratory flow termination can result in activate exhalation. A low SIMV rate is another cause of patient-ventilator dys-synchrony. Changing the mode, increasing the rate, or adding pressure support may be required. Proper adjustment of F_{IO_2} and PEEP will decrease the level of hypoxic drive and may improve synchrony.

Patient

Sudden respiratory distress may be a result of changes in the patient's physiologic status including the airways, lung parenchyma, pleural space, cardiovascular system and ventilatory drive (Table 37-4). Secretions, edema, and

Table 37-4 Patient causes of sudden respiratory distress

Airway	Cardiovascular dysfunction
Secretions	Acute myocardial infarction
Obstruction	Congestive heart failure
Mucosal edema	Fluid overload
Bronchospasm	Altered ventilatory drive
Lung parenchyma	Fever
Atelectasis	Pain
Consolidation	Anxiety
Edema	Delirium
Hyperinflation	Excessive carbohydrate load
Pleural space	Inadequate nutritional support
Pneumothorax	Metabolic acid-base imbalance
Bronchopleural fistula	Electrolyte imbalance
Pleural effusion	
Empyema	

bronchospasm can increase ventilatory demand. Atelectasis and consolidation can cause respiratory distress. Auto-PEEP increases trigger effort. When sudden respiratory distress develops, a pneumothorax should be considered. Increases in peak airway pressure with volume controlled ventilation (or decreases in tidal volume with pressure controlled ventilation), cardiovascular compromise, a tympanic chest percussion note, and shifting of the mediastinum are clinical findings following the development of a tension pneumothorax. Pleural effusion and empyema can also cause respiratory distress. Fluid overload, congestive heart failure, and acute myocardial infarction also lead to sudden respiratory distress. Acid-base, electrolyte, temperature, and nutritional imbalances can alter ventilatory drive. Pain, anxiety, and delirium can increase ventilatory drive and cause sudden distress.

Assessing the Problem

A sudden change in level of respiratory distress should be managed in a systematic manner. Manual ventilation with 100% oxygen assists in stabilizing the patient and eliminates the ventilator as a potential problem. This allows assessment for cuff leaks and increased impedance to ventilation. If a high pressure is needed to ventilate, passing a suction catheter will identify whether the problem is airway obstruction. Physical examination and chest X-ray can determine if a pneumothorax is present. Once the patient is stabilized with manual ventilation, a more careful analysis of the cause of the sudden distress is possible.

DRUGS USED TO CONTROL VENTILATION

Most patients requiring acute ventilatory support require sedation and analgesia. Mechanical ventilation produces fear and anxiety. The drugs most commonly used to facilitate mechanical ventilation are sedatives, neuroleptics, analgesics, and neuromuscular blocking agents.

Sedatives

Sedatives refer to the benzodiazepines (diazepam, lorazepam, midazolam), barbiturates, and propofol. These agents are anxiolytic and hypnotic, they produce muscle relaxation and amnesia, but they do not cause pain relief. Many are also anticonvulsants, but have little depressant effect on the cardiovascular system. The exceptions are midazolam and propofol, which may produce cardiovascular depression. Of concern is the long half-life of some of these agents. Diazepam (Valium) and the long-acting barbiturates are of particular concern because they have a half-life of one to three days. Because they are lipid-soluble and metabolized by the liver and kidney, accumulation and prolonged effects are common in elderly and critically ill patients. This is a particular concern during weaning from the ventilator. Because of its shorter half-life (6 to 15 hr), lorazepam (Ativan) is more appropriate than diazepam when the patient is ready for ventilator weaning. Midazolam (Versed) has a rapid onset of action and a short half-life (one hour). As a result, it allows fine control of the level of sedation compared to the other agents in this drug class. Benzodiazepines can be reversed with flumazenil. The use of this agent in critically ill mechanically ventilated patients has not been well evaluated. Moreover, its half-life is very short (one hour), requiring continuous infusion to avoid periodic respiratory depression. Propofol (Diprivan) is used for rapid induction of anesthesia in mechanically ventilated patients. It is particularly useful for minor surgical and other invasive procedures. It has a very rapid onset of action and short half-life (< 30 min). However, it frequently causes hypotension (occasionally profound) and it is expensive (Table 37-5).

Several sedation rating scales have been developed. The Ramsey Scale (Table 37-6) is the most simple and most frequently used scale. It evaluates patient response from agitated to deep sedation. The Ramsey Scale assigns a numerical value to observed patient behavior. In patients who are paralyzed, assurance of adequate anesthesia level and amnesia is extremely important, but sedation scoring systems cannot be used. The use of processed electroencephalographic monitoring (Bispectral Index or BIS monitoring) has been advocated to assess the level of sedation in these patients. The BIS monitor provides a numerical value indicating the level of sedation (range of 0 to 100, with 100 representing normal wakefulness and 0 represents flat line EEG). The role of BIS monitoring in mechanically ventilated patients is yet to be determined. Due to interference by muscular activity, its use in the ICU may be limited to patients who are paralyzed or when deep anesthesia is the goal.

Neuroleptics

Delirium is common in critically ill adults and manifests as reduced ability to appropriately respond to external stimuli. Disorganized thinking, rambling, incoherent or irrelevant speech, altered level of psychomotor activity, decreased level of consciousness, altered sensory perception, and disorientation are common clinical findings. Narcotics and sedatives generally worsen the symptoms of delir-

Table 37-5 Sedatives used in the ICU

	Lorazepam (Ativan)	Midazolam (Versed)	Diazepam (Valium)	Haloperidol (Haldol)	Propofol (Diprivan)
Onset of action	5–20 min	2–5 min	2–5 min	3–20 min	1–2 min
Intermittent Dose	0.02–0.06 mg/kg every 2–6 hr	0.02–0.08 mg/kg every 0.5–2 hr	0.03–0.01 mg/kg every 0.5–6 hr	0.03–0.15 mg/kg every 0.5–6 hr	—
Infusion rate	0.01–0.10 mg/kg/hr	0.04–0.20 mg/kg/hr	—	0.04–0.15 mg/kg/hr	5–80 µg/kg/min
Cost	Low	High	Low	Low	High

Table 37-6 Ramsey sedation scale

Level	Response
1	Anxious, agitated, restless
2	Cooperative, oriented, tranquil
3	Responds to commands only
4	Asleep, brisk response to stimulus
5	Asleep, sluggish response to stimulus
6	Unarousable

ium since these agents further alter sensory perception. Haloperidol (Haldol), a butyrophenone neuroleptic drug, is used to treat delirium. Haloperidol may cause QT prolongation of the electrocardiogram (ECG) and should be used with caution with other drugs that may prolong the QT interval.

Analgesics

Analgesics are used for pain control. Sedatives modify the emotional component of pain but do nothing to affect its physical component. Analgesics can be grouped into two categories – narcotics and non-narcotics. Narcotic analgesics affect the central nervous system (CNS) and bowel, whereas non-narcotic analgesics affect peripheral pain receptors. In addition to analgesia, narcotics cause sedation, drowsiness, mood changes (euphoria), mental clouding, sleep and respiratory depression. The non-narcotic analgesics do not affect the CNS and do not induce respiratory depression. In the acutely ill, mechanically ventilated patient, intravenous narcotic analgesics are the drugs of choice (Table 37-7). Three primary agents are used in this setting – morphine, fentanyl (Sublimaze), and hydromorphine (Dilaudid). Morphine is the preferred agent unless cardiovascular instability exists. Morphine is associated with transient hypotension due to histamine release. In the setting of hemodynamic instability, fentanyl is the drug of choice, although hydromorphine is an acceptable substitute. Narcotic analgesics can produce ileus, causing intolerance to enteral feeding and aggravation of pancreatic inflammation.

Paralytic Agents

These agents produce either competitive inhibition of acetylcholine (nondepolarizing agents) or prolonged depolarization of the postsynaptic receptors (depolarizing agents). The nondepolarizing agents include pancuronium bromide (Pavulon), vecuronium bromide (Norcuron), tubocurarine chloride (Curare), and cis-atracurium (Nimbex). Succinylcholine (Anectine) is a depolarizing agent. These drugs (Table 37-8) render patients paralyzed, but none has any analgesic or sedative properties. Accordingly, they must always be administered with appropriate levels of sedatives or narcotics. The depolarizing agents, because

Table 37-7 Narcotics used in the ICU

	Morphine	Fentanyl	Hydromorphine
Onset of action	Rapid	Rapid	Rapid
Intermittent dose	0.01–0.15 mg/kg	0.35–1.5 μ/kg	10–30 μg/kg
Infusion rate	0.07–0.5 mg/kg/hr	0.7–1 μg/kg/hr	7–15 μg/kg/hr
Cost	Low	Moderate	Moderate

of their short duration of action (five minutes), are only used for short-term paralysis to allow intubation, whereas the nondepolarizing agents may be used for prolonged paralysis to ensure controlled ventilation. Of concern with these agents are polyneuropathy or myopathy, prolonged neuromuscular blockade, and tolerance. Polyneuropathy has been reported, especially in patients with diabetes and those receiving large-dose steroid therapy. It is characterized by primary axonal degeneration of motor and sensory fibers, denervation atrophy of muscles, impaired tendon reflexes, and damaged muscle membranes. Weakness is prolonged for weeks or months and is not reversed by cholinesterase inhibitors. Prolonged nerve block without damage has been reported in patients receiving high-dose steroids and those with renal failure or sepsis. Increased dosing may be required due to tolerance. Use of paralytics in the ICU should be avoided and limited to situations in which sedatives and analgesics have failed to facilitate controlled ventilation.

Since there is wide individual variation in the response to neuromuscular blocking agents, careful monitoring of their effects is essential. Observation of the patient is the most direct method of evaluating the level of paralysis. Spontaneous breathing efforts, biting on the endotracheal tube, and coughing may indicate inadequate neuromuscular blockade. A more precise method is to assess motor nerve response to a supramaximal stimulus applied over the ulnar nerve at the wrist. This form of stimulation is referred to as a train-of-four, since four rapid and independent stimuli are applied. The response to the four stimuli indicates the magnitude of blockade. One or two twitches is the usual goal when paralysis is used during mechanical ventilation. Train-of-four monitoring may be unreliable in some critically ill patients, such as those who are very edematous.

Table 37-8 Neuromuscular blocking agents used in the ICU

	Pancuronium	Vecuronium	Tubocurarine	cis-Atracurium
Intubating dose	0.08–0.1 mg/kg	0.1–0.2 mg/kg	0.5–0.6 mg/kg	0.15–0.2 mg/kg
Infusion rate	1 μg/kg/min	1 μg/kg/min	0.08–0.12 mg/kg/hr	2 μg/kg/min
Cost	Low	High	Low	Moderate

PRACTICAL GUIDE TO PHARMACOLOGIC THERAPY

Patients receiving acute invasive ventilatory support require some level of sedation. Most patients can be adequately sedated with benzodiazepines or propofol. Those experiencing pain should also receive narcotics, titrated to the minimal level to produce patient comfort and ventilator synchrony. In patients experiencing delirium, haloperidol should be added. Dosages of sedatives and narcotics should be increased in patients who are dys-synchronous with the ventilator once other causes of respiratory distress have been eliminated. It is only in the exceptionally difficult-to-sedate patient, where patient activity is interfering with gas exchange and hemodynamics, that neuromuscular blocking agents should be considered. If paralytics are used, the duration of use should be limited.

POINTS TO REMEMBER

- Sudden respiratory distress is identified by changes in physiologic presentation.
- Sudden respiratory distress causes changes in airway pressure, flow and tidal volume.
- The airway, ventilator, or patient is the cause of sudden respiratory distress.
- Most ventilator-related problems are associated with malfunction or improper settings.
- Artificial airways may become obstructed, have malfunctioning cuffs, or move in the airway.
- Inappropriate matching of ventilator settings to patient demand results in dys-synchrony.
- Physiologic alterations in the airway, lung parenchyma, pleural space, cardiovascular system, and respiratory drive can cause sudden respiratory distress.
- Fear, pain, anxiety, and delirium may increase ventilatory drive and cause distress.
- Sedatives are anxiolytic and hypnotic, but do not produce pain relief.
- The Ramsey Scale is used to monitor level of sedation.
- Prolonged effects of sedatives are frequent in the elderly and critically ill.
- Analgesics relieve pain and cause sedation, but may cause ileus and hypotension.
- Neuromuscular blocking agents may result in prolonged weakness.
- Neuromuscular blocking agents should be used for short duration in critically ill patients.

ADDITIONAL READING

CAPUZZO M, PINAMONTI A, CINGOLANI E. Analgesia, sedation, and memory of intensive care. *J Crit Care* 2001; 16:83–89.

DEVLIN JW, BOLESKI G, MLYNAREK M, ET AL. Motor activity assessment scale: a valid and reliable sedation scale for use with mechanically ventilated patients in an adult surgical intensive care unit. *Crit Care Med* 1999; 27:1271–1275.

HURFORD WE. Neuromuscular blockade. In: HURFORD WE, BIGATELLO LM, HASPEL KL, HESS D, WARREN RL. *Critical Care Handbook of the Massachusetts General Hospital*. Philadelphia: Lippincott Williams & Wilkins; 2000:124–134.

HURFORD WE. Sedation and paralysis during mechanical ventilation. *Respir Care* 2002; 47:1–14.

JACOBI J, FRASER GL, COURSIN DB, ET AL. Clinical practice guidelines for the sustained use of sedatives and analgesics in the critically ill. *Crit Care Med* 2002; 30:119–141.

KRESS JP, POHLMAN AS, O'CONNOR MF, HALL JB. Daily interruption of sedative infusions in critically ill patients undergoing mechanical ventilation. *N Engl J Med* 2000; 342:1471–1477.

MURRAY MJ, COWEN J, DEBLOCK H, ET AL. Clinical practice guidelines for sustained neuromuscular blockade in the adult critically ill patient. *Crit Care Med* 2002; 30:142–156.

NASRAWAY SA, JACOBI J, MURRAY MJ, ET AL. Sedation, analgesia, and neuromuscular blockade of the critically ill adult: Revised clinical practice guidelines for 2002. *Crit Care Med* 2002; 30:117–118.

OSTERMANN ME, KEENAN SP, SEIFERLING RA, SIBBALD WJ. Sedation in the intensive care unit: a systematic review. *JAMA* 2000; 283:1451–1459.

THIRTY-EIGHT

HIGH FREQUENCY VENTILATION, PARTIAL LIQUID VENTILATION, AND TRACHEAL GAS INSUFFLATION

OBJECTIVES

1. Discuss approaches to high frequency ventilation and the rationale for their use.
2. Discuss the physiologic effects of partial liquid ventilation.
3. Describe the approaches to provide tracheal gas insufflation.
4. Discuss problems with the application of tracheal gas insufflation.
5. List indications for high frequency ventilation, partial liquid ventilation, and tracheal gas insufflation.

INTRODUCTION

Much interest has existed for alternate approaches to conventional mechanical ventilation that will improve gas exchange or decrease ventilator-induced lung injury. The techniques that have received the most interest are high frequency ventilation, partial liquid ventilation, and tracheal gas insufflation. The use of these techniques has primarily been recommended in settings where gas exchange is failing during conventional mechanical ventilation or the potential for lung injury from mechanical ventilation is high. However, the outcome data that is available regarding these techniques have failed to establish their superiority to conventional mechanical ventilation.

HIGH FREQUENCY VENTILATION

Approaches Available

Conventional mechanical ventilation is provided at rates < 2 Hz (1 Hz = 60 breaths/min). With high frequency ventilation (HFV), rates are provided at 2 to 15 Hz. The frequency range is determined by the specific technique and the size of the patient. Regardless of technique, adults are generally ventilated at the low end of the rate spectrum and neonates at the high end of the spectrum.

There are three techniques that have been classified as high frequency ventilation: high frequency positive pressure ventilation (HFPPV), high frequency jet ventilation (HFJV), and high frequency oscillation (HFO). With HFPPV, conventional ventilators are used to provide rates at the low end of the HFV spectrum (Table 38-1).

During HFJV (Figure 38-1), gas under high pressure is injected into the airway with a secondary gas source entrained to provide tidal volume. With HFJV, both a jet ventilator and conventional ventilator may be needed to establish gas delivery in the low to middle part of the HFV rate spectrum.

HFO has both an active inspiratory and expiratory phase. Oscillators establish gas flow by the movement of a diaphragm or piston, perpendicular to a bias flow that moves across the airway (Figure 38-2). With HFO, rates across the whole frequency spectrum are possible, but in general 10 to 15 Hz range are most common with neonates and 3 to 8 Hz range are used with adults. The most commonly used high frequency technique is HFO.

Table 38-1 Types of HFV

Type	Frequency range
High Frequency Positive Pressure Ventilation (HFPPV)	2–4 Hz
High Frequency Jet Ventilation (HFJV)	2–8 Hz
High Frequency Oscillation (HFO)	2–15 Hz

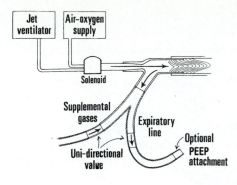

Figure 38-1 Design of a high-frequency jet ventilator. (From CARLTON GC: High-frequency jet ventilation: A prospective randomized evaluation. *Chest* 1983; 84:551–559.)

Factors Affecting Gas Exchange

At the rates provided with all three approaches to HFV, tidal volumes are smaller than those with conventional ventilation. The higher the respiratory rate, the lower the tidal volume. At moderate to high rates (≥ 8 Hz), tidal volumes can be less than anatomic dead space. Although numerous mechanisms are active during HFV to establish gas exchange (Figure 38-3), normal convection and molecular diffusion are the primary mechanisms affecting gas exchange. Other physical principles enhance molecule diffusion and the dispersion of gases in the airway.

Frequency, I:E ratio and pressure amplitude are the three variables affecting ventilation. Tidal volume during HFO is affected by rate. As rate is decreased, tidal volume increases and vice versa. Pressure amplitude (the pressure developed as the oscillator forces gas into the airway) and a longer inspiratory time also increase the tidal volume (Table 38-2). Neonates are generally ventilated at very high rates (10 to 15 Hz) but low-pressure amplitude (20 to 30 cm H_2O) that

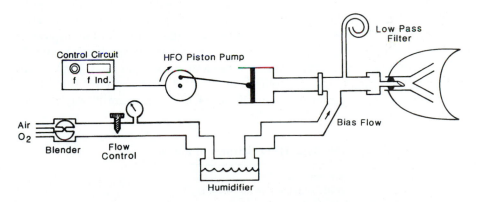

Figure 38-2 Essential parts of a HFO system. (From CHATBURN RL, BRANSON RD: High frequency ventilators. In BRANSON RD, HESS DR, CHATBURN RL: *Respiratory Care Equipment*. Philadelphia, Lippincott, Williams & Wilkins, 1995, pp. 458–469.)

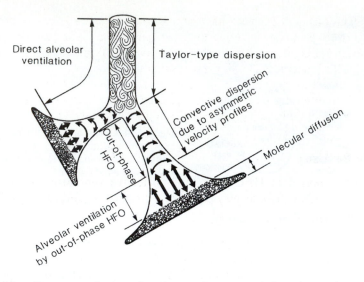

Figure 38-3 More than one mechanism of gas transport may operate in various regions of the lung during high-frequency ventilation. Moreover, mechanisms may act synergistically. Gas velocities decrease from the airway opening to alveolus. (From CHANG HF: Mechanisms of gas-transport during ventilation by high-frequency oscillation. *J Appl Physiol* 1984; 56:553–563.)

generates very small tidal volumes. Adults are ventilated at low rates (3 to 8 Hz) and high pressure amplitudes (60 to 90 cm H_2O). With neonates, bias flows are about 10 L/min, whereas with adults bias flows are in the 30 L/min range. In adults, tidal volumes approaching those delivered by conventional mechanical ventilation (5 to 6 mL/kg) are possible at 3 Hz and 90 cm H_2O pressure amplitude.

Oxygenation during HFO is determined by F_{IO_2} and mean airway pressure. During HFO, mean airway pressure is similar to PEEP in its effect on oxygenation since at the alveolar level there is minimal pressure change during HFO (particularly at high rates). It is estimated that as little as 15% of the inspiratory pressure amplitude is transmitted to the alveolar level through an 8 mm ID endotracheal tube at 8 Hz. With smaller tubes and more rapid rates, less pressure is transmitted. With a pressure amplitude of 60 cm H_2O (30 cm H_2O above mean airway pressure during inhalation and 30 cm H_2O below mean airway pressure

Table 38-2 HFO Settings in adults

Frequency: 3 to 8 Hz
Pressure amplitude: 60 to 90 cm H_2O
I:E ratio: 1:2
Bias flow: 30 L/min
Mean airway pressure: 25 to 35 cm H_2O

during exhalation) at 8 Hz with an 8 mm ID tube, the alveolar pressure would maximally rise 4.5 cm H_2O above the mean airway pressure and 4.5 cm H_2O below it. With HFO, a lung recruitment maneuver is often performed when HFO is initiated. This is accomplished by increasing the mean airway pressure to a level higher than expected to maintain oxygenation for a short period and then to the lowest level maintaining oxygenation. In adults, mean airway pressures during HFO are generally maintained between 25 and 35 cm H_2O.

Rationale for Use

Interest has increased in HFO as a lung-protective ventilatory strategy. With HFO, over-distending peak airway pressures and opening and closing of unstable lung units are theoretically avoided.

Indications for Use

The indication for the use of HFO in adults is severe ARDS. However, no data are available establishing the superiority of HFO to conventional ventilation. HFO can be safely applied to adults and outcomes are similar to those with conventional ventilation. Problems with the use of HFO are that the current devices are expensive, patients receiving HFO must be heavily sedated, and most clinicians lack familiarity with HFO.

PARTIAL LIQUID VENTILATION

Partial versus Full Liquid Ventilation

Partial liquid ventilation (PLV) was first described in 1991. Prior to this, attempts to provide liquid ventilation utilized total liquid ventilation systems. The difference between the two approaches relates to what is moved into the lungs with each breath. With total liquid ventilation, the fluid instilled into the lungs is the only liquid moved in and out of the lungs. No patient has ever been managed with total liquid ventilation. Partial liquid ventilation is accomplished by filling the lung to a fraction of the functional residual capacity (FRC) and providing conventional gas ventilation to the fluid-filled lung. All applications to date of liquid ventilation in humans have been by PLV.

The liquid used for PLV is the perfluorocarbon Perflubron (Alliance Pharmaceuticals, San Diego, CA). Perflubron has been used because of its physical properties (Table 38-3). It has an acceptable oxygen carrying capacity and has excellent carbon dioxide carrying capacity. Perflubron has a low surface tension, a high density, and a high spreading coefficient. These properties maintain gas exchange when used in patients with ARDS. Perflubron has a high vapor pressure and thus it rapidly evaporates from the lungs (about 90% in 24 hrs). However, its vapor pressure also means that the lungs need to be refilled on a

Table 38-3 Physical properties of Perflubron

- Colorless
- Odorless
- Insoluble in water
- Biologically inert
- Chemically stable
- Oxygen solubility: 63 mL/100 mL
- Carbon dioxide solubility: 210 mL/100 mL
- Surface tension: 18 dynes/cm
- Density: 1.92 g/mL
- Spreading coefficient: +2.7 dynes/cm
- Vapor pressure: 11 mm Hg

regular basis because of evaporation. In clinical trials, refilling has been necessary every 3 hours.

Physiologic Effects of Partial Liquid Ventilation

During PLV, a number of mechanisms for improving lung function and gas exchange have been proposed (Table 38-4). PLV has been called liquid PEEP because is causes alveolar recruitment. Due to its density, Perflubron distributes to the most gravity dependent aspects of the lung where it recruits collapsed alveoli. In addition, its density redistributes pulmonary blood flow to the non-dependent lung regions. With gas ventilation after instillation of Perflubron, gas is distributed primarily to the least gravity dependent lung regions where perfusion has been redistributed. Ventilation-perfusion matching is thus improved and both oxygenation and ventilation are enhanced. Because of its low surface tension, Perflubron has a surfactant effect. Secretions and cellular debris are moved from the lung periphery to central airways with PLV. This occurs because of the combined effect of density and the inability of Perflubron to mix with water. Although this improves the removal of secretions, care must be taken to avoid obstruction in large airways with this material. Perflubron also has an anti-inflammatory effect.

Table 38-4 Physiologic effects of PLV

- Lung recruitment
- Dependent PEEP effect
- Redistribution of pulmonary blood flow
- Improved ventilation/perfusion matching
- Improved oxygenation
- Improved ventilation
- Pulmonary lavage
- Anti-inflammatory effect

Gas Ventilation During Partial Liquid Ventilation

It was initially believed that PLV would protect the lung from ventilator-induced lung injury. However, it can be argued that a Perflubron-filled lung may be more susceptible to ventilator-induced lung injury than the non-Perflubron filled lung. In the most gravity-dependent part of the lungs, over-distension is caused not only by the pressure of the ventilating gas but also by the weight of the Perflubron. Thus, it is important to limit plateau pressure and use a small tidal volume during PLV. In addition, PEEP sufficient to move the Perflubron into distal airways and to stabilize non-dependent lung is necessary. Based on available data, 12 to 14 cm H_2O PEEP should be used during PLV. In addition, PEEP helps to avoid desaturation and hemodynamic compromise during initial and subsequent filling of the lung with Perflubron. Rate and I:E ratio during PLV should be set to avoid air trapping. Because of the density and inertia of Perflubron, auto-PEEP develops at high rates and a short expiratory time. Thus, a sufficient expiratory time should be provided.

Impact on ARDS

Randomized controlled trials comparing PLV to conventional ventilation have not shown a benefit for PLV. In the latest clinical trial, there was a trend to greater mortality in the low dose (10 mL/kg) PLV group than with conventional ventilation. It is unlikely that PLV will become available for the management of acute respiratory failure. Additional laboratory studies on the use of HFO with Perflubron and the use of Perflubron to assist in lung recruitment are ongoing.

TRACHEAL GAS INSUFFLATION

Physiologic Effects

With tracheal gas insufflation (TGI), a small diameter catheter is placed into the artificial airway until it projects just past the tip of the tube. Gas is then injected through the tube during conventional mechanical ventilation. CO_2 is normally present in the endotracheal tube and the mechanical dead space of the ventilator at end-exhalation (Figure 38-4). During the next breath, this CO_2 is moved into the alveolar space. With TGI, the injected flow of gas washes CO_2 from the endotracheal tube, the proximal trachea, and the mechanical dead space of the ventilator circuit. As a result, during the next breath gas that is moved into the alveoli from these areas is free of CO_2, decreasing arterial P_{CO_2}.

System Description

TGI should, ideally, only be active during the last part of the expiratory phase. In order to accomplish this, the TGI system must interact with the ventilator or it must be capable of identifying the beginning and end of exhalation. The system

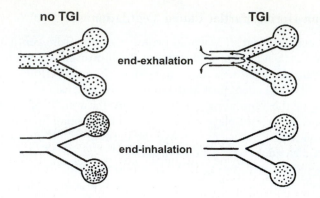

Figure 38-4 At end-exhalation, in the absence of TGI (upper left), central airways are laden with carbon dioxide (CO_2). This exhaled CO_2 is then recycled back into the alveoli during the next inspiration (lower left), thus limiting CO_2 elimination. With TGI, CO_2 is flushed out of the central airways during expiration, so less is recycled back to the alveoli, effectively decreasing anatomic dead space and increasing CO_2 elimination. (From RAVENSCRAFT SA. Tracheal gas insufflation: adjunct to conventional mechanical ventilation. *Respir Care* 1996; 41:105–111.)

must be appropriately monitored and alarmed so that TGI flow stops if an obstruction occurs between the point of injection and the mechanical ventilator. The secondary TGI flow makes it difficult to accurately measure tidal volume, plateau pressure, and auto-PEEP. A continuous flow TGI system can be constructed easily, but it increases tidal volume and plateau pressure. TGI flow can be directed toward the carina or toward the ventilator. With flow directed toward the carina, PEEP is increased, whereas PEEP is decreased with flow directed toward the ventilator.

Specific Indications

TGI is indicated when P_{CO_2} needs to be lowered but the limits of mechanical ventilation from a lung protective perspective have been reached. This may include patients with ARDS, asthma, and other diseases. Unfortunately, a system for TGI is not yet commercially available. Homemade systems provide too much patient risk to be recommended for use outside experimental protocols.

POINTS TO REMEMBER

- High frequency ventilation refers to systems providing rates between 2 and 15 Hz.
- HFO is the approach to high frequency ventilation most commonly used.
- During HFO, the higher the rate, the smaller the tidal volume.

- Most of the pressure amplitude during HFO is dissipated before reaching the alveolar level.
- HFO during ARDS results in outcomes similar to conventional mechanical ventilation.
- PLV is also referred to as liquid PEEP since it has a PEEP effect on dependent lung.
- PLV is not protective against large V_T and high plateau pressures.
- PLV has failed to show any clinical benefit during clinical trials.
- TGI should decrease CO_2 without increasing V_T or plateau pressure.
- TGI should ideally be provided during the last part of exhalation.
- Monitoring is difficult during TGI.
- TGI is not recommended because of the lack of a commercially available system.

ADDITIONAL READING

CHANG HF. Mechanisms of gas-transport during ventilation by high-frequency oscillation. *J Appl Physiol* 1984; 56:553–563.

CROCE MA, FABIAN TC, PATTON JH, ET AL. Partial liquid ventilation decreases the inflammatory response in the alveolar environment of trauma patients. *J Trauma* 1998; 45:273–282.

FORT P, FARMER C, WESTEMAN J, ET AL. High-frequency oscillatory ventilation for adult respiratory distress syndrome: a pilot study. *Crit Care Med* 1997; 25:937–947.

FUHRMAN BP, PACZAN PR, DEFRANCISIS M. Perfluorocarbon-associated gas exchange. *Crit Care Med* 1991; 19:712–722.

HIRSCHL RB, PRANIKOFF T, WISE C, ET AL. Initial experience with partial liquid ventilation in adult patients with the acute respiratory distress syndrome. *JAMA* 1996; 275:383–389.

IMANAKA H, KIRMSE M, MANG H, ET AL. Expiratory phase tracheal gas insufflation and pressure control in sheep with permissive hypercapnia. *Am J Respir Crit Care Med* 1999; 159:49–54.

KACMAREK RM. Complications of tracheal gas insufflation. *Respir Care* 2001; 46:167–176.

KACMAREK RM. Ventilatory adjuncts. *Respir Care* 2002; 47:319–333.

KIRMSE M, FUJINO Y, HROMI J, ET AL. Pressure-release tracheal gas insufflation reduces airway pressures in lung-injured sheep maintaining eucapnia. *Am J Respir Crit Care* 1999; 160:1462–1467.

MEHTA S, LAPINSKY SE, HALLETT DC, ET AL. Prospective trial of high-frequency oscillation in adults with acute respiratory distress syndrome. *Crit Care Med* 2001; 29:1360–1369.

RAVENSCRAFT SA. Tracheal gas insufflation: adjunct to conventional mechanical ventilation. *Respir Care* 1996; 41:105–111.

INDEX